Pediatric Body Imaging with Advanced MDCT and MRI

Editor

EDWARD Y. LEE

RADIOLOGIC CLINICS OF NORTH AMERICA

www.radiologic.theclinics.com

Consulting Editor
FRANK H. MILLER

July 2013 • Volume 51 • Number 4

ELSEVIER

1600 John F. Kennedy Boulevard • Suite 1800 • Philadelphia, Pennsylvania, 19103-2899

http://www.theclinics.com

RADIOLOGIC CLINICS OF NORTH AMERICA Volume 51, Number 4
July 2013 ISSN 0033-8389, ISBN 13: 978-0-323-18816-6

Editor: Adrianne Brigido

Radiologic Clinics of North America (ISSN 0033-8389) is published bimonthly by Elsevier Inc., 360 Park Avenue South, New York, NY 10010-1710. Months of issue are January, March, May, July, September, and November. Periodicals postage paid at New York, NY and additional mailing offices. Subscription prices are USD 438 per year for US individuals, USD 685 per year for US institutions, USD 210 per year for US students and residents, USD 511 per year for Canadian individuals, USD 858 per year for Canadian institutions, USD 630 per year for international individuals, USD 858 per year for international institutions, and USD 302 per year for Canadian and foreign students/residents. To receive student and resident rate, orders must be accompanied by name of affiliated institution, date of term and the signature of program/residency coordinatior on institution letterhead. Orders will be billed at individual rate until proof of status is received. Foreign air speed delivery is included in all *Clinics* subscription prices. All prices are subject to change without notice. **POSTMASTER:** Send address changes to *Radiologic Clinics of North America*, Elsevier Health Sciences Division, Subscription Customer Service, 3251 Riverport Lane, Maryland Heights, MO63043. **Customer Service: Telephone: 1-800-654-2452** (U.S. and Canada); **1-314-447-8871** (outside U.S. and Canada). **Fax: 1-314-447-8029. E-mail: journalscustomerservice-usa@elsevier.com** (for print support); **journalsonlinesupport-usa@elsevier.com** (for online support).

Reprints. For copies of 100 or more of articles in this publication, please contact the Commercial Reprints Department, Elsevier Inc., 360 Park Avenue South, New York, New York 10010-1710. Tel.: (+1) 212-633-3812; Fax: (+1) 212-462-1935; E-mail: reprints@elsevier.com.

Radiologic Clinics of North America also published in Greek Paschalidis Medical Publications, Athens, Greece.

Radiologic Clinics of North America is covered in *MEDLINE/PubMed (Index Medicus), EMBASE/Excerpta Medica, Current Contents/Life Sciences, Current Contents/Clinical Medicine, RSNA Index to Imaging Literature, BIOSIS, Science Citation Index,* and *ISI/BIOMED.*

Printed in the United States of America.

Contributors

CONSULTING EDITOR

FRANK H. MILLER, MD
Professor of Radiology; Chief, Body Imaging
Section and Fellowship Program and GI
Radiology; Medical Director MRI, Department
of Radiology, Feinberg School of Medicine,
Northwestern University, Chicago, Illinois

EDITOR

EDWARD Y. LEE, MD, MPH
Director and Chief, Division of Magnetic
Resonance and Thoracic Imaging; Associate
Professor of Radiology, Department of
Radiology and Pediatrics, Boston Children's
Hospital, Harvard Medical School, Boston,
Massachusetts

AUTHORS

TALISSA A. ALTES, MD
Associate Professor, Department of Radiology
and Medical Imaging, University of Virginia,
Charlottesville, Virginia

BEHRANG AMINI, MD, PhD
Department of Diagnostic Radiology, The
University of Texas MD Anderson Cancer
Center, Houston, Texas

PAUL S. BABYN, MD
Professor of Radiology and Head, Department
of Medical Imaging, Saskatoon Health Region,
Royal University Hospital, University of
Saskatchewan, Saskatoon, Canada

RICHARD BELLAH, MD
Division of Body Imaging, Department of
Radiology, The Children's Hospital of
Philadelphia, Perelman School of Medicine,
University of Pennsylvania, Philadelphia,
Pennsylvania

MARCELO F. BENVENISTE, MD
Department of Diagnostic Radiology,
The University of Texas MD Anderson
Cancer Center, Houston, Texas

PIERLUIGI CIET, MD
Radiologist and PhD Student, Departments of
Radiology and Pediatric Pulmonology,
Erasmus Medical Imaging Group (ELIG),
Erasmus Medical Center, Sophia Children's
Hospital, Rotterdam, The Netherlands

CESAR CORTES, MD
Department of Diagnostic Radiology,
University of Puerto Rico School of Medicine,
San Juan, Puerto Rico

KASSA DARGE, MD, PhD
Division of Body Imaging, Department of
Radiology, The Children's Hospital of
Philadelphia, Perelman School of Medicine,
University of Pennsylvania, Philadelphia,
Pennsylvania

JORGE DELGADO
Division of Body Imaging, Department of Radiology, The Children's Hospital of Philadelphia, Philadelphia, Pennsylvania

JONATHAN R. DILLMAN, MD
Assistant Professor of Radiology, Section of Pediatric Radiology, Department of Radiology, C.S. Mott Children's Hospital, University of Michigan Health System, Ann Arbor, Michigan

LAURA DINNEEN, MD
Assistant Professor, Department of Radiology, University of Missouri-Kansas City; Pediatric Radiologist, Children's Mercy Hospital and Clinics, Kansas City, Missouri

RICHARD L. EHMAN, MD
Department of Radiology, Center for Advanced Imaging Research, Mayo Clinic, Rochester, Minnesota

JOHN A.I. GROSSMAN, MD
Director of Brachial Plexus Program, Miami Children's Hospital, Miami, Florida

MATTHEW R. HAMMER, MD
Pediatric Radiology Fellow, Section of Pediatric Radiology, Department of Radiology, C.S. Mott Children's Hospital, University of Michigan Health System, Ann Arbor, Michigan

F. WILLIAM HERSMAN, PhD
Professor, Department of Physics, University of New Hampshire; CEO, Xemed LLC, Durham, New Hampshire

MIKHAIL HIGGINS, MD, MPH
Division of Body Imaging, Department of Radiology, The Children's Hospital of Philadelphia; Department of Radiology, Hospital of the University of Pennsylvania, Philadelphia, Pennsylvania

VICTOR M. HO-FUNG, MD
Assistant Professor of Radiology, The Children's Hospital of Philadelphia, Perelman School of Medicine, University of Pennsylvania, Philadelphia, Pennsylvania

STEVEN Y. HUANG, MD
Department of Diagnostic Radiology, The University of Texas MD Anderson Cancer Center, Houston, Texas

TIFFANY J. HWANG, BA
Division of Body Imaging, Department of Radiology, The Children's Hospital of Philadelphia, Philadelphia, Pennsylvania

DIEGO JARAMILLO, MD, MPH
Professor of Radiology and Radiologist-in-Chief, The Children's Hospital of Philadelphia, Perelman School of Medicine, University of Pennsylvania, Philadelphia, Pennsylvania

HEE KYUNG KIM, MD
Department of Radiology, Cincinnati Children's Hospital Medical Center, Cincinnati, Ohio

RAMYA KOLLIPARA, BA
University of Missouri-Kansas City SOM, Kansas City, Missouri

TAL LAOR, MD
Department of Radiology, Cincinnati Children's Hospital Medical Center, University of Cincinnati College of Medicine, Cincinnati, Ohio

EDWARD Y. LEE, MD, MPH
Director and Chief, Division of Magnetic Resonance and Thoracic Imaging; Associate Professor of Radiology, Department of Radiology and Pediatrics, Boston Children's Hospital, Harvard Medical School, Boston, Massachusetts

DIANA M. LINDQUIST, PhD
Department of Radiology, Imaging Research Center, Cincinnati Children's Hospital Medical Center, Cincinnati, Ohio

MARK C. LISZEWSKI, MD
Pediatric Radiology Fellow, Department of Radiology, Boston Children's Hospital, Harvard Medical School, Boston, Massachusetts

LISA H. LOWE, MD, FAAP
Professor and Chair, Department of Radiology, University of Missouri-Kansas City; Pediatric Radiologist, Children's Mercy Hospital and Clinics, Kansas City, Missouri

ROBERT D. MACDOUGALL, MSc
Clinical Medical Physicist, Department of Radiology, Boston Children's Hospital, Boston, Massachusetts

YOGESH K. MARIAPPAN, PhD
Department of Radiology, Centre for Advanced
Imaging Research, Mayo Clinic, Rochester,
Minnesota

KIARAN P. MCGEE, PhD
Department of Radiology, Center for Advanced
Imaging Research, Mayo Clinic, Rochester,
Minnesota

ARNOLD C. MERROW, MD
Department of Radiology, Cincinnati Children's
Hospital Medical Center, Cincinnati, Ohio

ASHIKA ODHAV, BA
University of Missouri-Kansas City SOM,
Kansas City, Missouri

YOSHIHARU OHNO, MD, PhD
Department of Radiology, Advanced
Biomedical Imaging Research Center, Kobe
University Graduate School of Medicine,
Chuo-ku, Kobe, Japan

DANIEL J. PODBERESKY, MD
Associate Professor of Clinical Radiology,
Department of Radiology, Cincinnati Children's
Hospital Medical Center, University of
Cincinnati College of Medicine, Cincinnati, Ohio

YANERYS RAMOS, MD
Department of Radiology, Cincinnati Children's
Hospital Medical Center, Cincinnati, Ohio

KENNY E. RENTAS, MD
Department of Radiology, Saint Luke's
Hospital and The University of Missouri-
Kansas City, Kansas City, Missouri

JOSE ANDRES RESTREPO, MD
Department of Rehabilitation Medicine,
Humana, CAC Florida Medical Center, Miami,
Florida

RICARDO RESTREPO, MD
Professor of Radiology, Department of
Radiology, Miami Children's Hospital, Miami,
Florida

DOUGLAS C. RIVARD, DO
Associate Professor, Department of Radiology,
University of Missouri-Kansas City; Chief of
Pediatric Radiology, Children's Mercy Hospital
and Clinics, Kansas City, Missouri

HECTOR H. ROBLEDO, MD
Department of Radiology, Córdoba Children's
Hospital, Córdoba, Argentina

SURAJ D. SERAI, MS, PhD
Department of Radiology, Cincinnati Children's
Hospital Medical Center, Cincinnati, Ohio

ASSEM SHUKLA, MD
Division of Urology, Department of Surgery,
The Children's Hospital of Philadelphia,
Perelman School of Medicine, University of
Pennsylvania, Philadelphia, Pennsylvania

KEITH J. STRAUSS, MSc, FAAPM, FACR
Clinical Imaging Physicist, Assistant Professor
of Radiology, Department of Radiology,
Cincinnati Children's Hospital Medical Center,
University of Cincinnati School of Medicine,
Cincinnati, Ohio

VY THAO TRAN, MD
Clinical Instructor, Department of Radiology,
Lucile Packard Children's Hospital, Stanford
University, Palo Alto, California

JASON TSAI, MD
Division of Diagnostic Imaging and Radiology,
Children's National Medical Center,
Washington, DC

SHREYAS VASANAWALA, MD, PhD
Associate Professor, Department of Radiology,
Lucile Packard Children's Hospital, Stanford
University, Palo Alto, California

LILY L. WANG, MBBS, MPH
Department of Radiology, Cincinnati Children's
Hospital Medical Center, Cincinnati, Ohio

SIMON K. WARFIELD, PhD
Professor of Radiology, Department of
Radiology, Boston Children's Hospital, Boston,
Massachusetts

Contents

Magnetic resonance (MR) imaging is a noninvasive imaging modality, particularly attractive for pediatric patients given its lack of ionizing radiation. Despite many advantages, the physical properties of the lung (inherent low signal-to-noise ratio, magnetic susceptibility differences at lung-air interfaces, and respiratory and cardiac motion) have posed technical challenges that have limited the use of MR imaging in the evaluation of thoracic disease in the past. However, recent advances in MR imaging techniques have overcome many of these challenges. This article discusses these advances in MR imaging techniques and their potential role in the evaluation of thoracic disorders in pediatric patients.

The main imaging modality of the urinary tract in children is ultrasound. When further cross-sectional morphologic examination and/or functional evaluation is required, magnetic resonance (MR) imaging is the logical and optimal second step, particularly in pediatric patients. There are two main exceptions to this. The first one is when after an ultrasound, additional diagnostic imaging for urolithiasis is needed. The second one involves severe polytrauma, including blunt abdominal trauma. In this review, an overview of the MR imaging and computed tomography examinations important for current and future daily pediatric uroradiologic practice is presented.

Magnetic resonance (MR) imaging is an effective and noninvasive modality for evaluating hepatobiliary pathologic conditions. This article provides an up-to-date review of anatomy, indications, and imaging goals and protocols, including patient preparation, pulse sequences, and contrast agents used in pediatric MR hepatobiliary imaging. This article also highlights some of the common MR features of pediatric liver pathologic conditions, including tumors, congenital biliary ductal plate malformations, trauma, fibrosis, and infection.

Advanced multidetector computed tomographic and magnetic resonance imaging techniques (CT and MR enterography, respectively), designed to provide detailed images of the bowel and mesentery, can be successfully performed in children of all ages, frequently without sedation. Cross-sectional enterography allows for noninvasive diagnosis, detection of various disease-related complications and extraintestinal manifestations, and monitoring of bowel-wall inflammation in pediatric inflammatory bowel disease (IBD). This article provides a contemporary review of CT and MR enterography in the pediatric population, including up-to-date techniques and clinical applications. A range of bowel abnormalities is illustrated, with an emphasis on IBD and its many abdominopelvic manifestations.

Multidetector computed tomography (MDCT) offers an important noninvasive imaging modality for confirmation and further characterization of primary lung and large airway neoplasms encountered in pediatric patients. Children represent a unique challenge in imaging, not only because of unique patient factors (eg, inability to follow instructions, motion, need for sedation) but because of the technical factors that must be optimized to reduce radiation dose. This article reviews an MDCT imaging algorithm, up-to-date imaging techniques, and clinical applications of MDCT for evaluating benign and malignant primary neoplasms of lung and large airway in infants and children.

Recent advances in knowledge regarding histopathology, cause, and treatment of pediatric vascular anomalies have led to substantial changes in classification and terminology. Over the past two decades, various subspecialists have adopted a new classification system proposed by the International Society for the Study of Vascular Anomalies (ISSVA). The ISSVA classification of vascular anomalies divides vascular anomalies into two categories: vascular neoplasms and malformations. It has been widely adopted by various pediatric subspecialists, because it reliably correlates patient presentation and disease progression, with more accurate histology, diagnosis, imaging, and treatment.

Magnetic resonance (MR) imaging is an excellent tool for the evaluation of peripheral nerves in children not only because of its excellent soft tissue contrast resolution but also because it is noninvasive and does not use ionizing radiation. In nonconclusive cases, MR neurography can be complementary to physical examination and electromyography in identifying a specific affected nerve and the site of the lesion. This article reviews the MR imaging technique used in the evaluation of peripheral nerves (ie, MR neurography), its major indications, and the common pathologic conditions encountered in the pediatric population.

Evaluation of hyaline cartilage in pediatric patients requires in-depth understanding of normal physiologic changes in the developing skeleton. Magnetic resonance (MR) imaging is a powerful tool for morphologic and functional imaging of the cartilage. In this review article, current imaging indications for cartilage evaluation pertinent to the pediatric population are described. In particular, novel surgical techniques for cartilage repair and MR classification of cartilage injuries are summarized. The authors also provide a review of the normal anatomy and a concise description of the advances in quantitative cartilage imaging (ie, T2 mapping, delayed gadolinium-enhanced MR imaging of cartilage, and T1rho).

The diagnosis of juvenile idiopathic arthritis (JIA) is based on clinical and laboratory findings. However, there is mounting evidence of the imaging potential to accurately stage and evaluate disease activity. With new medications offering more aggressive and effective treatments, monitoring response to treatment becomes increasingly important. The use of more sensitive imaging modalities such as ultrasound and more importantly magnetic resonance imaging is gaining favor. The time has come to consider the incorporation of imaging in the scoring and evaluation of disease activity in JIA.

This review describes various quantitative magnetic resonance imaging techniques that can be used to objectively analyze the composition (T2 relaxation time mapping, Dixon imaging, and diffusion-weighted imaging), architecture (diffusion tensor imaging), mechanical properties (magnetic resonance elastography), and function (magnetic resonance spectroscopy) of normal and pathologic skeletal muscle in the pediatric population.

This review includes an overview of the fundamental physics and dose metrics of multidetector computed tomography (MDCT), a brief summary of research concerning health effects of ionizing radiation with an emphasis on risks to children, research of dose optimization, and practical recommendations that can be implemented immediately at the radiologist's own center. It is hoped that by combining results of recent research, this review will provide valuable information for the practicing radiologist. The sections of this review were designed such that each section can be read independently or skipped depending on the level of expertise of the reader.

PROGRAM OBJECTIVE

The objective of the Radiologic Clinics of North America is to keep practicing radiologists and radiology residents up to date with current clinical practice in radiology by providing timely articles reviewing the state of the art in patient care.

TARGET AUDIENCE

Practicing radiologists, radiology residents, and other health care professionals who provide patient care utilizing radiologic findings.

LEARNING OBJECTIVES

Upon completion of this activity, participants will be able to:
1. Review recent advances and clinical applications of MR Imaging of pediatric muscular disorders.
2. Discuss MR and CT in pediatric urology and its current and future daily practice.
3. Recognize vascular anomalies in pediatric patients using updated classification, imaging, and therapies.

ACCREDITATION

The Elsevier Office of Continuing Medical Education (EOCME) is accredited by the Accreditation Council for Continuing Medical Education (ACCME) to provide continuing medical education for physicians.

The EOCME designates this enduring material for a maximum of 15 *AMA PRA Category 1 Credit*(s) ™. Physicians should claim only the credit commensurate with the extent of their participation in the activity.

All other health care professionals requesting continuing education credit for this enduring material will be issued a certificate of participation.

DISCLOSURE OF CONFLICTS OF INTEREST

The EOCME assesses conflict of interest with its instructors, faculty, planners, and other individuals who are in a position to control the content of CME activities. All relevant conflicts of interest that are identified are thoroughly vetted by EOCME for fair balance, scientific objectivity, and patient care recommendations. EOCME is committed to providing its learners with CME activities that promote improvements or quality in healthcare and not a specific proprietary business or a commercial interest.

The planning committee, staff, authors and editors listed below have identified no financial relationships or relationships to products or devices they or their spouse/life partner have with commercial interest related to the content of this CME activity:

Behrang Amini, MD, PhD; Paul S. Babyn, MD; Richard Bellah, MD; Marcelo F. Benveniste, MD; Adrianne Brigido; Pierluigi Ciet, MD; Nicole Congleton; Cesar Cortes, MD; Kassa Darge, MD, PhD; Jorge Delgado, MD; Jonathan R. Dillman, MD; Laura Dinneen, MD; John A.I. Grossman, MD; Matthew R. Hammer, MD; Mikhail Higgins, MD, MPH; Victor M. Ho-Fung, MD; Steven Y. Huang, MD; Diego Jaramillo, MD, MPH; Ramya Kollipara, BA; Tal Laor, MD; Sandy Lavery; Charles A. Lawrence, Jr, MD; Edward Y. Lee, MD, MPH; Diana M. Lindquist, PhD; Mark C. Liszewski, MD; Lisa H. Lowe, MD, FAAP; Robert D. MacDougall, MSc; Jill McNair; Frank H. Miller, MD; Ashika Odhav, BA; Yanerys Ramos, MD; Kenny E. Rentas, MD; Jose Andres Restrepo, MD; Ricardo Restrepo, MD; Douglas C. Rivard, DO; Hector H. Robledo, MD; Suraj D. Serai, MS, PhD; Aseem Shukla, MD; Keith J. Strauss, MSc, FAAPM, FACR; Karthikeyan Subramaniam; Vy Thao Tran, MD; Jason Tsai, MD; Lily L. Wang, MBBS, MPH; and Simon K. Warfield, PhD.

The planning committee, staff, authors and editors listed below have identified financial relationships or relationships to products or devices they or their spouse/life partner have with commercial interest related to the content of this CME activity:

Talissa A. Altes, MD has research grants from Vertex Pharmaceuticals, Novartis and Siemens Health Care.
Richard L. Ehman, MD has a research grant and stock ownership with Resoundant, Inc.
F. William Hersman, PhD has stock ownership, a research grant, employment affiliation and royalties/patents with Xemed LLC.
Tiffany J. Hwang, BA has a research grant from Siemens Healthcare.
Hee Kyung Kim, MD has a RSNA scholar grant and has an employment affiliation with a a CCHMC Trustee grant.
Yogesh K. Mariappan, PhD has royalties/patents with Resoundant, Inc.
Kiaran P. McGee, PhD has royalties/patents/intellectual property related to magnetic resonance elastography.
Arnold C. Merrow, MD has an employment affiliation and royalties/patents with Amirsys, Inc.
Yoshiharu Ohno, MD, PhD has research grants from Toshiba Medical Systems, Philips Healthcare and Guerbet.
Daniel J. Podberesky, MD is on the speaker's bureau for Toshiba of America Medical Systems and receives royalties/patents from Amirsys, Inc.
Shreyas S. Vasanawala, MD, PhD has a research grant from GE Healthcare.

UNAPPROVED/OFF-LABEL USE DISCLOSURE

The EOCME requires CME faculty to disclose to the participants:
1. When products or procedures being discussed are off-label, unlabelled, experimental, and/or investigational (not US Food and Drug Administration (FDA) approved); and

2. Any limitations on the information presented, such as data that are preliminary or that represent ongoing research, interim analyses, and/or unsupported opinions. Faculty may discuss information about pharmaceutical agents that is outside of FDA-approved labelling. This information is intended solely for CME and is not intended to promote off-label use of these medications. If you have any questions, contact the medical affairs department of the manufacturer for the most recent prescribing information.

TO ENROLL

To enroll in the *Radiologic Clinics of North America* Continuing Medical Education program, call customer service at 1-800-654-2452 or sign up online at http://www.theclinics.com/home/cme. The CME program is available to subscribers for an additional annual fee of USD 288.

METHOD OF PARTICIPATION

In order to claim credit, participants must complete the following:
1. Complete enrolment as indicated above.
2. Read the activity.
3. Complete the CME Test and Evaluation. Participants must achieve a score of 70% on the test. All CME Tests and Evaluations must be completed online.

CME INQUIRIES/SPECIAL NEEDS

For all CME inquiries or special needs, please contact elsevierCME@elsevier.com.

RADIOLOGIC CLINICS OF NORTH AMERICA

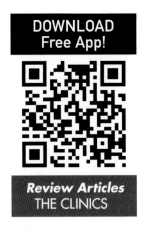

Preface

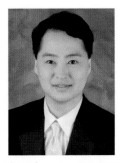

Edward Y. Lee, MD, MPH
Editor

Technical advancement and clinical utilization of pediatric body computed tomography (CT) and magnetic resonance imaging (MRI) have undergone substantial and rapid growth over the past decade. The introduction and continued advances in the multidetector CT (MDCT) technology have revolutionized the cross-sectional imaging evaluation in the pediatric population. For example, the faster scanning time and increased anatomic coverage that can be afforded by MDCT are particularly beneficial to pediatric patients. Additionally, MDCT provides high-quality multiplanar 2-dimensional, 3-dimensional, and dynamic 4-dimensional imaging, especially beneficial for evaluating small anatomic structures in infants and young children. During the same period of time, MRI, which is a powerful imaging modality that combines anatomic information and functional data without the use of ionizing radiation exposure, has also undergone a major revolution. The advancement to 3T magnets, many newer and faster MRI sequences, and multichannel coils with parallel imaging capabilities have substantially improved image quality of MRI and allowed 3D imaging while reducing image acquisition time, all of which contribute to the improved diagnosis and characterization. These advances have enabled MDCT and MRI to become the current primary noninvasive imaging modality of choice for the diagnosis, treatment planning, and follow-up evaluation of various congenital and acquired disorders in infants and children.

As the guest editor for this issue, I have selected topics that are considered to be of current importance and of potential widespread clinical relevance in pediatric body imaging with MDCT and MRI. The major aim of this issue is to introduce some new MDCT and MRI techniques that have a great potential for clinical use particularly in pediatric patients and also to facilitate the reader's ability to successfully employ these imaging techniques for evaluating disorders affecting various organ systems in pediatric patients. A clear understanding of the up-to-date techniques of MDCT and MRI combined with practical knowledge of proper clinical utilization is essential for optimal pediatric patient care.

I had the great privilege and pleasure of working with highly experienced and talented contributing authors—all of whom are experts in the field of pediatric body imaging with MDCT and MRI. Their invaluable efforts and extraordinary expertise have helped create a resource of information that should facilitate the understanding of pediatric body imaging with MDCT and MRI. I would also like to thank Richard Robertson, MD, my department chair, and Caroline Robson, MD and Kirsten Ecklund, MD, my department vice-chairs, for their support; my colleagues at Boston Children's Hospital, for their encouragement; Adrianne Brigido and her colleagues at Elsevier for their administrative and editorial assistance; and my family for their constant encouragement and support.

Edward Y. Lee, MD, MPH
Division of Magnetic Resonance and
Thoracic Imaging
Department of Radiology and Pediatrics
Boston Children's Hospital
Harvard Medical School
330 Longwood Avenue
Boston, MA 02115, USA

E-mail address:
Edward.Lee@childrens.harvard.edu

Radiol Clin N Am 51 (2013) xiii
http://dx.doi.org/10.1016/j.rcl.2013.04.008
0033-8389/13/$ – see front matter © 2013 Published by Elsevier Inc.

radiologic.theclinics.com

Magnetic Resonance Imaging of Pediatric Lung Parenchyma, Airways, Vasculature, Ventilation, and Perfusion
State of the Art

Mark C. Liszewski, MD[a], F. William Hersman, PhD[b,c], Talissa A. Altes, MD[d], Yoshiharu Ohno, MD, PhD[e], Pierluigi Ciet, MD[f,g], Simon K. Warfield, PhD[h], Edward Y. Lee, MD, MPH[i,*]

KEYWORDS

- Magnetic resonance imaging • Pediatric patients • Lungs • Airways • Vasculature • Ventilation
- Perfusion

KEY POINTS

- Magnetic resonance (MR) imaging has been increasingly used particularly for evaluating pediatric thoracic disorders in recent years.
- Adoption of MR imaging for assessing diseases of the thorax has lagged behind MR imaging in other organ systems because of the technical challenges posed by low proton density within the lungs, magnetic susceptibility differences at lung-air interfaces, and respiratory and cardiac motion.
- New techniques in fast scanning, respiratory triggering, spirometer control, electrocardiography gating, nonenhanced and contrast-enhanced MR angiography, O_2-enhanced imaging, and hyperpolarized gas imaging allow MR imaging to be used to evaluate many pediatric thoracic diseases.
- Understanding proper MR techniques and the characteristic MR imaging appearance of various thoracic diseases in pediatric patients is essential to arrive at an early and accurate diagnosis, which in turn, leads to optimal patient care.

INTRODUCTION

In recent years, magnetic resonance (MR) imaging, a noninvasive imaging modality, has been receiving a lot of attention and is particularly attractive for children, mainly because pediatric patients have greater sensitivity to the potentially harmful effects of ionizing radiation associated

[a] Department of Radiology, Boston Children's Hospital, Harvard Medical School, 330 Longwood Avenue, Boston, MA 02115, USA; [b] Department of Physics, University of New Hampshire, 105 Main Street, Durham, NH 03824, USA; [c] Xemed LLC, 16 Strafford Avenue, Durham, NH 03824, USA; [d] Department of Radiology and Medical Imaging, University of Virginia, Box 800170, Lane Road, Charlottesville, VA 22901, USA; [e] Department of Radiology, Advanced Biomedical Imaging Research Center, Kobe University Graduate School of Medicine, 7-5-2 Kusunoki-cho, Chuo-ku, Kobe 650-0017, Japan; [f] Erasmus Medical Imaging Group (ELIG), Department Radiology, Erasmus Medical Center, Sophia Children's Hospital, WK 331, Westzeedijk 118, 3015 GJ Rotterdam, The Netherlands; [g] Erasmus Medical Imaging Group (ELIG), Departments Pediatric Pulmonology, Erasmus Medical Center, Sophia Children's Hospital, WK 331, Westzeedijk 118, 3015 GJ Rotterdam, The Netherlands; [h] Department of Radiology, Boston Children's Hospital, 330 Longwood Avenue, Boston, MA 02115, USA; [i] Division of Thoracic Imaging, Magnetic Resonance Imaging, Boston Children's Hospital, Harvard Medical School, 330 Longwood Avenue, Boston, MA 02115, USA
* Corresponding author.
E-mail address: edward.lee@childrens.harvard.edu

Radiol Clin N Am 51 (2013) 555–582
http://dx.doi.org/10.1016/j.rcl.2013.04.004
0033-8389/13/$ – see front matter © 2013 Elsevier Inc. All rights reserved.

with other imaging modalities.[1,2] However, the physical properties of the lungs and thorax present many challenges to obtaining diagnostic quality MR images, which have limited the clinical use of MR imaging in pediatric patients with various thoracic disorders. Fortunately, many new MR imaging techniques have recently been developed that aim to overcome these challenges. Clear understanding of these new MR imaging techniques and knowledge of their clinical use are paramount. Therefore, the goal of this article is to provide up-to-date information about these techniques, including patient preparation and imaging protocols for the evaluation of lung parenchyma, airways, and thoracic vasculature. Ventilation imaging techniques using hyperpolarized (HP) gas (helium, xenon, and oxygen enhanced) and perfusion imaging techniques using arterial spin labeling (ASL) and contrast-enhanced imaging are also discussed. The potential role for these innovative MR imaging techniques in the evaluation of several pediatric thoracic diseases is highlighted and examples are presented.

IMAGING TECHNIQUES
Patient Preparation

Imaging of children can pose unique challenges to obtaining diagnostic quality MR images, including patient motion and difficulty or inability to follow breathing instructions. These challenges can be magnified when imaging the lungs and airways with MR imaging because complex breathing instructions are often required. Several techniques can be used to minimize these problems, including coaching patients on breathing techniques and the use of sedation and intubation in appropriate situations.[3] In general, sedation is necessary when imaging infants and uncooperative young children (≤6 years old) with MR imaging, but can often be avoided in older children (>6 years old) who are able to perform the necessary respiratory maneuvers with adequate coaching. It is essential that adequate time is devoted to practicing breath-hold techniques with children before MR imaging to reduce patient anxiety and improve diagnostic quality.

Imaging Protocols

Lung parenchymal evaluation
Although computed tomography (CT) remains the reference standard for evaluation of the lung parenchyma, advances in MR imaging have made imaging of infiltrative and solid lung pathologies possible with high sensitivity[4–9] and interstitial lung disease with fair sensitivity and specificity.[7] Protocol recommendations have

been published[3,4,10] and a standard 15-minute examination is usually sufficient to answer many clinical scenarios (**Table 1**).[4] Additional sequences can be included depending on the specific clinical question to be answered.[3,4,10]

The basic evaluation of the lung can consist of 5 non–contrast-enhanced sequences, including 3-plane gradient recalled echo (GRE) localizer for planning, coronal T2-weighted half Fourier acquisition single-shot turbo spin echo (HASTE) for evaluation of pulmonary consolidation, single breath-hold axial T1-weighted three-dimensional (3D)-GRE (VIBE) for evaluation of smaller parenchymal lesions, free-breathing coronal steady-state free precession (TrueFISP) for basic evaluation of pulmonary and cardiac motion and exclusion of large central pulmonary embolism (PE), and multiple breath-hold axial T2 weighted-short tau inversion recovery (STIR) (T2-TIRM) to evaluate for lymphadenopathy and osseous lesions.[4] An additional contrast-enhanced 3D-GRE (VIBE) sequence is also useful in some situations, including evaluation of malignancy, infection, and inflammatory disease.[4] In patients who are unable to cooperate with breathing instructions, free-breathing Propeller (BLADE + navigator) sequences[11] can be used

Table 1		
Basic MR imaging protocol for evaluation of lung parenchyma		
Sequence	Imaging Plane	Weighting
Gradient recalled echo (GRE) localizer	3-plane	T1
Single-shot half Fourier turbo spin echo (HASTE)	Coronal	T2
3-D GRE volumetric interpolated breath-hold (VIBE)	Axial	T1
Steady-state free precession (TrueFISP)	Coronal	PD/T1/T2[a]
Short tau inversion recovery (STIR)	Axial	(STIR)
Optional		
Postcontrast 3D-GRE VIBE with fat saturation	Axial	T1
Propeller (BLADE + navigator) free breathing[b]	Axial	T2

[a] Combination of proton density and T1 and T2 contrast.
[b] Can be used in place of STIR in patients who cannot perform breath-hold.

instead of breath-hold axial T2-weighted-STIR (T2-TIRM) sequences.

This basic protocol can be expanded to include additional sequences tailored to the specific clinical questions[3,4,10] and several of these specialized sequences are described in the following sections. These protocols have been proposed mainly for use in adults, but they are equally well suited to the pediatric patient population after appropriate patient preparation.[3]

Large airway evaluation

Although CT has been the mainstay of airway evaluation,[12–16] recent advances have allowed for the evaluation of large airways using MR imaging.[3,12,15,17–19] Using the basic MR sequences described earlier, it is now possible to image most static diseases of the large airways including bronchiectasis, bronchial wall thickening, mucous plugging, large airway neoplasms, and large airway branching anomalies.[6] Until recently, dynamic imaging of the large airways to evaluate for tracheobronchomalacia (TBM) was only feasible using CT. However, new techniques in spirometer-controlled MR imaging now provide promising imaging alternatives to CT.[20]

Using a spirometer compatible with MR imaging (Fig. 1) and a team comprising a lung function technician, MR imaging technologist, and a radiologist, spirometer-controlled MR imaging can be performed to evaluate for dynamic airway collapse seen in TBM. Approximately 30 minutes before imaging, the patient meets with a lung function technician and practices breathing maneuvers using a spirometer compatible with MR imaging (custom made Masterscope, CareFusion, Houten, The Netherlands). Patients are trained to perform maximum breath-hold times of 15 seconds at at least 95% inspiratory vital capacity (IVC) and 90% expiratory vital capacity (EVC). They are also trained to perform full forced expiration and cough maneuvers starting at IVC. After training, patients are moved to the MR imaging scanner where the lung function technician and MR imaging technologist monitor and communicate with the patient throughout the examination.

The standard protocol to evaluate for dynamic airway changes of TBM begins with a 3-plane GRE localizer sequence performed at IVC. Next, 3D radiofrequency-spoiled gradient echo (SPGR) sequences are performed at IVC and EVC covering the complete thorax to evaluate lung anatomy and measure central airway dimensions. The field of view (FOV) is then narrowed to include only the trachea and main stem bronchi and 3D SPGR sequences are obtained at IVC and EVC. Finally, four-dimensional (4D) temporally resolved imaging of contrast kinetics (TRICKS) acquisitions of the same limited FOV are obtained during forced expiration and cough to image real-time movements of the trachea and main stem bronchi. The scan time to perform these maneuvers is approximately 12 minutes (range 7–15 minutes). Spirometer-controlled MR imaging is only feasible in older children who are able to follow breathing instructions. Dynamic MR evaluation of the airway is a promising new tool that can help to minimize the number of CT scans in pediatric patients suspected of having TBM for an initial diagnosis and follow-up assessment after treatment.

Thoracic vasculature evaluation

Typical indications for imaging of the thoracic vasculature in children include evaluation of

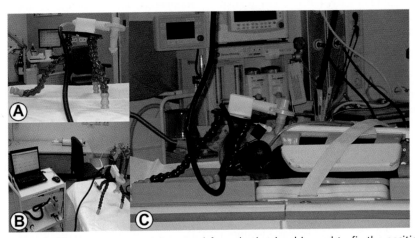

Fig. 1. MR imaging spirometer apparatus. (A) A metal free plastic tripod is used to fix the position of the MR imaging–compatible spirometer and mouthpiece. (B) The spirometer is connected to the mouthpiece by a plastic tube to measure differential pressure for computation of flow, which is introduced into the Faraday cage. (C) The complete apparatus is shown, including a nose clip.

vascular anomalies, investigation of lesions with associated abnormal vascular supply, and the study of PE. Imaging protocols include basic T1-weighted and T2-weighted sequences described in detail earlier[4] along with electrocardiography (ECG)-gated black blood single-shot fast spin echo (SSFSE) with double inversion recovery, bright blood 2D or 3D balanced steady-state free precession (SSFP) sequences, and MR angiography. MR angiography sequences can be used with or without contrast. Noncontrast MR angiography sequences rely on SSFP-GRE, double inversion recovery, or time of flight techniques and have been used in the evaluation of the thoracic vasculature and PE.[3,21–25] These noncontrast techniques can be repeated numerous times without concern about contrast dose. However, many consider contrast-enhanced MR angiography (CEMRA) to be the preferred method for pulmonary MR angiography given its high spatial and contrast resolution.[3,4,26,27] CEMRA requires breath-hold times of approximately 15 seconds, and is therefore not possible in young pediatric patients who cannot follow breathing instructions. The basic principle behind CEMRA is the acquisition of a heavily T1-weighted sequence after intravenous administration of a paramagnetic contrast agent.[4,28] Short relaxation times (TR) of less than 5 milliseconds allow for minimization of breath-hold times and short echo times (TE) of less than 2 milliseconds and high flip angles decrease background signal and susceptibility artifacts.[4,26] 3D techniques can be used to allow for multiplanar reformation. To achieve high contrast between vascular branches and surrounding structures, it is essential to administer the contrast bolus using an automatic power injector with flow rates between 2 and 5 mL/s followed by a saline flush (**Table 2**).[4] Because patients in need of thoracic vasculature imaging often have varied flow

dynamics, optimum timing should be individually adjusted using a test bolus. If the timing is incorrectly calculated and images are obtained in a later phase, enhancement of the pulmonary veins can impair the assessment of the arteries. In cases of arterial/venous superimposition, several postprocessing strategies can be used to differentiate arteries from veins, including cine or stack-mode viewing, continuous rotation, multiplanar reformation (MPR), and maximum intensity projection (MIP).[4] One strategy to avoid the issue of superimposition uses high temporal resolution multiphasic acquisitions, which begin at the time of contrast administration and continue through the venous phase, although these sequences have lower spatial resolution.[4,29,30]

Ventilation evaluation: HP gas and oxygen-enhanced imaging

HP gas imaging One of the primary technical challenges of lung MR imaging is an inherent low signal-to-noise ratio, because most of the lung is composed of gas-filled spaces where the concentration of water molecules is approximately 1000 times less than that in solid tissue.[6] Given this physical property, there will always be challenges to obtaining signal from lung parenchyma using standard proton MR. Over the past decade, an alternative to proton MR has been developed that obtains signal from inhaled HP ^{129}Xe or ^{3}He, which serve as positive contrast agents as they move through the airways, thus providing a method for imaging ventilation.[6,31–35]

To perform HP gas MR imaging, the patient is fitted with an radiofrequency (RF) coil that is tuned to operate at the resonant frequency of ^{129}Xe or ^{3}He, a function that can be performed on most commercial MR scanners. A bag of HP gas is generated in a noble gas polarizer, and the patient inhales the HP gas immediately before imaging (**Fig. 2**). A static breath-hold, fast, 2D, multislice GRE sequence is then acquired at end inspiration to assess the distribution of ventilated gas (**Fig. 3**).[6,31,33,35] Excellent image quality can be obtained with both ^{129}Xe or ^{3}He. Gaseous ^{129}Xe has a much higher molecular weight and lower coefficient than ^{3}He, which may result in differences in the flow and distribution of the gases during inhalation. This may make ^{129}Xe more sensitive to airflow abnormalities in obstructive lung diseases (**Fig. 4**).[36]

Diffusion-weighted imaging (DWI) can also be performed to evaluate the lung microstructure at the alveolar level.[37–40] Because HP gas molecules move randomly through the airways and alveoli as a result of Brownian motion, the average distance that an HP gas molecule moves in a given period of

Table 2
Intravenous catheter size, injection rate, and method for MR imaging

Intravenous Catheter Size (Gauge)	Maximum Injection Rate (mL/s)	Injection Method
24	1.0	Hand injection
22	2.0	Power injection
20	2.0–3.0[a]	Power injection
18	3.0–4.0[a]	Power injection

[a] In pediatric patients, diagnostic thoracic MR imaging and MR angiography examinations can usually be performed with injection rates of ~2 mL/s.

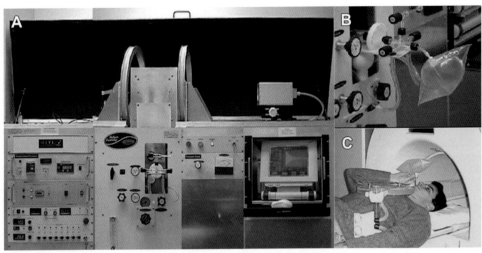

Fig. 2. HP ³He or ¹²⁹Xe generation and administration. (A) ³He or ¹²⁹Xe is polarized using a noble gas polarizer (IGI-9600, MITI, Durham, NC). (B) HP gas is dispensed into an inert plastic bag. (C) The patient inhales the gas immediately before imaging. (Adapted from Mugler JP, Altes TA. Hyperpolarized 129Xe MRI of the human lung. J Magn Reson Imaging 2013;37(2):313–31; with permission.)

time is determined by the alveolar microstructure. Therefore, the random movements of HP gas molecules are influenced by disease processes that cause the alveoli to be abnormally expanded (Fig. 5). Using the same principles used in DWI of the brain and body, apparent diffusion coefficient (ADC) maps can be obtained, providing an assessment of lung microstructure including alveoli and acini, with larger airspaces leading to higher ADC values (Fig. 6).[41] DWI has been performed with both ¹²⁹Xe or ³He, and qualitatively similar results have been obtained with both gases (Fig. 7).[36] An increase in mean ³He ADC has been observed with increasing age in children from 4 years old to adulthood, suggesting that HP gas DWI can detect the known age-related increase in alveolar size during childhood

(Fig. 8).[42] Furthermore, increased ADC values have been detected in children with a history of preterm birth and subsequent bronchopulmonary dysplasia compatible with histologic evidence that these children have enlarged alveoli, which are reduced in number (Fig. 9). Thus, HP gas DWI is a noninvasive technique that can be used to evaluate normal alveolar development and the alterations in lung development caused by pediatric lung diseases.

Although most clinical MR scanners have the ability to perform HP gas imaging, it is not in widespread use because ¹²⁹Xe and ³He are not readily available in most centers. Global supplies of ³He are limited and expensive because the market price of ³He is partially determined by governmental and political considerations.[6,43] Therefore,

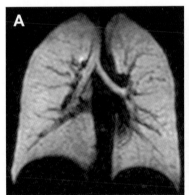
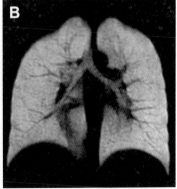

Fig. 3. HP gas MR lung ventilation imaging in normal individuals. (A) ³He MR imaging. (B) ¹²⁹Xe MR imaging. (Adapted from Mugler JP, Altes TA. Hyperpolarized 129Xe MRI of the human lung. J Magn Reson Imaging 2013;37(2):313–31; with permission.)

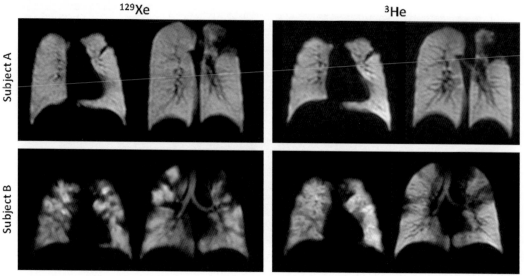

Fig. 4. Coronal HP ^{129}Xe and ^{3}He ventilation images from 2 patients with CF. Imaging for each patient was completed on the same day. Note that excellent image quality was obtained with both ^{129}Xe and ^{3}He. In subject A, the ventilation defects with the 2 gases are similar. In subject B, the ventilation defects are larger and more conspicuous with ^{129}Xe. This difference observed in subject B is possibly attributable to the different physical properties of ^{129}Xe and ^{3}He gases. All images were acquired at 1.5 T using a single-channel chest RF coil and a low-flip-angle gradient echo (FLASH) pulse sequence. (*Adapted from* Mugler JP, Altes TA. Hyperpolarized 129Xe MRI of the human lung. J Magn Reson Imaging 2013;37(2):313–31; with permission.)

^{129}Xe has been adopted by many as the imaging agent of choice because it is more readily available and less expensive[6,35] than ^{3}He. New ^{129}Xe generators, such as the XeBox-E10 produced by Xemed (**Fig. 10**) are currently in development and may make widespread implementation of HP gas imaging feasible in the near future.[44]

In addition to the greater availability and affordability of ^{129}Xe, the physical characteristics of ^{129}Xe provide certain imaging advantages over ^{3}He. Unlike ^{3}He, ^{129}Xe is soluble in tissue and blood, allowing it to be used in imaging of gas exchange at the level of the alveolar capillary bed and provide information about diffusion capacity.[33,45–47] This can be performed using a chemical shift saturation recovery method using ^{129}Xe magnetization[6,34,43,48] or using xenon transfer contrast.[6,49,50]

Oxygen-enhanced imaging O_2-enhanced MR imaging was first proposed when shortening of the T_1 of lung parenchyma was noted in patients breathing 100% oxygen.[51–53] Although oxyhemoglobin is diamagnetic, O_2 is paramagnetic and it therefore modulates the signal emitted from protons in adjacent fluid and tissues.[6,32] This dissolved paramagnetic free molecular O_2 causes a reduction in the T_1 relaxation time in oxygenated tissues.[32] When imaging the lung while a patient is breathing room air, the partial pressure of O_2

Normal Alveolus   **Emphysematous Alveolus**

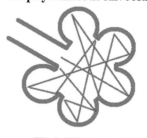

Low HP Gas ADC   High HP Gas ADC

Fig. 5. HP gas diffusion MR imaging. ADC is determined by random Brownian motion of HP gas molecules within the alveoli. When the alveolus is expanded, molecules travel a greater distance, leading to larger ADC values.

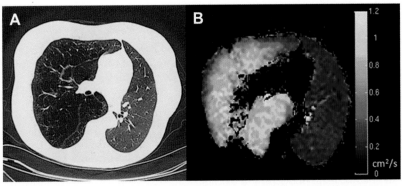

Fig. 6. Axial CT and [3]He ADC map of a patient after left lung transplant. (*A*) Axial CT demonstrates hyperexpansion of the native right lung, with a relatively normal transplanted left lung. (*B*) The ADC map demonstrates increased ADC values within hyperexpanded portions of the native right lung and normal ADC values within the transplanted left lung. (*Adapted from* Altes TA, Salerno M. Hyperpolarized gas MR imaging of the lung. J Thorac Imaging 2004;19(4):250–8; with permission.)

within the pulmonary venous and systemic arterial blood (Pa$_{O_2}$) is equal to the partial pressure of O_2 within the alveoli (PA$_{O_2}$), each measuring approximately 100 mm Hg. However, when a patient breathes 100% oxygen, the alveolar PA$_{O_2}$ is approximately 600 mm Hg, leading to a 6-fold increase in the concentration of dissolved O_2 in arterial blood.[32,54] This 6-fold increase results in a reduction in the T_1 relaxation time by approximately 9%,[39] and this change in T_1 relaxation time is used to perform O_2-enhanced MR imaging. Because this is a small change in the T_1 relaxation time, separate sequences are performed with the patient breathing both room air and 100% O_2, allowing for better quantification of signal changes.

MR imaging is performed while the patient wears a nonrebreathing mask or mouthpiece with a nose clamp and alternates between breathing room air and 100% oxygen. A subtraction map is generated, and the difference between the 2 image sets results in the O_2-enhanced ventilation images.[32] T1-weighted inversion recovery (IR) single-shot turbo spin echo (TSE), HASTE, and rapid acquisition with relaxation enhancement (RARE) sequences are usually used, with TE kept as sort as possible.[32] Background subtraction can be optimized by suppressing signal from thoracic fat and muscle using IR HASTE sequences[55] or applying inversion pulses to the surrounding tissues.[56] Imaging can be performed in quiet breathing, but respiratory and cardiac motion can often degrade the quality of the subtracted O_2 ventilation image so respiratory triggering and ECG gating are often helpful.[57,58]

Because O_2-enhanced MR imaging assesses oxygen delivery at the alveolar level, several studies

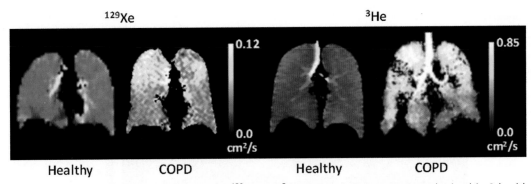

Fig. 7. Comparison of diffusion imaging using [129]Xe and [3]He. Coronal ADC maps were obtained in 2 healthy individuals and in 2 patients with chronic obstructive pulmonary disease (COPD) using [129]Xe (*2 images on the left*) or [3]He (*2 images on the right*). For both gases, the ADC values are relatively low and spatially uniform in the healthy individuals. In contrast, the ADC values for the COPD patients are markedly inhomogeneous and generally increased compared with those for the healthy individuals, particularly in the apices. (*Adapted from* Mugler JP, Altes TA. Hyperpolarized 129Xe MRI of the human lung. J Magn Reson Imaging 2013;37(2):313–31; with permission.)

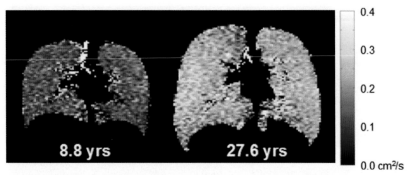

Fig. 8. Coronal HP ^{3}He ADC maps from 2 healthy individuals aged 8.8 years and 27.6 years. The ADC maps of both individuals are relatively homogeneous but the ADC values of the older individual are higher (mean ADC 0.236 cm^2/s) than those of the younger individual (mean ADC 0.146 cm^2/s), demonstrating the ability of imaging to detect growth of the lung microstructure during childhood. (*Adapted from* Altes TA, Mata J, de Lange EE, et al. Assessment of lung development using hyperpolarized helium-3 diffusion MR imaging. J Magn Reson Imaging 2006;24(6):1277–83; with permission.)

have demonstrated its usefulness in the evaluation of a large number of pulmonary diseases.[59–66] Diagnostic studies combining O$_2$-enhanced MR imaging and contrast-enhanced perfusion imaging (described in the next section) have been described, and may be well suited to replace nuclear medicine V/Q studies in the future.[67,68]

Perfusion evaluation
Numerous different pulmonary disease processes in both pediatric and adult patients cause alterations in lung perfusion. Perfusion can be evaluated on MR imaging with or without contrast enhancement. Alterations in perfusion can be related to ventilation, as when hypoxic vasoconstriction leads to regional hypoperfusion. Decreases in perfusion can also be independent of ventilation, such as in the case of PE. Perfusion imaging can be performed alone or along with ventilation imaging to create ventilation/perfusion MR imaging.[31]

Contrast-enhanced perfusion imaging Several techniques to image lung perfusion have been

described, but the most commonly used method is known as dynamic contrast-enhanced (DCE) imaging.[69] In this technique, a paramagnetic contrast agent such as gadolinium diethylenetraminepentaacetic acid (Gd-DTPA) is administered intravenously and time-resolved dynamic MR imaging is performed. Several imaging sequences have been described, including 3D fast low-angle shot (FLASH), time-resolved echo-shared angiographic technique (TREAT), TRICKS, and time-resolved angiography with interleaved stochastic trajectories (TWIST).[31,69–71] Dynamic imaging allows for visualization of the contrast as it circulates through the body and diffuses into the extravascular extracellular space of the lung.[31] Visual assessment of regional perfusion is facilitated by subtraction of the precontrast images from the images obtained during peak enhancement. More sophisticated analyses can also be performed to evaluate the kinetics of contrast enhancement. This can include evaluation of the signal curve and analysis of time to peak enhancement, bolus arrival time, and maximum enhancement.[72] Statistical analysis and automatic lung segmentation

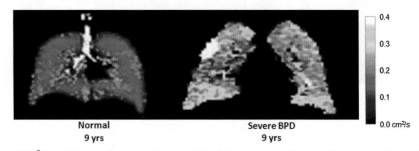

Fig. 9. Coronal HP ^{3}He ADC maps from two 9-year-old children: one healthy and the other with a history of preterm birth and severe bronchopulmonary dysplasia (BPD). The healthy child has homogeneous low ADC values (mean ADC 0.17 cm^2/s). The child with BPD has markedly increased and heterogeneous ADC values (mean ADC 0.23 cm^2/s).

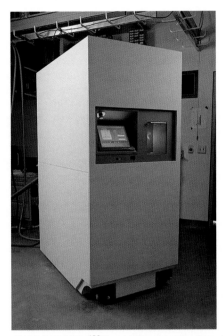

Fig. 10. XeBox-E10 [129]Xe generator, produced by Xemed. This portable automated [129]Xe generator is about the size of a household refrigerator and is currently available to research collaborators. (*Adapted from* Mugler JP, Altes TA. Hyperpolarized 129Xe MRI of the human lung. J Magn Reson Imaging 2013;37(2):313–31; with permission.)

can be applied and percent perfusion per lung region can be estimated. Using the indicator dilution theory, quantitative estimations of pulmonary blood volume, pulmonary blood flow, and mean transit time can be performed.[69,73–75] A greater signal-to-noise ratio is achieved on 1.5-T systems compared with 3.0-T systems as a result of higher susceptibility effects at greater magnetic field strengths.[76]

Most of the research on DCE MR imaging of the lung has been performed in adults to evaluate for PE,[77,78] chronic obstructive pulmonary disease,[79–81] pulmonary hypertension,[82,83] and postoperative lung function,[84] but perfusion imaging has also been described in the evaluation of cystic fibrosis in children.[85]

Non–contrast-enhanced perfusion imaging Using techniques that mark a fraction of blood by selective RF excitation, it is possible to obtain perfusion information without the use of intravenous contrast.[86–91] This technique is called arterial spin labeling (ASL). Two ASL techniques called flow-sensitive alternating inversion recovery (FAIR) and flow-sensitive alternating inversion recovery with an extra RF pulse (FAIRER) have been developed, and allow for quantification of

pulmonary perfusion.[88,91] Detailed descriptions of image acquisition are described elsewhere.[92,93] FAIR sequences apply a spatially selective inversion pulse before acquiring one image set and a nonselective inversion pulse before a second image set, and perfusion-weighted images are obtained from the subtraction of the 2 image sets.[91,93] FAIRER sequences are slightly different because they apply an additional spatially selective 90° RF pulse followed by a dephasing gradient before or after the inversion pulse.[88] A major advantage of ASL is the ability to repeat sequences as many times as needed without the need to wait for contrast clearance or limitation by the maximum volume of contrast that can be administered per day. ASL is particularly sensitive to motion artifacts because it is a subtraction technique, and variation between images can lead to ghosting artifacts and the appearance of bright-dark pairs of blood vessels.[91] ECG gating is often used to mitigate these artifacts. Although studies of pulmonary ASL have been largely performed in the adult population, it has potential benefits in older pediatric patients who are able to follow breathing instructions.

SPECTRUM OF THORACIC DISORDERS IN PEDIATRIC PATIENTS

Using the imaging techniques described earlier, MR imaging provides a powerful diagnostic tool for the evaluation of a large number of thoracic disorders in pediatric patients without the use of ionizing radiation. The use of MR imaging in the diagnosis and management of these disorders is described and examples are presented.

Disorders of Lung Parenchyma

Congenital lung malformations
Congenital pulmonary malformations are a heterogeneous group of disorders that affect the lung parenchyma as well as the arterial supply and the venous drainage of the lung. These anomalies include, but are not limited to, bronchial atresia, congenital pulmonary airway malformation (CPAM; formerly known as congenital cystic adenomatoid malformation), and bronchopulmonary sequestration. These lesions are increasingly diagnosed prenatally with ultrasonography and MR imaging[94–97]; however, they can also present as a cause of respiratory distress in the newborn or as recurrent infection in older children. CT has been the mainstay of postnatal diagnosis and presurgical planning,[98–100] but use of MR has been described in the evaluation of congenital pulmonary malformations.[101,102]

MR imaging with MR angiography is well suited to imaging of bronchopulmonary sequestration, because a region of abnormal lung parenchyma is often easily identified on T2-weighted sequences and an aberrant vessel can be identified on MR angiography (**Figs. 11** and **12**).[103] Solid and microcystic CPAMs are also easily identified on MR images but macrocystic CPAMs can be more difficult to assess, given the lack of associated signal on MR, and CT is usually required for preoperative planning (**Fig. 13**).[98–100,103] MR evaluation of bronchial atresia has been described[101,102] and can be diagnosed based on the observation of high signal on T1-weighted and T2-weighted sequences within an atretic bronchus due to impacted mucus,[101] but the associated hyperinflation that is easily identified on radiographs and CT may be more difficult to assess on MR. Ventilation sequences may be helpful in this setting, although this requires further investigation.

A suggested MR protocol for the evaluation of a nonvascular congenital pulmonary malformation includes axial fast relaxation fast spin echo (FRFSE) T2 fat saturation, axial T1 or double inversion recovery (DIR) with breath-hold and ECG gating, coronal FRFSE T2 fat saturation, coronal 3D MR angiography, SPGR with gadolinium, and postcontrast axial and coronal T1 fat saturation using an 8-channel cardiac coil. When evaluating a vascular congenital pulmonary malformation, the addition of axial, sagittal, and coronal oblique fast spin echo (FSE) DIR sequences with breath-hold and ECG gating and contrast-enhanced sagittal 3D SPGR MR angiography is useful.

Pulmonary infection

The first-line imaging modality for evaluating pulmonary infection is radiography, but cross-sectional imaging is often needed in cases of immunocompromised patients and complicated pneumonia. A recent prospective study of 40 consecutive pediatric patients evaluated the efficacy of chest MR imaging with fast imaging sequences at 1.5 T for evaluating pneumonia by comparing MR imaging findings with those of chest radiographs. In this study, the investigators found that MR imaging with fast imaging sequences is comparable with chest radiographs for evaluating pulmonary consolidation, bronchiectasis, necrosis, abscess, and pleural effusion often associated with pneumonia in children.[104]

CT has a well-established role in the evaluation of pulmonary infection,[105–109] but MR is playing an increasing role[8,104,110–113] mainly because of concern about radiation exposure in children. Although CT may detect subtle early changes of pulmonary infection with greater sensitivity, MR has been proved useful in evaluation of abnormalities of the parenchyma, pleura, and lymph nodes in suspected complicated lung infection in children (**Fig. 14**).[8,110–113] A recent prospective study of 71 consecutive pediatric patients investigated the efficacy of thoracic MR imaging with fast imaging sequences without contrast at 1.5 T for evaluating thoracic abnormalities by comparing MR findings with those of contrast-enhanced multidetector computed tomography (MDCT). Gorkem and colleagues[114] found that MR imaging with fast imaging sequences without contrast is comparable with contrast-enhanced MDCT for detecting

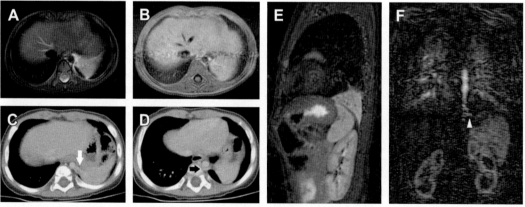

Fig. 11. A 20-month-old male infant with left lower extralobar pulmonary sequestration. (*A*) Axial T2-weighted fast relaxation fast spin echo with fat saturation. (*B*) Axial T1-weighted. (*C, D*) Consecutive axial images from contrast-enhanced CT. (*E*) Sagittal fast STIR. (*F*) Coronal contrast-enhanced TRICKS MR angiography. Wedge-shaped mass adjacent to the left lower lobe and superior to the diaphragm demonstrates hyperintensity on T1-weighted and T2-weighted images. Arterial supply from the descending aorta is seen on CT (*white arrow*) and MR angiography (*white arrowhead*) and venous drainage to the hemiazygous vein (*black arrow*) is seen on CT. Venous drainage is not well demonstrated on this MR image.

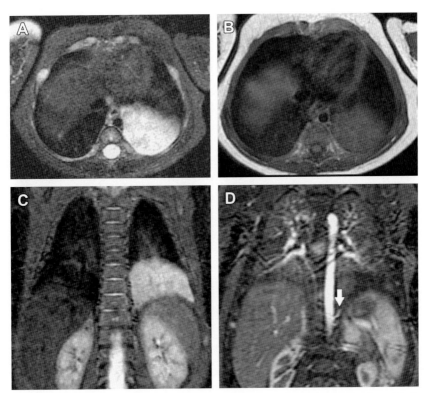

Fig. 12. A 48-day-old female infant with prenatal imaging demonstrating a chest mass, found to have left lower extralobar pulmonary sequestration. (*A*) Axial T2-weighted FSE with fat saturation. (*B*) Axial T1-weighted spin echo. (*C*) Coronal IR FSE. (*D*) Coronal CEMRA. Wedge-shaped mass adjacent to the left lower lobe and superior to the diaphragm demonstrates hyperintensity on T1-weighted and T2-weighted images. Arterial supply from the descending aorta is seen on MR angiography (*white arrow*). Venous drainage is not well demonstrated.

thoracic abnormalities in pediatric patients. They suggested that the use of MR imaging with fast imaging sequences without contrast as a first-line cross-sectional imaging study in lieu of contrast-enhanced MDCT has the potential to benefit this patient population because of reduced radiation exposure and intravenous contrast administration.[114]

A suggested MR protocol for the evaluation of suspected complicated lung infection includes axial T2-weighted, coronal T2-weighted, coronal STIR, and postcontrast axial and coronal fat-suppressed T1-weighted sequences,[110] although this new research suggests that contrast-enhanced sequences may be avoided in many cases.[114]

Neoplasm

Because primary lung tumors are rare in children, no systematic studies evaluating the use of MR imaging in primary pediatric malignancy have been conducted. The evaluation of pulmonary nodules and pulmonary metastases by MR has been investigated in adults,[5,115] and there is broad consensus that pulmonary metastases of 5 mm

or more can be reliably detected[103] and animal models have suggested that lesions of 4 mm or more could feasibly be identified using 3D and 2D GRE sequences.[116] Recently, Gorkem and colleagues[114] showed that the diagnostic accuracy of MR imaging with fast imaging sequences without contrast is high for detecting pulmonary nodules (>4 mm) in pediatric patients using contrast-enhanced MDCT as the reference standard. Because early identification of even small pulmonary metastasis ($\leq$4 mm) is clinically important, contrast-enhanced CT is currently the preferred method for initial evaluation of metastatic disease. However, MR imaging may be used to monitor known pulmonary metastases during therapy or as an alternative to CT when iodinated contrast is contraindicated (**Figs. 15** and **16**).[103,117] Such practice has great potential for decreasing overall radiation exposure in pediatric patients who require multiple imaging evaluations.

A proposed MR protocol for the evaluation of pulmonary nodules includes coronal T2-weighted HASTE, axial T1-weighted 3D-GRE (VIBE) during breath-hold, coronal steady-state free precession (SS-GRE, TrueFISP) in free-breathing, and axial

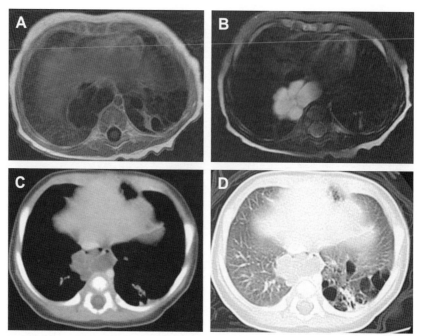

Fig. 13. A 6-year-old boy with macrocystic left lower lobe CPAM and right paraspinal complex esophageal duplication cyst. (*A*) Axial T1-weighted spin echo. (*B*) Axial T2-weighted FRFSE with fat saturation. (*C, D*) Axial contrast-enhanced CT in soft tissue and lung windows. Left lower lobe macrocystic CPAM is not as well seen on MR imaging as on CT in lung windows given the large air-filled spaces. However, the fluid-filled right paraspinal esophageal duplication cyst is easily seen on both MR and CT images.

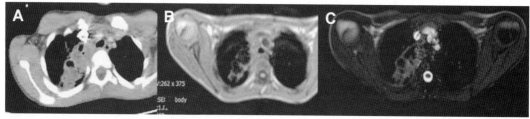

Fig. 14. A 5-year-old girl with recurrent right upper lobe pneumonia. Posterior right upper lobe consolidation and bronchiectasis are seen on CT (*A*) and are well visualized on MR images (*B, C*). (*Courtesy of* Sureyya B. Gorkem, MD, Department of Radiology, Erciyes Medical School, Kayseri, Turkey.)

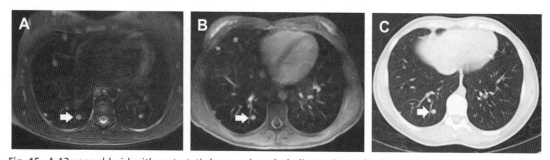

Fig. 15. A 12-year-old girl with metastatic hemangioendothelioma. Several pulmonary nodules are well seen on MR imaging and CT, including a 10-mm right lower lobe nodule (*arrows*). (*A*) Axial T2-weighted FRFSE with fat saturation. (*B*) Axial contrast-enhanced T1-weighted lung acquisition with volume acceleration. (*C*) Axial noncontrast CT in lung windows.

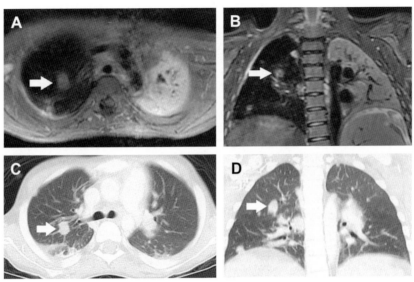

Fig. 16. A 14-year-old boy with lymphoma. Several pulmonary nodules are well seen on MR imaging and subsequent CT performed 4 days later, including a 13-mm right upper lobe nodule (*arrows*). Left lung collapse seen on MR imaging had resolved by the time of CT. (*A*) Axial contrast-enhanced T1-weighted. (*B*) Coronal IR FSE. (*C, D*) Axial and coronal contrast-enhanced CT in lung windows.

T2-weighted STIR (T2-TIRM) in a multi breath-hold technique. When motion artifact is an issue, the T2-weighted STIR sequence can be replaced by a fat-saturated T2-weighted FSE with Propeller acquisition and reconstruction (T2 TSE BLADE), which significantly reduces motion artifact although the acquisition time is longer.[5] Contrast-enhanced sequences may not improve nodule detection but they are generally preferred for clearer depiction of vessels, hilar structures, and pleural enhancement. Therefore, a postcontrast 3D-GRE (VIBE) sequence has also been recommended.[5]

Interstitial lung disease
Over the past 3 decades, CT has served as the primary imaging modality for the assessment of interstitial lung disease (ILD) in both adults and children.[117] With recent advances in MR imaging, it is now comparable with CT in many instances. However, a limited number of studies investigating MR in ILD have been performed and no systematic studies have been performed on children.

Findings in diseases of the lung interstitium involve abnormalities of the interstitium itself and/or the airspaces.[103,117] Airspace disease manifests as a hyperintense signal on T2-weighted sequences adjacent to hypointense air-filled normal lung parenchyma. This is akin to ground glass opacities seen on CT when the pulmonary vascular markings are not obscured by the T2 signal[117–119] and akin to consolidation seen

on CT when the vasculature is obscured by the T2 signal.[110,117,120] Interstitial abnormalities also appear as hyperintensity on T2-weighted images but are seen as curvilinear bands, nodules, reticulation, or parenchymal distortion (**Fig. 17**).[117,121–123] Given its superior contrast resolution over CT, MR imaging has the potential to differentiate active interstitial inflammation from fibrosis, which has significant clinical implications for predicting treatment response in ILD.

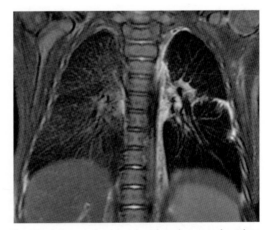

Fig. 17. A 6-month-old girl with pulmonary lymphangiectasia and persistent tachypnea after left chylothorax drainage. Coronal T2-weighted FRFSE with fat saturation demonstrates diffuse bilateral linear hyperintensity within the interstitium, which is greater on the right, and trace left pleural effusion.

Increased T2 signal within the interstitium has been shown to correlate with active inflammation, whereas an isointense signal correlates with fibrosis.[117,121,124] DCE perfusion MR imaging has also been used to evaluate active inflammation in ILD, and earlier peak enhancement times were shown to correlate with disease activity.[124]

The previously described standard MR protocol for evaluation of lung parenchyma[4] is also well suited for the evaluation of ILD. Imaging on a 3-T system is preferred.[121,124] DCE perfusion sequences can also be added to evaluate for active inflammation.[124]

Disorders of the Large Airways

Disorders of the pediatric large airway can be divided into static and dynamic processes. The static processes account for most airway abnormalities and include anomalies of tracheobronchial branching (**Fig. 18**), bronchial atresia, congenital tracheal stenosis, neoplasm, infection, and acquired tracheobronchial stenosis from previous instrumentation or surgery (**Fig. 19**). MR imaging is well suited to the evaluation of these disorders. The main dynamic disease process of the pediatric airway is TBM, which is characterized by weakening of the tracheal and bronchial walls or supporting cartilage leading to excessive collapse of the airway during expiration.[125] MR imaging is also well suited to the evaluation of this dynamic disease process, although specific patient preparation and MR imaging sequences are required (see **Fig. 1; Fig. 20**).

Static large airway abnormalities
MR imaging is well suited to evaluate the static large airway abnormalities described earlier because the air-filled tracheobronchial tree appears as a low signal outlined by the higher signal tracheal and bronchial walls, mediastinum, and lungs.[3,12,15,17–19] Airways smaller than 3 mm in diameter cannot be reliably visualized unless filled with hyperintense material.[3,126,127] This is particularly important in the evaluation of young children; MR imaging has been shown to reliably depict airways to the first subsegmental level in regions without artifact, although it is more limited in areas with cardiac pulsation and motion artifact.[3,128]

The previously described standard non–contrast-enhanced protocol for evaluation of lung parenchyma[4] with the addition of a 3D SPGR sequence is well suited for the evaluation of anomalies of tracheobronchial branching, bronchial atresia, congenital tracheal stenosis, and acquired tracheobronchial stenosis. The addition of a contrast-enhanced 3D GRE (VIBE) sequence is useful when evaluating neoplasms, infection, and inflammation affecting the large airway.[4]

Dynamic large airway abnormalities
TBM is a relatively common dynamic disease process of the pediatric large airway. Because the major imaging finding in this disorder is excessive collapse of the airway during expiration,[125] imaging must be performed at end expiration in addition to end inspiration (see **Fig. 20**). Dynamic imaging obtained during breathing can be used to visualize airway collapse. Until recently, CT

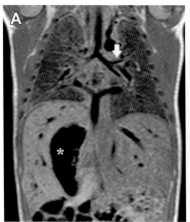
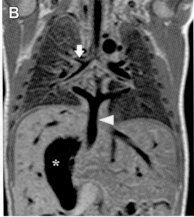
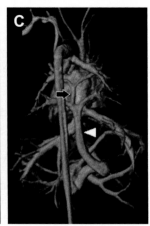

Fig. 18. A 2-day-old boy with heterotaxy, right-sided branching pattern of bilateral bronchi (*white arrows*), right-sided stomach (*asterisk*), midline liver, asplenia, and total anomalous pulmonary venous connection (*black arrow* and *white arrowhead*). TAPVC is characterized by small left and right upper pulmonary veins that join to form a small vertical confluence (*black arrow*), which then joins the left and right lower pulmonary veins to form a larger confluence (*white arrowhead*) that crosses the diaphragm and connects with the portal vein. (*A, B*) Coronal bright blood proton density TSE. (*C*) Volume-rendered reconstruction of CEMRA.

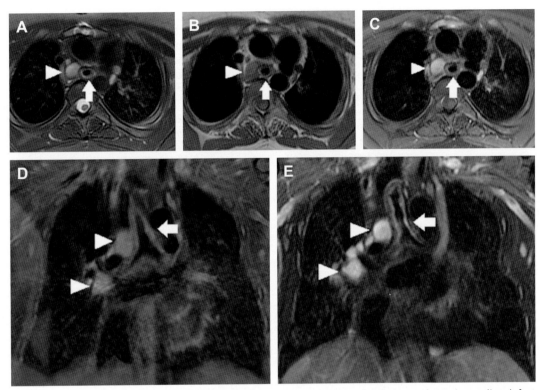

Fig. 19. A 16-year-old girl with a history of VACTERL association (vertebral defects, anal atresia, cardiac defects, tracheoesophageal fistula, renal anomalies, and limb abnormalities) with tracheoesophageal fistula and left pulmonary artery sling leading to severe subglottic stenosis, after tracheal transplant and left pulmonary artery plasty. The tracheal transplant is diffusely thickened, edematous, and hyperenhancing (*arrows*). Reactive right paratracheal and hilar lymph nodes are also noted (*arrowheads*). (*A*) Axial T2-weighted FRFSE with fat saturation. (*B*) Axial ECG-gated T1-weighted. (*C*) Axial contrast-enhanced ECG-gated T1-weighted with fat saturation. (*D*) Coronal T2-weighted FRFSE with fat saturation. (*E*) Coronal contrast-enhanced ECG-gated T1-weighted with fat saturation.

has been the mainstay of evaluation[12–16] although emerging techniques in spirometer-controlled MR imaging provide a method for dynamic evaluation of the airway without the use of ionizing radiation. This technique, described in detail previously, may play an important role in the evaluation of TBM in the near future.

Diseases of Small and Medium Airways

Two major diseases of the small and medium airways in children are asthma and cystic fibrosis (CF). These diseases lead to characteristic changes within the airway including narrowing, wall thickening, smooth muscle contraction, and/or dilation. Functional and morphologic evaluation

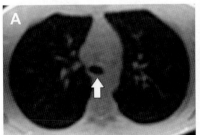
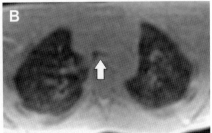

Fig. 20. Patient with TBM. Images obtained during inspiration (*A*) and expiration (*B*) demonstrate dynamic tracheal collapse (*arrow*) during expiration. (*A*) Spirometry-gated 3D SPGR during inspiration. (*B*) Spirometry-gated 3D SPGR during expiration.

of these changes can be evaluated using MR techniques including standard nonenhanced and contrast-enhanced sequences, HP gas imaging, and O_2-enhanced imaging.

Asthma

Asthma is a chronic inflammatory disorder of the lungs that is fairly common in the pediatric patient population. Asthma affects small and medium airways and causes smooth muscle hyperresponsiveness and hypertrophy, increased mucous production, and subepithelial fibrosis. Many of these findings are not evident on standard MR sequences, but investigational techniques in HP gas imaging using ^3He and ^{129}Xe and O_2-enhanced MR have shown promise in the evaluation of patients with asthma.

During HP gas MR imaging, ^3He or ^{129}Xe is inhaled and acts as a positive contrast agent, filling the airspaces. When inhaled by a healthy patient, the HP gas distributes evenly within the lung (see Fig. 3). When the HP gas is inhaled by a patient with obstruction of medium and small airways caused by asthma, the airspaces distal to the obstruction do not fill with the positive contrast agent. Therefore, the lungs of healthy patients demonstrate a uniform high signal, whereas the lungs of patients with asthma show wedge-shaped regions of low signal intensity (Fig. 21).[24,33,35,45,47–50,129–135] In patients with asthma, these defects have been shown to increase with provocation by exercise or administration of a bronchoconstrictor (methacholine) and

decrease with albuterol[133,134,136] (Figs. 22 and 23) and often persist after symptoms have resolved.[136] Using fast acquisition techniques, ventilation images can be obtained in nonsedated infants and young children (Fig. 24). Ventilation imaging with ^3He and ^{129}Xe operate on this same principle; however, ^{129}Xe has the additional property of being soluble in tissue and blood. Therefore, ^{129}Xe has the potential to evaluate gas delivery and transport within the lung (Fig. 25).[33,34,36,43,45,47,49,50] Recent advances in ^{129}Xe production technology[44] may allow this investigative technique to gain more widespread use in the evaluation of asthma in the future.

O_2-enhanced MR imaging is another investigational technique that uses the paramagnetic properties of O_2 to image oxygen delivery at the alveolar level. In asthmatics, obstruction of small and medium airways leads to patchy areas of lower oxygenation which appear as patchy regions of low signal on O_2-enhanced MR images (Fig. 26).[6] This technique has demonstrated usefulness in the assessment of asthma in adult patients[66] and may play a role in the evaluation of asthma in pediatric patients in the future.

Cystic fibrosis

CF is a multisystem disorder caused by a mutation of the CFTR gene that results in abnormal viscosity of mucous and impaired mucociliary clearance. Recent progress in the management of CF has led to a significant increase in the life expectancy of patients with CF but it remains one of the

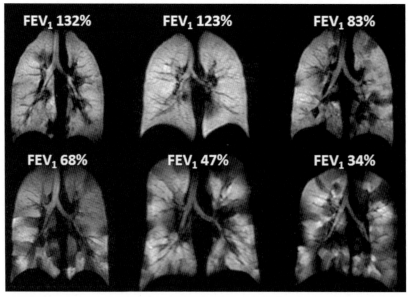

Fig. 21. HP ^3He MR lung ventilation imaging in a patient with asthma. Images obtained at variable forced expiratory volume in first second of expiration (FEV_1) demonstrate numerous regions of signal hypointensity reflecting regions of hypoventilation, which increase as FEV_1 decreases.

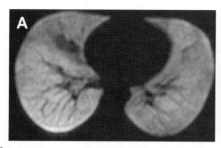
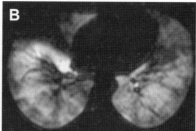

Fig. 22. HP ^{3}He MR lung ventilation imaging in a patient with asthma at baseline at $FEV_1 = 103\%$ (A) and after exercise at $FEV_1 = 40\%$ (B). Postexercise image demonstrates regions of hypointensity reflecting inducible regions of hypoventilation.

most frequent lethal inherited diseases in the United States and Europe. Lung involvement is the main cause of morbidity and mortality,[137] and imaging findings can include air trapping, bronchiectasis, bronchial wall thickening, mucus plugging, cetrilobular tree-in-bud nodules, and superimposed infection.[138] CT is considered the gold standard for evaluation of CF,[139–141] but advances in MR imaging have allowed it to play an increasing role.[142]

Previously described standard T1-weighted and T2-weighted nonenhanced and contrast-enhanced MR sequences used for the evaluation of lung parenchyma[4] have variable accuracy in the evaluation of bronchiectasis and bronchial wall thickening. The accuracy depends on the bronchial level, bronchial diameter, wall thickness, wall signal, and signal within the lumen.[6] Central bronchi and bronchiectasis are well visualized but bronchi at the third to fourth generation are not as well seen.[142] T2 prolongation within the bronchial walls and enhancement on postcontrast imaging can be seen and are related to edema and inflammation. Mucus plugging is well demonstrated to the level of small peripheral airways on T2-weighted sequences and can be differentiated from T2 hyperintense edematous bronchial walls based on lack of enhancement.[142] Consolidation is also well visualized on T2-weighted sequences (see **Fig. 14; Fig. 27**).[112,142]

HP gas, O_2-enhanced, and DCE perfusion MR imaging have also been investigated in the evaluation of CF. Airway obstruction leads to ventilatory defects on ^{3}He imaging (see **Fig. 4; Fig. 28**),[143,144] regions of decreased oxygenation on O_2-enhanced imaging,[60] and perfusion defects are seen within these regions as a result of reflex hypoxic vasoconstriction or tissue destruction.[85] With increased investigation, it is anticipated that MR imaging will play a larger role in the evaluation of patients with CF[6,142] in the future.

Abnormalities of the Thoracic Vasculature

Common indications for imaging of the thoracic vasculature in children include vascular anomalies

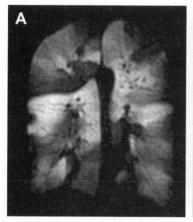
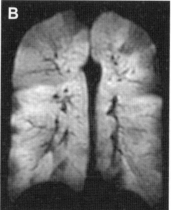

Fig. 23. HP ^{3}He MR lung ventilation imaging in a patient with asthma at baseline at $FEV_1 = 36\%$ (A) and after albuterol at $FEV_1 = 57\%$ (B). Postalbuterol image demonstrates increased signal reflecting improvement in regional hypoventilation.

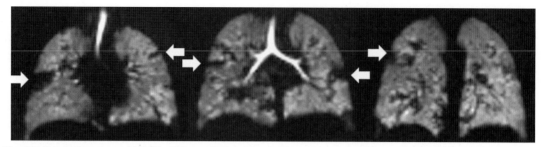

Fig. 24. Successive coronal HP ³He MR ventilation images from a nonsedated, marginally cooperative 4-year-old child with asthma demonstrates multiple small ventilation defects throughout the lungs (eg, *arrows*). This spiral-based sequence has an acquisition time of less than 0.15 seconds per slice, which is adequate to freeze lung motion.

such as vascular rings and slings and partial and total anomalous pulmonary venous connection (PAPVC and TAPVC), lesions with associated abnormal vascular supply such as bronchopulmonary sequestration (see **Figs. 11** and **12**) and scimitar syndrome, and PE. By using nonenhanced and contrast-enhanced techniques, these entities are well evaluated with MR imaging.

Vascular rings and slings
Vascular rings and slings are causes of respiratory distress and dysphagia in children that are often treated surgically.[145] Entities include double aortic arch, right aortic arch with aberrant left subclavian artery with left ligamentum arteriosum, right aortic arch with mirror-image branching and right (retroesophageal) ligamentum arteriosum, left aortic

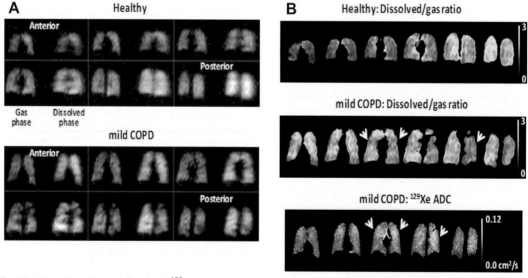

Fig. 25. Direct imaging of dissolved ¹²⁹Xe in the human lung. (*A*) Three-dimensional acquisitions depicting gas-phase ¹²⁹Xe in the lung airspaces (*left side of each section*) and dissolved-phase ¹²⁹Xe in the tissue and blood (*right side of each section*) from a healthy individual (*top*) and a patient with mild (GOLD stage 1) COPD (*bottom*). Although the signal intensity distributions for the gas-phase and dissolved-phase components were generally uniform for the healthy individual, except for noticeably higher dissolved-phase signal intensity in the posterior portion of the lung, both gas-phase and dissolved-phase components showed nonuniform signal distributions in the patient with COPD, with some regions of mismatch between corresponding gas-phase and dissolve-phase signal variations. Acquisition parameters are described in Ref.[36] (*B*) Maps showing the ratio of dissolved-phase to gas-phase ¹²⁹Xe in the healthy individual (*top row*) and the patient with COPD (*middle row*), and showing the ADC for ¹²⁹Xe (b values of 0 and 10 s/cm²) for the patient with COPD (*lower row*). In the anterior portion of the lung, the ratio of dissolved-phase to gas-phase ¹²⁹Xe for the patient with COPD was substantially higher than that for the healthy individual. Regions of relatively low ratio values for the patient with COPD were generally associated with increased ADC values (eg, *arrowheads*). (*Adapted from* Mugler JP, Altes TA. Hyperpolarized 129Xe MRI of the human lung. J Magn Reson Imaging 2013;37(2):313–31; with permission.)

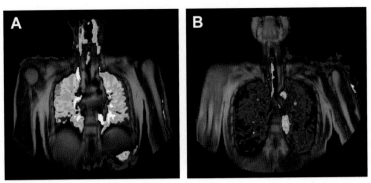

Fig. 26. Oxygen-enhanced coronal MR images in a normal patient (*A*) and a patient with severe asthma (*B*). In the normal patient, the O_2-enhanced signal is uniform throughout the lungs. In the patient with severe asthma, the O_2-enhanced signal is diffusely decreased with patchy regions of more decreased signal in the right lower lobe and left midlung.

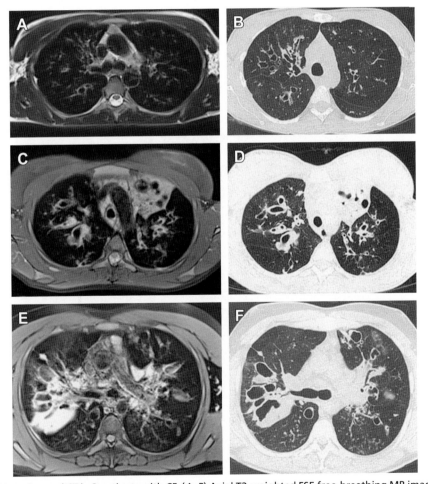

Fig. 27. MR imaging and CT in 3 patients with CF. (*A, B*) Axial T2-weighted FSE free-breathing MR imaging (*A*) and axial noncontrast CT in lung windows demonstrate bilateral upper lobe bronchiectasis and bronchial wall thickening. (*C, D*) Axial T2-weighted BLADE PD + navigator MR imaging and noncontrast CT in lung windows demonstrate bilateral bronchiectasis, bronchial wall thickening, and left upper lobe consolidation. (*E, F*) Axial T2-weighted BLADE PD + navigator MR imaging and noncontrast CT in lung windows demonstrate bilateral bronchiectasis, bronchial wall thickening, and bilateral perihilar consolidation.

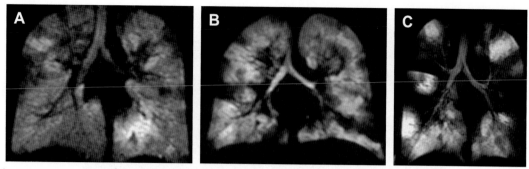

Fig. 28. Hyperpolarized ³He MR lung ventilation imaging in 3 patients with CF causing mild (*A*, FEV₁ = 89%), moderate (*B*, FEV₁ = 67%), and severe (*C*, FEV₁ = 34%) respiratory disease. Wedge-shaped regions of hypointensity increase in number and size as disease severity increases.

arch with aberrant right subclavian artery, left aortic arch with right descending aorta and right ligamentum arteriosum, anomalous innominate artery, cervical aortic arch, and pulmonary artery sling.[146] Vascular rings and slings can be reliably identified using nonenhanced MR angiography[25] or CEMRA[26] (**Fig. 29**).

Suggested protocols include basic T1-weighted and T2-weighted sequences described in detail earlier,[4] ECG-gated black blood SSFSE with DIR, bright blood 2D or 3D SSFP, and MR angiography sequences with or without contrast. Noncontrast MR angiography can be performed using ECG-gated high-resolution free-breathing 3D double-slab fast imaging with steady precession MR angiography (3D FISP MRA) sequences,[25] and are preferable in nonsedated less cooperative patients in whom motion artifact may necessitate multiple image acquisitions. CEMRA is obtained using an ultrafast 3D gradient echo pulse

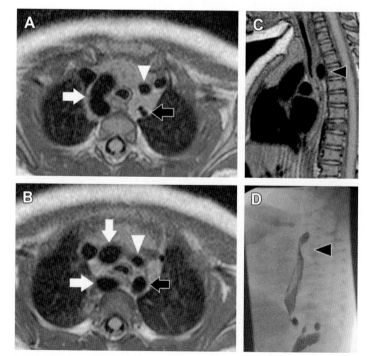

Fig. 29. An 11-month-old girl with vascular ring due to a double aortic arch. (*A, B*) Two contiguous axial proton density-weighted TSE images of the upper chest. (*C*) Sagittal proton density-weighted TSE image of the upper chest. (*D*) Lateral fluoroscopic image from barium swallow. MR imaging and fluoroscopic images demonstrate a double aortic arch characterized by a right aortic arch (*white arrow*) and a partially atretic left arch giving rise to left common carotid (*white arrowhead*) and subclavian arteries (*black arrow*). The vascular ring causes a mass effect on the esophagus (*black arrowhead*).

sequence with short TE and TR (TE/TR/α = 0.9/ 2.3 ms/25° or TE/TR/α = 1.0 m/2.2 ms/40°) during and after the intravenous injection of 0.2 mmol/kg body weight Gd-DTPA at a rate of 2 mL/s using an automatic power injector.[26] CEMRA requires a breath-hold of approximately 15 seconds and is therefore more suitable for intubated and cooperative older patients (>6 years).

Partial anomalous pulmonary venous connection

In PAPVC, 1 or more (but not all) of the pulmonary veins is abnormally connected to a systemic vein. Depending on the degree of shunting, hemodynamic sequelae can develop as a result of increased pulmonary circulation and can lead to pulmonary hypertension and right heart failure. PAPVC can be associated with several other anomalies including pulmonary developmental anomalies in the spectrum of congenital pulmonary venolobar syndrome (including scimitar syndrome and bronchopulmonary sequestration) and sinus venosis defect. In TAPVC, all the pulmonary veins are abnormally connected to a systemic vein. CEMRA is an excellent imaging test for the evaluation of PAPVC and TAPVC (see **Fig. 18**; **Fig. 30**) and several studies have shown it to be superior to cardiac catheterization and transesophageal echocardiography (TEE) in the evaluation of the abnormal pulmonary venous connections.[27,147,148]

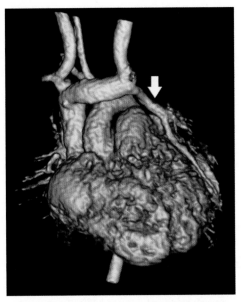

Fig. 30. A 3-year-old girl with PAPVC. 3D volume-rendered reconstruction of CEMRA demonstrates an anomalous connection (*arrow*) between the left upper pulmonary vein and the brachiocephalic vein.

MR protocols to evaluate for PAPVC should include basic T1-weighted and T2-weighted sequences,[4] ECG-gated black blood, bright blood, and CEMRA sequences[27,147,148] described in detail previously. Phase contrast sequences can also be obtained to quantify flow across the shunt and determine the pulmonary-to-systemic flow ratio and differential pulmonary blood flow.

Pulmonary embolism

The current reference standard technique to diagnose PE is contrast-enhanced MDCT.[149] However, given the significant radiation exposure associated with CT, MR angiography has been investigated as an alternative. Several studies have shown CEMRA to be a sensitive and specific modality for the diagnosis of PE in adults (**Fig. 31**),[150–153] although these findings were not reproduced in a large multicenter study (PIOPED III).[154] Therefore, MR angiography should only be considered for the diagnosis of PE in cases when contrast-enhanced MDCT is contraindicated. For these patients, a 2-step protocol has been suggested, combining noncontrast and contrast-enhanced MR techniques.[3]

The suggested protocol begins with a free-breathing TrueFISP sequence[21,153] acquired in 2 or 3 planes in the first 5 minutes of imaging. Kluge and colleagues[153] report that this technique has a sensitivity of 85% and a specificity of 98% for the detection of central PE. If a central PE is identified, the examination can be stopped and the patient can be immediately referred for treatment. If no PE is identified, the protocol can be continued with contrast-enhanced sequences, including DCE perfusion[77,78,153,155] sequences and CEMRA of the pulmonary arteries using a fat-suppressed 3D-FLASH sequence with breath-hold.[153] Kluge and colleagues[153] report that this combined protocol has a sensitivity of 100% and specificity of 93% for the detection of PE. The addition of MR ventilation imaging may also be useful in the diagnosis of PE.[156–160]

FUTURE DIRECTION

Recent advances in MR imaging have allowed for its increased use in the evaluation of thoracic diseases of children. In the future, MR imaging may replace CT for many indications and reduce children's exposure to ionizing radiation. Because MR imaging is more susceptible to motion artifacts than CT, advances in fast scanning techniques and cardiac and respiratory gating continue to improve the diagnostic quality of thoracic MR imaging. With further study and more widespread availability, DCE perfusion, O_2-enhanced imaging,

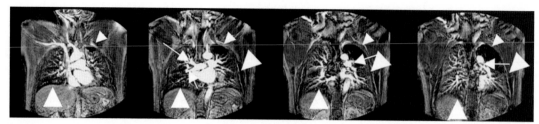

Fig. 31. A 45-year-old woman with acute PE. Images from CEMRA using SENSE demonstrate multiple PEs (*arrows*) and a perfusion defect (*small arrowheads*) in the superior segment of the left lower lobe. Reduced pulmonary blood flow (*large arrowheads*) in bilateral lower lobes and in the right middle lobe are also high probability indicators for PE. (*Adapted from* Ohno Y, Higashino T, Takenaka D, et al. MR angiography with sensitivity encoding (SENSE) for suspected pulmonary embolism: comparison with MDCT and ventilation-perfusion scintigraphy. AJR Am J Roentgenol 2004;183(1):91–8; with permission.)

and HP gas MR imaging may play an increased role in the evaluation of pediatric thoracic diseases including asthma, CF, and PE in the future. New advances in CEMRA using vastly undersampled imaging with projection sequences, which produce 3D data sets by using spherical k-space coverage, have been described in cardiac imaging[161] and show great promise in imaging of the pulmonary vasculature in the future. Additional newer techniques using Fourier decomposition MR imaging allow for ventilation and perfusion scanning without intravenous or inhaled contrast agents and are in the early stages of development.[157,162–164] With these and other advances, MR imaging will continue to play an increasing role in the evaluation of pediatric thoracic disease.

SUMMARY

Mainly as a result of concern about the effects of ionizing radiation in children[1,2] MR imaging has been increasingly used for evaluating pediatric disease in recent years. Adoption of MR imaging for imaging diseases of the thorax has lagged behind MR imaging in other organ systems because of the technical challenges posed by low proton density within the lungs, magnetic susceptibility differences at lung-air interfaces, and respiratory and cardiac motion. However, along with appropriate use of sedation and patient preparation, new techniques in fast scanning, respiratory triggering, spirometer control, ECG gating, MR angiography with and without contrast, O_2-enhanced imaging, and HP gas imaging allow MR imaging to be used to evaluate many pediatric thoracic diseases. Understanding proper MR techniques and the characteristic MR imaging appearance of various thoracic diseases in pediatric patients is essential to arrive at early and accurate diagnoses, which, in turn, leads to optimal patient care.

REFERENCES

1. Brenner DJ. Estimating cancer risks from pediatric CT: going from the qualitative to the quantitative. Pediatr Radiol 2002;32:228–31 [discussion: 242–4].
2. Mayo JR, Aldrich J, Muller NL. Radiation exposure at chest CT: a statement of the Fleischner Society. Radiology 2003;228:15–21.
3. Biederer J, Beer M, Hirsch W, et al. MRI of the lung (2/3). Why… When… How? Insights Imaging 2012;3:355–71.
4. Puderbach M, Hintze C, Ley S, et al. MR imaging of the chest: a practical approach at 1.5T. Eur J Radiol 2007;64:345–55.
5. Biederer J, Hintze C, Fabel M. MRI of pulmonary nodules: technique and diagnostic value. Cancer Imaging 2008;8:125–30.
6. Ohno Y, Koyama H, Yoshikawa T, et al. Pulmonary magnetic resonance imaging for airway diseases. J Thorac Imaging 2011;26:301–16.
7. Rajaram S, Swift AJ, Capener D, et al. Lung morphology assessment with balanced steady-state free precession MR imaging compared with CT. Radiology 2012;263:569–77.
8. Rizzi EB, Schinina V, Cristofaro M, et al. Detection of pulmonary tuberculosis: comparing MR imaging with HRCT. BMC Infect Dis 2011;11:243.
9. Sieren JC, Ohno Y, Koyama H, et al. Recent technological and application developments in computed tomography and magnetic resonance imaging for improved pulmonary nodule detection and lung cancer staging. J Magn Reson Imaging 2010;32:1353–69.
10. Wielputz M, Kauczor HU. MRI of the lung: state of the art. Diagn Interv Radiol 2012;18:344–53.
11. Serra G, Milito C, Mitrevski M, et al. Lung MRI as a possible alternative to CT scan for patients with primary immune deficiencies and increased radiosensitivity. Chest 2011;140:1581–9.
12. Yedururi S, Guillerman RP, Chung T, et al. Multimodality imaging of tracheobronchial disorders in children. Radiographics 2008;28:e29.

13. Lee EY, Siegel MJ. MDCT of tracheobronchial narrowing in pediatric patients. J Thorac Imaging 2007;22:300–9.

14. Lee EY, Siegel MJ, Hildebolt CF, et al. MDCT evaluation of thoracic aortic anomalies in pediatric patients and young adults: comparison of axial, multiplanar, and 3D images. AJR Am J Roentgenol 2004;182:777–84.

15. Lee EY. Advancing CT and MR imaging of the lungs and airways in children: imaging into practice. Pediatr Radiol 2008;38(Suppl 2):S208–12.

16. Lee EY, Zurakowski D, Bastos M, et al. Evaluation of image quality and patient safety: paired inspiratory and expiratory MDCT assessment of tracheobronchomalacia in paediatric patients under general anaesthesia with breath-hold technique. J Med Imaging Radiat Oncol 2012;56:151–7.

17. Freeman SJ, Harvey JE, Goddard PR. Demonstration of supernumerary tracheal bronchus by computed tomographic scanning and magnetic resonance imaging. Thorax 1995;50:426–7.

18. Zylak CJ, Eyler WR, Spizarny DL, et al. Developmental lung anomalies in the adult: radiologic-pathologic correlation. Radiographics 2002; 22(Spec No):S25–43.

19. Berrocal T, Madrid C, Novo S, et al. Congenital anomalies of the tracheobronchial tree, lung, and mediastinum: embryology, radiology, and pathology. Radiographics 2004;24:e17.

20. Ciet P, Wielopolski P, Manniesing R, et al. Spirometer controlled cine-magnetic resonance imaging to diagnose tracheobronchomalacia in pediatric patients. Eur Respir J 2013. [Epub ahead of print].

21. Kluge A, Muller C, Hansel J, et al. Real-time MR with TrueFISP for the detection of acute pulmonary embolism: initial clinical experience. Eur Radiol 2004;14:709–18.

22. Xu J, McGorty KA, Lim RP, et al. Single breathhold noncontrast thoracic MRA using highly accelerated parallel imaging with a 32-element coil array. J Magn Reson Imaging 2012;35:963–8.

23. Moody AR, Liddicoat A, Krarup K. Magnetic resonance pulmonary angiography and direct imaging of embolus for the detection of pulmonary emboli. Invest Radiol 1997;32:431–40.

24. Wild JM, Paley MN, Kasuboski L, et al. Dynamic radial projection MRI of inhaled hyperpolarized 3He gas. Magn Reson Med 2003;49:991–7.

25. Greil GF, Kramer U, Dammann F, et al. Diagnosis of vascular rings and slings using an interleaved 3D double-slab FISP MR angiography technique. Pediatr Radiol 2005;35:396–401.

26. Eichhorn J, Fink C, Delorme S, et al. Rings, slings and other vascular abnormalities. Ultrafast computed tomography and magnetic resonance angiography in pediatric cardiology. Z Kardiol 2004;93:201–8.

27. Greil GF, Powell AJ, Gildein HP, et al. Gadolinium-enhanced three-dimensional magnetic resonance angiography of pulmonary and systemic venous anomalies. J Am Coll Cardiol 2002;39: 335–41.

28. Prince MR. Gadolinium-enhanced MR aortography. Radiology 1994;191:155–64.

29. Goyen M, Laub G, Ladd ME, et al. Dynamic 3D MR angiography of the pulmonary arteries in under four seconds. J Magn Reson Imaging 2001; 13:372–7.

30. Schoenberg SO, Bock M, Floemer F, et al. High-resolution pulmonary arterio- and venography using multiple-bolus multiphase 3D-Gd-mRA. J Magn Reson Imaging 1999;10:339–46.

31. Bauman G, Eichinger M. Ventilation and perfusion magnetic resonance imaging of the lung. Pol J Radiol 2012;77:37–46.

32. Mosbah K, Ruiz-Cabello J, Berthezene Y, et al. Aerosols and gaseous contrast agents for magnetic resonance imaging of the lung. Contrast Media Mol Imaging 2008;3:173–90.

33. Mugler JP 3rd, Altes TA, Ruset IC, et al. Simultaneous magnetic resonance imaging of ventilation distribution and gas uptake in the human lung using hyperpolarized xenon-129. Proc Natl Acad Sci U S A 2010;107:21707–12.

34. Patz S, Hersman FW, Muradian I, et al. Hyperpolarized (129)Xe MRI: a viable functional lung imaging modality? Eur J Radiol 2007;64:335–44.

35. Fain SB, Gonzalez-Fernandez G, Peterson ET, et al. Evaluation of structure-function relationships in asthma using multidetector CT and hyperpolarized He-3 MRI. Acad Radiol 2008;15:753–62.

36. Mugler JP 3rd, Altes TA. Hyperpolarized (129) Xe MRI of the human lung. J Magn Reson Imaging 2013;37:313–31.

37. Saam BT, Yablonskiy DA, Kodibagkar VD, et al. MR imaging of diffusion of (3)He gas in healthy and diseased lungs. Magn Reson Med 2000;44:174–9.

38. Yablonskiy DA, Sukstanskii AL, Woods JC, et al. Quantification of lung microstructure with hyperpolarized 3He diffusion MRI. J Appl Phys 2009;107:1258–65.

39. Sukstanskii AL, Conradi MS, Yablonskiy DA. (3)He lung morphometry technique: accuracy analysis and pulse sequence optimization. J Magn Reson 2010;207:234–41.

40. Sukstanskii AL, Yablonskiy DA. Lung morphometry with hyperpolarized 129Xe: theoretical background. Magn Reson Med 2012;67:856–66.

41. Altes TA, Salerno M. Hyperpolarized gas MR imaging of the lung. J Thorac Imaging 2004;19:250–8.

42. Altes TA, Mata J, de Lange EE, et al. Assessment of lung development using hyperpolarized helium-3 diffusion MR imaging. J Magn Reson Imaging 2006;24:1277–83.

43. Fain S, Schiebler ML, McCormack DG, et al. Imaging of lung function using hyperpolarized helium-3 magnetic resonance imaging: review of current and emerging translational methods and applications. J Magn Reson Imaging 2010;32:1398–408.

44. Hersman FW, Ruset IC, Ketel S, et al. Large production system for hyperpolarized 129Xe for human lung imaging studies. Acad Radiol 2008; 15:683–92.

45. Muradyan I, Butler JP, Dabaghyan M, et al. Single-breath xenon polarization transfer contrast (SB-XTC): implementation and initial results in healthy humans. J Magn Reson Imaging 2013; 37(2):457–70.

46. Dregely I, Ruset IC, Wiggins G, et al. 32-channel phased-array receive with asymmetric birdcage transmit coil for hyperpolarized xenon-129 lung imaging. Magn Reson Med 2012. http://dx.doi.org/10.1002/mrm.24482.

47. Dregely I, Mugler JP 3rd, Ruset IC, et al. Hyperpolarized Xenon-129 gas-exchange imaging of lung microstructure: first case studies in subjects with obstructive lung disease. J Magn Reson Imaging 2011;33:1052–62.

48. Patz S, Muradian I, Hrovat MI, et al. Human pulmonary imaging and spectroscopy with hyperpolarized 129Xe at 0.2T. Acad Radiol 2008;15:713–27.

49. Ruppert K, Brookeman JR, Hagspiel KD, et al. Probing lung physiology with xenon polarization transfer contrast (XTC). Magn Reson Med 2000;44:349–57.

50. Ruppert K, Mata JF, Brookeman JR, et al. Exploring lung function with hyperpolarized (129)Xe nuclear magnetic resonance. Magn Reson Med 2004;51:676–87.

51. Edelman RR, Hatabu H, Tadamura E, et al. Noninvasive assessment of regional ventilation in the human lung using oxygen-enhanced magnetic resonance imaging. Nat Med 1996;2:1236–9.

52. Chen Q, Jakob PM, Griswold MA, et al. Oxygen enhanced MR ventilation imaging of the lung. MAGMA 1998;7:153–61.

53. Stock KW, Chen Q, Morrin M, et al. Oxygen-enhanced magnetic resonance ventilation imaging of the human lung at 0.2 and 1.5 T. J Magn Reson Imaging 1999;9:838–41.

54. Tadamura E, Hatabu H, Li W, et al. Effect of oxygen inhalation on relaxation times in various tissues. J Magn Reson Imaging 1997;7:220–5.

55. Mai VM, Chen Q, Bankier AA, et al. Multiple inversion recovery MR subtraction imaging of human ventilation from inhalation of room air and pure oxygen. Magn Reson Med 2000;43:913–6.

56. Ohno Y, Hatabu H, Higashino T, et al. Centrically reordered inversion recovery half-Fourier single-shot turbo spin-echo sequence: improvement of the image quality of oxygen-enhanced MRI. Eur J Radiol 2004;52:200–5.

57. Vaninbroukx J, Bosmans H, Sunaert S, et al. The use of ECG and respiratory triggering to improve the sensitivity of oxygen-enhanced proton MRI of lung ventilation. Eur Radiol 2003;13:1260–5.

58. Molinari F, Gaudino S, Fink C, et al. Simultaneous cardiac and respiratory synchronization in oxygen-enhanced magnetic resonance imaging of the lung using a pneumotachograph for respiratory monitoring. Invest Radiol 2006;41:476–85.

59. Ohno Y, Chen Q, Hatabu H. Oxygen-enhanced magnetic resonance ventilation imaging of lung. Eur J Radiol 2001;37:164–71.

60. Jakob PM, Wang T, Schultz G, et al. Assessment of human pulmonary function using oxygen-enhanced T(1) imaging in patients with cystic fibrosis. Magn Reson Med 2004;51:1009–16.

61. Ohno Y, Hatabu H, Takenaka D, et al. Oxygen-enhanced MR ventilation imaging of the lung: preliminary clinical experience in 25 subjects. AJR Am J Roentgenol 2001;177:185–94.

62. Ohno Y, Sugimura K, Hatabu H. Clinical oxygen-enhanced magnetic resonance imaging of the lung. Top Magn Reson Imaging 2003;14:237–43.

63. Ohno Y, Hatabu H, Higashino T, et al. Oxygen-enhanced MR imaging: correlation with postsurgical lung function in patients with lung cancer. Radiology 2005;236:704–11.

64. Ohno Y, Koyama H, Nogami M, et al. Dynamic oxygen-enhanced MRI versus quantitative CT: pulmonary functional loss assessment and clinical stage classification of smoking-related COPD. AJR Am J Roentgenol 2008;190:W93–9.

65. Ohno Y, Iwasawa T, Seo JB, et al. Oxygen-enhanced magnetic resonance imaging versus computed tomography: multicenter study for clinical stage classification of smoking-related chronic obstructive pulmonary disease. Am J Respir Crit Care Med 2008;177:1095–102.

66. Ohno Y, Koyama H, Matsumoto K, et al. Oxygen-enhanced MRI vs. quantitatively assessed thin-section CT: pulmonary functional loss assessment and clinical stage classification of asthmatics. Eur J Radiol 2011;77:85–91.

67. Mai VM, Bankier AA, Prasad PV, et al. MR ventilation-perfusion imaging of human lung using oxygen-enhanced and arterial spin labeling techniques. J Magn Reson Imaging 2001;14:574–9.

68. Nakagawa T, Sakuma H, Murashima S, et al. Pulmonary ventilation-perfusion MR imaging in clinical patients. J Magn Reson Imaging 2001;14:419–24.

69. Hatabu H, Gaa J, Kim D, et al. Pulmonary perfusion: qualitative assessment with dynamic contrast-enhanced MRI using ultra-short TE and inversion recovery turbo FLASH. Magn Reson Med 1996;36:503–8.

70. Korosec FR, Frayne R, Grist TM, et al. Time-resolved contrast-enhanced 3D MR angiography. Magn Reson Med 1996;36:345–51.

71. Fink C, Ley S, Kroeker R, et al. Time-resolved contrast-enhanced three-dimensional magnetic resonance angiography of the chest: combination of parallel imaging with view sharing (TREAT). Invest Radiol 2005;40:40–8.

72. Risse F, Eichinger M, Kauczor HU, et al. Improved visualization of delayed perfusion in lung MRI. Eur J Radiol 2011;77:105–10.

73. Ingrisch M, Dietrich O, Attenberger UI, et al. Quantitative pulmonary perfusion magnetic resonance imaging: influence of temporal resolution and signal-to-noise ratio. Invest Radiol 2010;45:7–14.

74. Levin DL, Chen Q, Zhang M, et al. Evaluation of regional pulmonary perfusion using ultrafast magnetic resonance imaging. Magn Reson Med 2001; 46:166–71.

75. Nikolaou K, Schoenberg SO, Brix G, et al. Quantification of pulmonary blood flow and volume in healthy volunteers by dynamic contrast-enhanced magnetic resonance imaging using a parallel imaging technique. Invest Radiol 2004; 39:537–45.

76. Nael K, Michaely HJ, Lee M, et al. Dynamic pulmonary perfusion and flow quantification with MR imaging, 3.0T vs. 1.5T: initial results. J Magn Reson Imaging 2006;24:333–9.

77. Amundsen T, Torheim G, Kvistad KA, et al. Perfusion abnormalities in pulmonary embolism studied with perfusion MRI and ventilation-perfusion scintigraphy: an intra-modality and inter-modality agreement study. J Magn Reson Imaging 2002; 15:386–94.

78. Kluge A, Gerriets T, Lange U, et al. MRI for short-term follow-up of acute pulmonary embolism. Assessment of thrombus appearance and pulmonary perfusion: a feasibility study. Eur Radiol 2005;15:1969–77.

79. Ley-Zaporozhan J, Ley S, Eberhardt R, et al. Assessment of the relationship between lung parenchymal destruction and impaired pulmonary perfusion on a lobar level in patients with emphysema. Eur J Radiol 2007;63:76–83.

80. Ley-Zaporozhan J, van Beek EJ. Imaging phenotypes of chronic obstructive pulmonary disease. J Magn Reson Imaging 2010;32:1340–52.

81. Ley-Zaporozhan J, Ley S, Kauczor HU. Morphological and functional imaging in COPD with CT and MRI: present and future. Eur Radiol 2008;18: 510–21.

82. Nikolaou K, Schoenberg SO, Attenberger U, et al. Pulmonary arterial hypertension: diagnosis with fast perfusion MR imaging and high-spatial-resolution MR angiography–preliminary experience. Radiology 2005;236:694–703.

83. Ley S, Mereles D, Risse F, et al. Quantitative 3D pulmonary MR-perfusion in patients with pulmonary arterial hypertension: correlation with invasive pressure measurements. Eur J Radiol 2007;61: 251–5.

84. Molinari F, Fink C, Risse F, et al. Assessment of differential pulmonary blood flow using perfusion magnetic resonance imaging: comparison with radionuclide perfusion scintigraphy. Invest Radiol 2006;41:624–30.

85. Eichinger M, Puderbach M, Fink C, et al. Contrast-enhanced 3D MRI of lung perfusion in children with cystic fibrosis–initial results. Eur Radiol 2006;16: 2147–52.

86. Fan L, Liu SY, Sun F, et al. Assessment of pulmonary parenchyma perfusion with FAIR in comparison with DCE-MRI–initial results. Eur J Radiol 2009;70:41–8.

87. Fan L, Liu SY, Xiao XS, et al. Demonstration of pulmonary perfusion heterogeneity induced by gravity and lung inflation using arterial spin labeling. Eur J Radiol 2010;73:249–54.

88. Mai VM, Berr SS. MR perfusion imaging of pulmonary parenchyma using pulsed arterial spin labeling techniques: FAIRER and FAIR. J Magn Reson Imaging 1999;9:483–7.

89. Arai TJ, Prisk GK, Holverda S, et al. Magnetic resonance imaging quantification of pulmonary perfusion using calibrated arterial spin labeling. J Vis Exp 2011;30(51). http://dx.doi.org/10.3791/2712.

90. Hopkins SR, Prisk GK. Lung perfusion measured using magnetic resonance imaging: new tools for physiological insights into the pulmonary circulation. J Magn Reson Imaging 2010;32: 1287–301.

91. Ley S, Ley-Zaporozhan J. Pulmonary perfusion imaging using MRI: clinical application. Insights Imaging 2012;3:61–71.

92. Martirosian P, Boss A, Schraml C, et al. Magnetic resonance perfusion imaging without contrast media. Eur J Nucl Med Mol Imaging 2010; 37(Suppl 1):S52–64.

93. Bolar DS, Levin DL, Hopkins SR, et al. Quantification of regional pulmonary blood flow using ASL-FAIRER. Magn Reson Med 2006;55:1308–17.

94. Biyyam DR, Chapman T, Ferguson MR, et al. Congenital lung abnormalities: embryologic features, prenatal diagnosis, and postnatal radiologic-pathologic correlation. Radiographics 2010;30: 1721–38.

95. Liu YP, Chen CP, Shih SL, et al. Fetal cystic lung lesions: evaluation with magnetic resonance imaging. Pediatr Pulmonol 2010;45:592–600.

96. Santos XM, Papanna R, Johnson A, et al. The use of combined ultrasound and magnetic resonance imaging in the detection of fetal anomalies. Prenat Diagn 2010;30:402–7.

97. Epelman M, Kreiger PA, Servaes S, et al. Current imaging of prenatally diagnosed congenital lung lesions. Semin Ultrasound CT MR 2010;31:141–57.

98. Lee EY, Tracy DA, Mahmood SA, et al. Preoperative MDCT evaluation of congenital lung anomalies in children: comparison of axial, multiplanar, and 3D images. AJR Am J Roentgenol 2011;196:1040–6.

99. Lee EY, Boiselle PM, Cleveland RH. Multidetector CT evaluation of congenital lung anomalies. Radiology 2008;247:632–48.

100. Yikilmaz A, Lee EY. CT imaging of mass-like nonvascular pulmonary lesions in children. Pediatr Radiol 2007;37:1253–63.

101. Ko SF, Lee TY, Kao CL, et al. Bronchial atresia associated with epibronchial right pulmonary artery and aberrant right middle lobe artery. Br J Radiol 1998;71:217–20.

102. Naidich DP, Rumancik WM, Ettenger NA, et al. Congenital anomalies of the lungs in adults: MR diagnosis. AJR Am J Roentgenol 1988;151:13–9.

103. Hirsch W, Sorge I, Krohmer S, et al. MRI of the lungs in children. Eur J Radiol 2008;68:278–88.

104. Yikilmaz A, Koc A, Coskun A, et al. Evaluation of pneumonia in children: comparison of MRI with fast imaging sequences at 1.5T with chest radiographs. Acta Radiol 2011;52:914–9.

105. Wheeler JH, Fishman EK. Computed tomography in the management of chest infections: current status. Clin Infect Dis 1996;23:232–40.

106. Lahde S, Jartti A, Broas M, et al. HRCT findings in the lungs of primary care patients with lower respiratory tract infection. Acta Radiol 2002;43:159–63.

107. Syrjala H, Broas M, Suramo I, et al. High-resolution computed tomography for the diagnosis of community-acquired pneumonia. Clin Infect Dis 1998;27:358–63.

108. Katz DS, Leung AN. Radiology of pneumonia. Clin Chest Med 1999;20:549–62.

109. Tan Kendrick AP, Ling H, Subramaniam R, et al. The value of early CT in complicated childhood pneumonia. Pediatr Radiol 2002;32:16–21.

110. Peltola V, Ruuskanen O, Svedstrom E. Magnetic resonance imaging of lung infections in children. Pediatr Radiol 2008;38:1225–31.

111. Peprah KO, Andronikou S, Goussard P. Characteristic magnetic resonance imaging low T2 signal intensity of necrotic lung parenchyma in children with pulmonary tuberculosis. J Thorac Imaging 2012;27:171–4.

112. Hebestreit A, Schultz G, Trusen A, et al. Follow-up of acute pulmonary complications in cystic fibrosis by magnetic resonance imaging: a pilot study. Acta Paediatr 2004;93:414–6.

113. Wagner M, Bowing B, Kuth R, et al. Low field thoracic MRI–a fast and radiation free routine imaging modality in children. Magn Reson Imaging 2001;19:975–83.

114. Gorkem S, Coskun A, Yikilmaz A, et al. Evaluation of Pediatric Thoracic Disorders: Comparison of Unenhanced Fast-Imaging-Sequence 1.5-T MRI and contrast enhanced MDCT. AJR Am J Roentgenol 2013;200(6). Available at: http://www.ajronline.org/page/future/200/6.

115. Kono R, Fujimoto K, Terasaki H, et al. Dynamic MRI of solitary pulmonary nodules: comparison of enhancement patterns of malignant and benign small peripheral lung lesions. AJR Am J Roentgenol 2007;188:26–36.

116. Regier M, Kandel S, Kaul MG, et al. Detection of small pulmonary nodules in high-field MR at 3 T: evaluation of different pulse sequences using porcine lung explants. Eur Radiol 2007;17:1341–51.

117. Biederer J, Mirsadraee S, Beer M, et al. MRI of the lung (3/3)-current applications and future perspectives. Insights Imaging 2012;3:373–86.

118. Eibel R, Herzog P, Dietrich O, et al. Pulmonary abnormalities in immunocompromised patients: comparative detection with parallel acquisition MR imaging and thin-section helical CT. Radiology 2006;241:880–91.

119. Muller NL, Mayo JR, Zwirewich CV. Value of MR imaging in the evaluation of chronic infiltrative lung diseases: comparison with CT. AJR Am J Roentgenol 1992;158:1205–9.

120. Rieger C, Herzog P, Eibel R, et al. Pulmonary MRI–a new approach for the evaluation of febrile neutropenic patients with malignancies. Support Care Cancer 2008;16:599–606.

121. Lutterbey G, Grohe C, Gieseke J, et al. Initial experience with lung-MRI at 3.0T: comparison with CT and clinical data in the evaluation of interstitial lung disease activity. Eur J Radiol 2007;61:256–61.

122. Lutterbey G, Gieseke J, von Falkenhausen M, et al. Lung MRI at 3.0 T: a comparison of helical CT and high-field MRI in the detection of diffuse lung disease. Eur Radiol 2005;15:324–8.

123. Shioya S, Tsuji C, Kurita D, et al. Early damage to lung tissue after irradiation detected by the magnetic resonance T2 relaxation time. Radiat Res 1997;148:359–64.

124. Yi CA, Lee KS, Han J, et al. 3-T MRI for differentiating inflammation- and fibrosis-predominant lesions of usual and nonspecific interstitial pneumonia: comparison study with pathologic correlation. AJR Am J Roentgenol 2008;190:878–85.

125. Carden KA, Boiselle PM, Waltz DA, et al. Tracheomalacia and tracheobronchomalacia in children and adults: an in-depth review. Chest 2005;127:984–1005.

126. Puderbach M, Eichinger M, Haeselbarth J, et al. Assessment of morphological MRI for pulmonary changes in cystic fibrosis (CF) patients: comparison to thin-section CT and chest x-ray. Invest Radiol 2007;42:715–25.

127. Puderbach M, Eichinger M, Gahr J, et al. Proton MRI appearance of cystic fibrosis: comparison to CT. Eur Radiol 2007;17:716–24.

128. Biederer J, Reuter M, Both M, et al. Analysis of artefacts and detail resolution of lung MRI with breath-hold T1-weighted gradient-echo and T2-weighted fast spin-echo sequences with respiratory triggering. Eur Radiol 2002;12:378–84.

129. Wild JM, Woodhouse N, Paley MN, et al. Comparison between 2D and 3D gradient-echo sequences for MRI of human lung ventilation with hyperpolarized 3He. Magn Reson Med 2004;52:673–8.

130. Salerno M, Altes TA, Brookeman JR, et al. Dynamic spiral MRI of pulmonary gas flow using hyperpolarized (3)He: preliminary studies in healthy and diseased lungs. Magn Reson Med 2001;46:667–77.

131. Holmes JH, O'Halloran RL, Brodsky EK, et al. 3D hyperpolarized He-3 MRI of ventilation using a multi-echo projection acquisition. Magn Reson Med 2008;59:1062–71.

132. Holmes JH, O'Halloran RL, Brodsky EK, et al. Three-dimensional imaging of ventilation dynamics in asthmatics using multiecho projection acquisition with constrained reconstruction. Magn Reson Med 2009;62:1543–56.

133. Samee S, Altes T, Powers P, et al. Imaging the lungs in asthmatic patients by using hyperpolarized helium-3 magnetic resonance: assessment of response to methacholine and exercise challenge. J Allergy Clin Immunol 2003;111:1205–11.

134. de Lange EE, Altes TA, Patrie JT, et al. The variability of regional airflow obstruction within the lungs of patients with asthma: assessment with hyperpolarized helium-3 magnetic resonance imaging. J Allergy Clin Immunol 2007;119:1072–8.

135. Altes TA, Powers PL, Knight-Scott J, et al. Hyperpolarized 3He MR lung ventilation imaging in asthmatics: preliminary findings. J Magn Reson Imaging 2001;13:378–84.

136. de Lange EE, Altes TA, Patrie JT, et al. Changes in regional airflow obstruction over time in the lungs of patients with asthma: evaluation with 3He MR imaging. Radiology 2009;250:567–75.

137. O'Sullivan BP, Freedman SD. Cystic fibrosis. Lancet 2009;373:1891–904.

138. Garcia-Pena P, Boixadera H, Barber I, et al. Thoracic findings of systemic diseases at high-resolution CT in children. Radiographics 2011;31:465–82.

139. Davis SD, Fordham LA, Brody AS, et al. Computed tomography reflects lower airway inflammation and tracks changes in early cystic fibrosis. Am J Respir Crit Care Med 2007;175:943–50.

140. Davis SD, Brody AS, Emond MJ, et al. Endpoints for clinical trials in young children with cystic fibrosis. Proc Am Thorac Soc 2007;4:418–30.

141. Sly PD, Brennan S, Gangell C, et al. Lung disease at diagnosis in infants with cystic fibrosis detected by newborn screening. Am J Respir Crit Care Med 2009;180:146–52.

142. Eichinger M, Heussel CP, Kauczor HU, et al. Computed tomography and magnetic resonance imaging in cystic fibrosis lung disease. J Magn Reson Imaging 2010;32:1370–8.

143. Mentore K, Froh DK, de Lange EE, et al. Hyperpolarized HHe 3 MRI of the lung in cystic fibrosis: assessment at baseline and after bronchodilator and airway clearance treatment. Acad Radiol 2005;12:1423–9.

144. van Beek EJ, Hill C, Woodhouse N, et al. Assessment of lung disease in children with cystic fibrosis using hyperpolarized 3-Helium MRI: comparison with Shwachman score, Chrispin-Norman score and spirometry. Eur Radiol 2007;17:1018–24.

145. Sebening C, Jakob H, Tochtermann U, et al. Vascular tracheobronchial compression syndromes– experience in surgical treatment and literature review. Thorac Cardiovasc Surg 2000;48:164–74.

146. Kussman BD, Geva T, McGowan FX. Cardiovascular causes of airway compression. Paediatr Anaesth 2004;14:60–74.

147. Ferrari VA, Scott CH, Holland GA, et al. Ultrafast three-dimensional contrast-enhanced magnetic resonance angiography and imaging in the diagnosis of partial anomalous pulmonary venous drainage. J Am Coll Cardiol 2001;37:1120–8.

148. Beerbaum P, Parish V, Bell A, et al. Atypical atrial septal defects in children: noninvasive evaluation by cardiac MRI. Pediatr Radiol 2008;38:1188–94.

149. Stein PD, Fowler SE, Goodman LR, et al. Multidetector computed tomography for acute pulmonary embolism. N Engl J Med 2006;354:2317–27.

150. Meaney JF, Weg JG, Chenevert TL, et al. Diagnosis of pulmonary embolism with magnetic resonance angiography. N Engl J Med 1997;336:1422–7.

151. Oudkerk M, van Beek EJ, Wielopolski P, et al. Comparison of contrast-enhanced magnetic resonance angiography and conventional pulmonary angiography for the diagnosis of pulmonary embolism: a prospective study. Lancet 2002;359:1643–7.

152. Ohno Y, Higashino T, Takenaka D, et al. MR angiography with sensitivity encoding (SENSE) for suspected pulmonary embolism: comparison with MDCT and ventilation-perfusion scintigraphy. AJR Am J Roentgenol 2004;183:91–8.

153. Kluge A, Luboldt W, Bachmann G. Acute pulmonary embolism to the subsegmental level: diagnostic accuracy of three MRI techniques compared with 16-MDCT. AJR Am J Roentgenol 2006;187:W7–14.

154. Stein PD, Chenevert TL, Fowler SE, et al. Gadolinium-enhanced magnetic resonance angiography

for pulmonary embolism: a multicenter prospective study (PIOPED III). Ann Intern Med 2010; 152:434–43, W142–3.

155. Kluge A, Gerriets T, Stolz E, et al. Pulmonary perfusion in acute pulmonary embolism: agreement of MRI and SPECT for lobar, segmental and subsegmental perfusion defects. Acta Radiol 2006;47:933–40.

156. Altes TA, Mai VM, Munger TM, et al. Pulmonary embolism: comprehensive evaluation with MR ventilation and perfusion scanning with hyperpolarized helium-3, arterial spin tagging, and contrast-enhanced MRA. J Vasc Interv Radiol 2005;16:999–1005.

157. Bauman G, Scholz A, Rivoire J, et al. Lung ventilation- and perfusion-weighted Fourier decomposition magnetic resonance imaging: in vivo validation with hyperpolarized (3) He and dynamic contrast-enhanced MRI. Magn Reson Med 2013;69:229–37.

158. Hong C, Leawoods JC, Yablonskiy DA, et al. Feasibility of combining MR perfusion, angiography, and 3He ventilation imaging for evaluation of lung function in a porcine model. Acad Radiol 2005;12:202–9.

159. Lipson DA, Roberts DA, Hansen-Flaschen J, et al. Pulmonary ventilation and perfusion scanning using hyperpolarized helium-3 MRI and arterial spin tagging in healthy normal subjects and in pulmonary embolism and orthotopic lung transplant patients. Magn Reson Med 2002;47:1073–6.

160. Zheng J, Leawoods JC, Nolte M, et al. Combined MR proton lung perfusion/angiography and helium ventilation: potential for detecting pulmonary emboli and ventilation defects. Magn Reson Med 2002;47:433–8.

161. Xie J, Lai P, Bhat H, et al. Whole-heart coronary magnetic resonance angiography at 3.0T using short-TR steady-state free precession, vastly undersampled isotropic projection reconstruction. J Magn Reson Imaging 2010;31:1230–5.

162. Bauman G, Puderbach M, Deimling M, et al. Non-contrast-enhanced perfusion and ventilation assessment of the human lung by means of Fourier decomposition in proton MRI. Magn Reson Med 2009;62:656–64.

163. Suga K, Ogasawara N, Okada M, et al. Lung perfusion impairments in pulmonary embolic and airway obstruction with noncontrast MR imaging. J Appl Phys 2002;92:2439–51.

164. Bauman G, Lutzen U, Ullrich M, et al. Pulmonary functional imaging: qualitative comparison of Fourier decomposition MR imaging with SPECT/CT in porcine lung. Radiology 2011;260:551–9.

Magnetic Resonance and Computed Tomography in Pediatric Urology
An Imaging Overview for Current and Future Daily Practice

Kassa Darge, MD, PhD[a],*, Mikhail Higgins, MD, MPH[b,c],
Tiffany J. Hwang, BA[b], Jorge Delgado[b],
Assem Shukla, MD[d], Richard Bellah, MD[a]

KEYWORDS

- Children • Urinary tract • MR imaging • MR urography • CT • CT cystography

KEY POINTS

- Ultrasound is the primary imaging modality for the pediatric urinary tract.
- Magnetic resonance (MR) imaging needs to be the second imaging option after ultrasound in children.
- Functional MR urography (fMRU) provides comprehensive morphologic and functional information.
- Computed tomography (CT) is the imaging choice in children only in the following circumstances: (1) inadequate ultrasound for urolithiasis, and (2) blunt abdominal trauma in the setting of polytrauma.
- The choice of CT over MR for uroradiologic imaging is mainly for ancillary reasons: availability, fast speed, no sedation, and low cost.
- In children, CT angiography (CTA) of the urinary tract is primarily performed for evaluation of the renal arteries for suspected stenosis. Direct CT cystography may be necessary for evaluation of bladder rupture.

INTRODUCTION

Ultrasound (US) is the most widely used and primary imaging modality for the urinary tract in children.[1,2] With the introduction of contrast-enhanced voiding urosonography (ceVUS) for diagnosis of vesicoureteric reflux, the spectrum of US applications has substantially broadened.[3] When further cross-sectional morphologic examination and/or functional evaluation are required, magnetic resonance (MR) imaging, including functional MR urography (fMRU), becomes the logical and optimal second step, particularly in pediatric patients. Thus, in an advanced pediatric radiology unit with state-of-the-art imaging, most routine uroradiologic examinations can be performed with US and MR imaging.[4] There are 2 main exceptions to

[a] Division of Body Imaging, Department of Radiology, The Children's Hospital of Philadelphia, Perelman School of Medicine, University of Pennsylvania, 34th Street and Civic Center Boulevard, Philadelphia, PA 19104, USA; [b] Division of Body Imaging, Department of Radiology, The Children's Hospital of Philadelphia, 34th Street and Civic Center Boulevard, Philadelphia, PA 19104, USA; [c] Department of Radiology, Hospital of the University of Pennsylvania, 3400 Spruce Street, Philadelphia, PA 19104, USA; [d] Division of Urology, Department of Surgery, The Children's Hospital of Philadelphia, Perelman School of Medicine, University of Pennsylvania, 34th Street and Civic Center Boulevard, Philadelphia, PA 19104, USA
* Corresponding author. Department of Radiology, The Children's Hospital of Philadelphia, 34th Street and Civic Center Boulevard, Philadelphia, PA 19104.
E-mail address: darge@email.chop.edu

Radiol Clin N Am 51 (2013) 583–598
http://dx.doi.org/10.1016/j.rcl.2013.03.004
0033-8389/13/$ – see front matter © 2013 Elsevier Inc. All rights reserved.

this.[5,6] The first exception is when, following an US, additional diagnostic imaging for urolithiasis is needed, and the second is in the case of severe polytrauma, including blunt abdominal trauma. The need for computed tomography (CT) in the former instance is because of the higher diagnostic yield that CT provides, and, in the latter instance, it is the accessibility and short duration of CT. The overarching goal of this review article was to present an up-to-date overview of the MR imaging and CT studies important for current and future daily pediatric uroradiologic practice with emphasis on clinical indications, techniques, and imaging findings.

MR IMAGING OF THE URINARY TRACT: URO-MR

Introduction

MR imaging is an important and valuable diagnostic modality for evaluating the pediatric urinary tract. It provides comprehensive morphologic and functional information (Fig. 1). There is no exposure to radiation. Despite its high diagnostic utility, the need for sedation in infants and small children, availability of MR scanners, and cost are ancillary factors that restrict the widespread use of MR in pediatric uroradiology.

Indications

In daily pediatric practice, the primary indications for using urinary tract MR imaging are congenital anomalies, mainly pelvicaliectasis and/or ureterectasis, and renal and bladder tumors. Infections and vascular anomalies of the urinary tract are less frequent indications for MR imaging. The MR imaging conducted for these indications are mainly 3 types: precontrast, postcontrast, and dynamic postcontrast studies.[4,5] The precontrast sequences are optimal for depicting the urine-filled pelvicalyceal system and ureter and provide exquisite morphologic detail. After administering intravenous (IV) contrast, performing dynamic sequences is a better choice for the kidneys, as it provides the information of a nondynamic contrast study in addition to functional information with depiction of the arterial, venous, nephrographic, and urographic phases. The postcontrast dynamic study can be conducted as MR angiography (MRA) and/or fMRU. The latter will provide some MRA information.

Procedure

The most comprehensive uro-MR imaging examination is fMRU, which provides detailed morphologic and functional information. It is primarily used for congenital anomalies of the urinary tract.

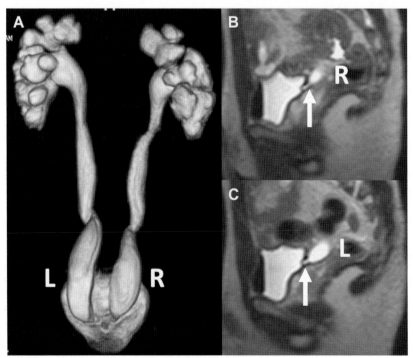

Fig. 1. Precontrast MR urography demonstrating bilateral ureterovesical junction obstruction. The posterior view of 3D volumetric maximum intensity projection (*A*) shows the bilateral moderate pelvicalyceal and ureteric dilatation. The T2 sagittal plane (*B, C*) reveals the 6-mm-long to 10-mm-long markedly narrow distal ureteric segments (*arrow*) on the right (R) and left (L) sides.

Modifications of the fMRU can be applied for other indications, which are described as follows.

fMRU

The protocols for fMRU have been rather long, which have hampered its widespread use.[7-11] We have now started using much more focused imaging protocols without compromising the yield of critical information delivered by the study.

Procedure

Preparation Before the MR scan, a few preparatory measures are necessary.[4,5,9-11] Hydration with IV fluid administration starting a half hour before the scan is essential. A bladder catheter is placed. An age-appropriate large enough catheter size is needed to allow continuous emptying of the bladder. A distended bladder may have a negative effect on the excretion of urine.[12] This is of even greater importance if the patient will be deeply sedated, has high-grade reflux, or has ureteral dilatation. When ectopic ureter is suspected, having a bladder catheter may improve delineation of the urethra and the potential ectopic insertion site. The bladder is emptied before going into the scanner. The urine bag is placed below the level of the scanner table. The catheter should not be kinked or pressed under the thigh of the patient. Furosemide (Lasix) is administered IV at a dose of 1 mg/kg (maximum 20 mg), 10 minutes before the patient is placed on the examination table.[13,14] This allows enough time for the furosemide to reach its peak effect before starting the 3-dimensional (3D) sequence to depict the urine-filled structures. It also makes it possible to begin the dynamic sequences at the peak of the diuretic effect. Furosemide belongs to a class of sulfa-containing drugs and, within this class, sulfa antibiotics are frequent causes of drug reactions. However, cross-sensitivity with sulfa-nonantibiotics is rare.[15,16] It is best to place the patient in the prone position if we are evaluating the contrast excretion into the ureters.[17] Prone position is even more important in those with pelvicalyceal dilatation.[18,19] The MR contrast agent that we currently use, gadolinium-DTPA (Magnevist), has higher (1.208) specific gravity than urine (1.002–1.030) and settles in the dependent position.[20] Consequently, with the patient in prone position, the contrast collects around the area of the pelvi-ureteric junction and, thus, passage into the ureters is facilitated. In a dilated pelvicalyceal system with the patient supine, it takes more time for the contrast to reach the normally more anterior pelvi-ureteric junction (**Fig. 2**).

Scan After a localizer scan, a sagittal T2 sequence follows.[4,5,10] This plane is necessary for properly setting the oblique coronal planes along the long axis of the kidneys. An axial T2 with fat saturation through the kidneys and/or pelvis allows exquisite morphologic depiction. A 3D T2 with fat saturation with 1-mm slice thickness makes postprocessing of the fluid-filled structures possible. These precontrast sequences are followed by the IV injection of gadolinium-DTPA, using a power injector at a slow rate (0.1–0.25 mL/s).[4,5,10] The T1 fat-saturated dynamic scan is started, allowing for a few initial noncontrast scans. The scan may be stopped when the ureters are contrasted. Thus, in most cases, the dynamic scan should not be longer than 5 minutes (**Fig. 3**).

Postprocessing This includes multiplanar reconstructions and 3D maximum intensity projection from the 3D precontrast scan (see **Fig. 3**D). In addition, a functional analysis is performed. This is

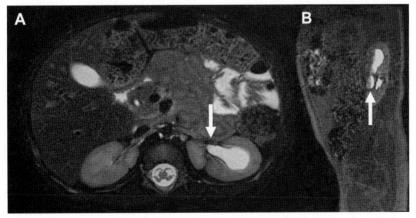

Fig. 2. On the axial plane in T2 with fat saturation (*A*), the pelviureteric junction (*arrow*) on the left is directed anteriorly. The postcontrast dynamic scan was performed with the patient in supine position. The sagittal T1 sequence with fat saturation through the left kidney (*B*) demonstrates the contrast-urine level (*arrow*) in the dilated renal pelvis in the absence of contrast in the ureter.

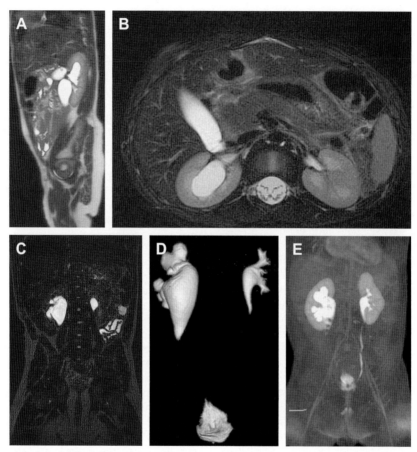

Fig. 3. Right pelvicalyceal dilatation with loss of corticomedullary differentiation and delayed excretion with the right to left Patlak differential function (pDRF) of 40% and 60%, respectively. The finding is compatible with uretero-pelvic junction obstruction (UPJO) with functional compromise of the kidney. Focused fMRU with a sagittal T2 (*A*), axial T2 with fat saturation (*B*), 3D T2 fat saturation (*C*), and postcontrast T1 with fat saturation dynamic sequences (*E*). Postprocessing of the 3D T2 data results in clear morphologic presentation in 3D volume rendering of the right UPJO (*D*). The functional analysis using the "chop-fmru" freeware produces the table with the results of the various parameters (*F*), the enhancement curve (*G*), and the excretion curve (*H*).

possible using freewares like the "chop-fmru," available at www.chop-fmru.com.[10,21] The results generated by the different freewares are comparable.[22] A detailed description of the "chop-fmru" freeware has been published.[10] The functional analysis provides mainly 4 types of results.[22–28] The first one is about transit times of the contrast, taking the starting point in the aorta, and encompassing the following: (1) time-to-peak (TTP), which is time to reach maximum contrast concentration in the renal parenchyma; (2) calyceal transit time (CTT), which is time until the contrast appears for the first time in the calyces; and (3) renal transit time (RTT), which is the time for the contrast to reach the proximal ureter at the level of the lower pole of the kidney (see **Fig. 3**G). Of the 3 parameters, renal transit time is influenced by a number of factors, such as position of the patient, position of the pelvi-ureteric junction, and extent of

pelvicalyceal dilation.[17–19] The prone positioning described previously not only shortens the time for the dynamic postcontrast sequence, but also eliminates some of the factors that artificially prolong the RTT, falsely making the result look like an obstruction. The second set of results deals with differential renal function (ie, split renal function) in percentage. To calculate the differentials, the enhanced renal parenchyma is segmented, and for each kidney the parenchymal volume calculated. Furthermore, using the "Patlak equation," the Patlak number of each kidney is generated.[10,29–32] The Patlak serves as an index of the glomerular filtration rate (GFR). The parenchymal volumes and the Patlak numbers are used to generate the differential renal functions after being converted to percentages. Thus, we have the volumetric differential renal function (vDRF), based on the renal parenchymal volumes, and the Patlak

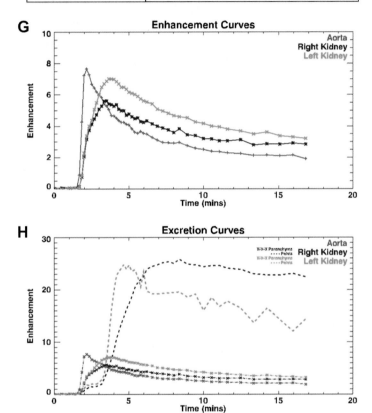

F	Right Kidney	Left Kidney
1. CTT	1min(s) 39sec(s)	1min(s) 59sec(s)
2. RTT	4min(s) 19sec(s)	2min(s) 19sec(s)
3. TTP	1min(s) 49sec(s)	1min(s) 59sec(s)
4. Whole Volume(mL)	X	X
5. Parenchymal Vol(mL)	35.16mL	25.27mL
6a. vDRF	58.18%	41.81%
6b. pDRF	39.51%	60.48%
6c. vpDRF	47.61%	52.38%

Fig. 3. (*continued*)

differential renal function (pDRF), based on the Patlak numbers. A combination of the parenchymal volumes and Patlak numbers allows the calculation of the volumetric Patlak differential renal function (vpDRF) (see **Fig. 3**G). A third set of results are the graphic presentations over time of the renal parenchymal contrast enhancement and the excretion of contrast (see **Fig. 3**G, H). The former is generated by segmenting the contrasted renal parenchyma for each time point and plotting them against the contrast concentration (**Fig. 4**). For the latter, only the contrast in the pelvicalyceal system is segmented. The form of the curves is greatly influenced by the length of the dynamic series. The shorter it is, we still find the end of the curves to be at a relatively high contrast concentration.

For the calculation of the transit times, differential functions, and generation of curves, a dynamic sequence of about 5 minutes will suffice. The curves do not go as flat as the curves from nuclear medicine studies, in which the scan time may go up to 40 minutes after injection of the radionuclide. It is possible to stretch the dynamic scan to comparable time and generate similar curves, but there is no diagnostic gain in the case of fMRU. The fourth and last set of information provided by "chop-fmru" is the "Patlak map." This is a color-coded mapping of the Patlak numbers per unit of renal parenchyma (see **Fig. 4**). The Patlak map does not provide additional diagnostic information, but it presents in a very visual manner the functional distribution in the kidneys. It is most useful in duplex kidneys

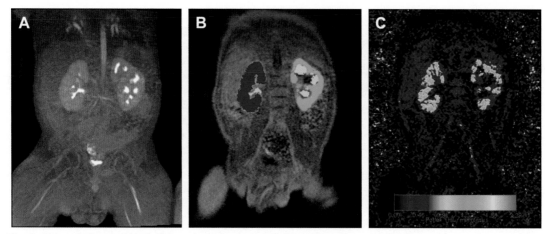

Fig. 4. Coronal planes of both kidneys in postcontrast: (*A*) excretory phase in the dynamic series demonstrating the delay of excretion on the left, (*B*) segmentation of the contrasted renal parenchyma and the contrast in the renal pelvis, and (*C*) the Patlak map showing comparable functional distribution bilaterally.

and pyelonephritis/scarring, in which there are focal or regional differences in function.

Procedural and scan modifications Depending on the specific indication, some procedural and scan modifications are necessary. These are as follows:

1. Ectopic ureter: the precontrast series may suffice to depict the morphologic findings and the postcontrast part needs to be added only if functional evaluations of the kidneys are requested (**Fig. 5**).[33,34] If the bladder is completely empty and the ectopic

insertion is difficult to evaluate, clamping the bladder and waiting for it to fill or simply administering normal saline into the bladder may be helpful. This is followed by a rescan using a T2 fat-saturated sequence in the optimal plane for depicting the ectopic ureter.

2. Cyst versus diverticulum: The differentiation between a renal cyst and a calyceal diverticulum may be difficult.[35,36] The definitive visualization of contrast ensures the diagnosis of calyceal diverticulum and excludes a renal cyst (**Fig. 6**). Calyceal diverticulum fills with contrast in a retrograde

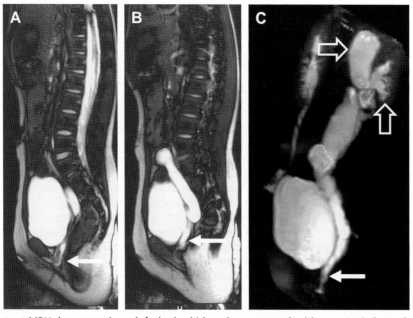

Fig. 5. Precontrast MRU demonstrating a left duplex kidney (*open arrows*) with an ectopic (*arrow*) upper moiety ureter. Sagittal T2 (*A*, *B*) and 3D volumetric rendering (*C*) from the 3D T2 sequences.

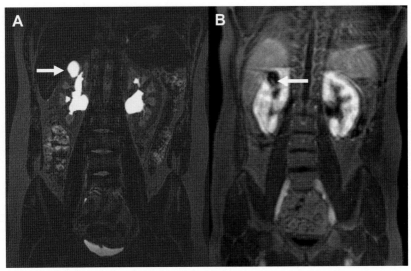

Fig. 6. Calyceal diverticulum (*arrow*) in the upper pole of the right kidney in the coronal 3D T2 (*A*) and postcontrast dynamic T1 with fat saturation (*B*) sequences. Starting in the early postcontrast dynamic sequence, whisp of contrast are seen on multiple images (*B*), compatible with reflux from the calyx into the diverticulum.

manner later than the calyces or renal pelvis. If contrast is not detected in the dynamic series, it is of paramount importance to perform delayed images. The patient can be taken out of the scanner and returned at a later time to be rescanned in sagittal plane using only a single run from the postcontrast T1 dynamic series. This sequence usually lasts less than 10 seconds. If the patient had been sedated, additional sedation will not be necessary. The sequence can be easily repeated if image degradation due to movement becomes a problem. The sagittal plane allows better depiction of small amounts of contrast in the dependent position in a calyceal diverticulum. The delay needs to be 1 hour or longer.[35,36]

Assessment When evaluating the fMRU studies, it is important to carefully assess at least the following basic parameters: precontrast images: corticomedullary differentiation, parenchymal signal intensity, cortical thickness, degree of pelvicalyceal and ureteric dilatation; postcontrast images: renal arteries, parenchymal enhancement, contrast excretion; precontrast and postcontrast images; kidney type, position, and size: ureteric insertion; bladder morphology (**Fig. 7**). The functional results described need to be interpreted taking into account all the morphologic findings.

Diagnostic utility The fMRU supersedes other diagnostic modalities in the morphologic evaluation of the urinary tract. It has been shown to have significant influence in management

decisions when compared with conventional diagnostic algorithms for obstructive uropathy.[37] Not only does it provide a panoramic view in different planes, but it is also capable of depicting little or nonfunctioning renal units or moieties and their ureters.[23] With regard to the functional evaluations, a prospective comparison with the scintigraphic MAG-3 study demonstrated in 62 patients a significant correlation (0.92) for the differential renal function and a strong agreement (0.67) for the excretion. Another prospective comparative study in 71 children yielded a comparable correlation coefficient for the differential renal functions.[38]

CONTRAST-ENHANCED MR IMAGING WITH OR WITHOUT FUNCTIONAL EVALUATION

The full fMRU scan is not necessary for all diagnostic questions.

Indications

This is primarily for renal and bladder masses or infections/abscesses.

Procedure

If evaluation of a urinary obstruction associated with a mass is not planned, one can forgo the hydration, IV diuretic administration, and bladder catheterization. The core sequences coronal and axial T2 fat-saturated, sagittal T2, axial T1, and axial diffusion-weighted imaging suffice as precontrast sequences. Diffusion-weighted imaging for renal masses is a recent addition with results

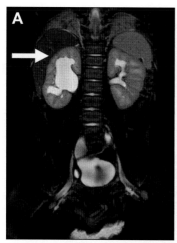
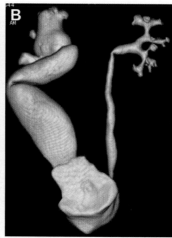
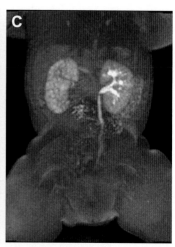

Fig. 7. Coronal plane of the kidneys in (*A*) T2 with fat saturation sequence demonstrating the marked pelvicaly-ceal dilatation, reduced corticomedullary differentiation, and focal cortical thinning (*arrow*) in the upper part of the right kidney; normal left kidney. (*B*) The right megaureter is conspicuously depicted in the 3D volumetric rendering from the T2 sequence. (*C*) In the postcontrast dynamic sequence, a dense nephrogram on the right signals decreased function.

that further enhance the MR diagnostic capability (**Fig. 8**).[39–41] It is optimal to do the postcontrast scan in a dynamic manner for renal masses, as described previously, and thus keep the option for functional evaluation (**Fig. 9**). A 3D T1 sequence is necessary if a 3D volumetric analysis or 3D visualization for surgical planning is envisaged.[42,43] An axial T1 with fat saturation is added after the dynamic scan. For a bladder mass, the dynamic sequence is not necessary and can be replaced with axial and sagittal T1 fat-saturated postcontrast sequences.

Assessment

The parameters to be evaluated described for the fMRU also apply to a large extent here. In addition, for a mass, the T1 and T2 signals, enhancement pattern, and relation to the surrounding structures need to be described. Presence or absence of vascular involvement or invasion is to be noted. Measurement of the diameter or volume of the mass is necessary. Functional analysis provides information about the normal renal tissue and/or kidney and potentially about the mass. The 3D reconstruction of renal or bladder masses allows active 3D visualization, virtual surgical planning, or virtual cystoscopy for the bladder.[42,43]

Diagnostic Utility

The limitations to using MR are not of a diagnostic nature, but ancillary ones. There are no large comparative studies for indications such as tumor or infection of the urinary tract, particularly in

children. However, the advantages of imaging renal tumors with MR imaging in children have been long touted.[44,45] Similarly, the use of MR imaging for pediatric pelvic tumors, including bladder tumors, has been described and is also increasing in adults.[46–51] In many European centers, after an US, only MR imaging is used for evaluation of tumors of the urinary tract in children.

CT OF THE URINARY TRACT: URO-CT
Introduction

In routine practice, the main attractions for using uro-CT in pediatrics are not necessarily a higher diagnostic yield, but rather relate to its availability, fast speed, less frequent/no need for sedation, and lesser cost.[6] In addition, CT may be used as a confirmatory secondary modality, as in the case of CT for urolithiasis. Here it is used when the result yielded by US proves inadequate or non-diagnostic, which is the case in just a small fraction of pediatric patients.[1] It is well-known and widely accepted that CT exposes a patient to high doses of radiation, and that children have a much higher risk of developing radiation-induced cancer.[52] Thus, initiatives, such as the "Image Gently" campaign, focus on eliminating or lowering the radiation exposure in children.[53] More information on these initiatives can be found at http://www.pedrad.org/associations/5364/ig/. All these apply to uro-CT, too. The most important step in this direction is to try to find alternative modalities, completely avoiding potential radiation exposure.[53–55] The alternatives for many or most

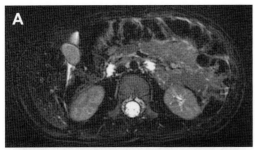

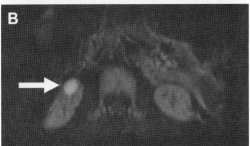

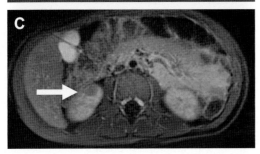

Fig. 8. MR imaging depicting a right upper pole Wilms tumor (*arrow*) in axial planes precontrast T2 (*A*), diffusion-weighted (b = 1000) (*B*), and postcontrast dynamic T1 fat-saturated (*C*) sequences. The mass is not visible on the T2-weighted sequence and is most conspicuous in the diffusion-weighted image (*B*).

indications for uro-CT may be US and/or MR imaging. If these are not possible to perform and uro-CT has to be done, care has to be taken to adhere strictly to the ALARA (as low as reasonably achievable) principle. The uro-CT is tailored based on the

information provided by already conducted imaging studies and the specific indication. Dedicated age-specific, size-specific, and/or weight-specific pediatric CT protocols must be used.[2,56–58]

Indications

As mentioned previously, in daily practice the main reasons for requesting a uro-CT are primarily ancillary. From a diagnostic standpoint, uro-CT needs to be considered as a secondary option if US and/or MR imaging are inadequate, unavailable, or cannot be performed and the clinical suspicion warrants further imaging clarification. In this context, it can be used to image congenital anomalies, tumors, infections, and stones of the urinary tract. The difficulty to visualize on US one or both kidneys in a child with severe scoliosis having hematuria and flank pain is an appropriate indication for conducting a CT for urolithiasis. Similarly, if a child with spinal fusion hardware has a renal mass and requires further evaluation after the US, and MR imaging cannot be done because of potential unwarranted consequences of the hardware, uro-CT needs to be considered. Even the information regarding calcification, which is better depicted on CT than MR imaging, can adequately be provided for diagnostic purposes by US.

The one indication in which ancillary issues override all other considerations is evaluation of severe blunt abdominal trauma directly or in the setting of polytrauma (**Fig. 10**). The considerations here are beyond just diagnostics: first, CT is much more widespread; practically, it is much easier with all the emergency support devices and personnel to accommodate a polytrauma patient in a CT suite; and finally, and in terms of throughput, CT is much faster in providing the comprehensive information of the whole or multiple parts of the body needed by the trauma team. It is important to note that in blunt abdominal trauma in children, renal lesions are more frequent

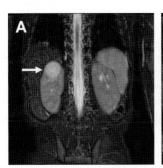

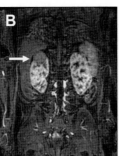

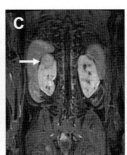

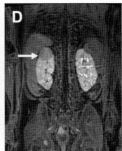

Fig. 9. MR imaging depicting a right upper pole Wilms tumor (*arrow*) in a coronal plane precontrast T2 (*A*) and postcontrast dynamic T1 fat-saturated sequences (*B–D*) from early to late phases.

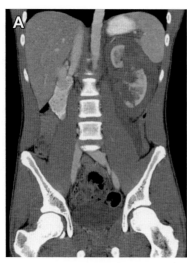
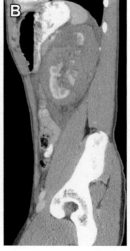
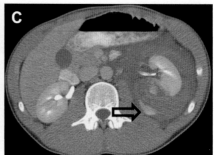

Fig. 10. Postcontrast CT for blunt abdominal trauma demonstrating a fractured left kidney on the coronal (A) and sagittal (B) reconstructions of the early-phase scan. The delayed axial scan (C) shows the contrast extravasation (open arrow) in the large hematoma.

than in adults because of a nonossified thoracic cage, thin abdominal wall, and paucity of perirenal fat.[2,56,57] Despite these advantages, one has to exhaust the full utility of US imaging and try not to overdo CT.[59,60] The CT radiation dose, even in the setting of pediatric trauma, still remains a concern.[61]

Procedure

It may be necessary to sedate uncooperative children. With advancing CT technology, and as a result of increasingly shorter scan times, it is expected for the sedation need to decline further.[58] Restraining techniques or devices may be necessary in some cases. In most cases, uro-CT is preceded at least by US. Consequently, the CT examination needs to be adapted in light of the already existing diagnostic information and the specific clinical indication. A multiphase study has rarely any place in pediatric uro-CT. It is more important to select the phase that is expected to deliver most results. To do so, the appropriate postinjection delay needs to be chosen.[6] The postinjection delays will depend on age, scan duration, contrast amount, injection type and speed, and diuresis. For the arterial phase, a bolus triggering can be performed or a delay of 8 to 20 seconds selected. For the nephrographic phase, a delay of 70 to 100 seconds is necessary, and for the excretory phase, the delay can be 5 to 15 minutes. Additional CT angiography and/or urography are not routinely performed. For renal trauma, mostly a nephrographic phase acquisition will suffice. If there are findings, however, suggesting urine (contrast) extravasation/

leakage, additional limited delayed excretory views should be obtained (see Fig. 10C). Alternatively, rather than a repeat CT scan for the excretory phase, either early or late, plain-film radiography of the abdomen, which has lesser radiation dose, may be considered. The technique of splitting the contrast bolus and injecting at 2 different time points can produce both nephrographic and urographic phases simultaneously on one scan.[62] Postprocessing with multiplanar reformatting in coronal and sagittal planes need to be automatically added, and 3D volume rendering whenever applicable and necessary.

Diagnostic Utility

Uro-CT does have high diagnostic yield, but the combination of high radiation exposure and availability of radiation-free alternatives with comparable or better diagnostic possibilities places it as a second alternative. In trauma cases, a meticulously conducted abdominal US and Doppler study is adequate to exclude major renal injury in children.[12] In the follow-up of traumatic renal findings, US is also the imaging modality of choice.[7] In a prospective study encompassing 1500 children who sustained blunt abdominal trauma, CT was performed and the decision for surgical or conservative management noted.[63] In 74% of the patients, the CT scan was normal. Of the 388 CT scans with abnormal findings, 286 were solid viscus injuries and the remaining 102 had other CT abnormalities. The decision for laparotomy was based on the CT in only 5.7% of the abnormal cases. Thus, CT rarely influenced the decision for operative intervention in children who sustained blunt abdominal trauma.[15] On the other hand, in a review of studies looking at the prevalence of intra-abdominal injuries and the negative predictive value (NPV) of an abdominal CT in children who present with blunt abdominal trauma, the NPV was found to be 99.8% with a 95% confidence interval of 99.6% to 99.9%. The study showed that it may be safe to discharge a stable child home after a negative abdominal CT. This has, of course, a major ancillary consequence with regard to the overall flow of patients in a hospital setting.

CT FOR UROLITHIASIS

A noncontrast CT of the kidneys, ureters, and bladder is performed in search of stones. This is probably the most common indication for CT in pediatric uro-imaging.

Indications

Suspected stone of the urinary tract when an US with color Doppler does not depict a stone, but secondary signs are present, or an US is inconclusive/negative, and high clinical suspicion remains (**Figs. 11 and 12**).[2]

Procedure

Having a well-hydrated patient is optimal. The patient is placed in prone position to be able to differentiate an impacted stone at the ureterovesical junction from that of a mobile bladder calculus.[64] The scan extends from the top of the kidneys to

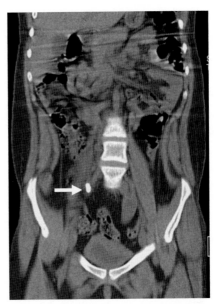

Fig. 12. CT for urolithiasis in a patient with a high clinical suspicion for urolithiasis, but a negative US for stones. A single right ureteral stone (*arrow*) is clearly depicted.

the bladder base in 3-mm to 5-mm slice thickness. The CT parameter settings need to be such that the radiation dose will be as low as reasonably possible. The influence of the actual or reconstructed slice thickness and/or the mA setting on the detection of stones needs to be kept in mind.[65–67] Multiplanar reformatted images are obtained in the coronal and sagittal planes.

Assessment

The search for stones should start with the coronal reformatted images, as they have a higher yield. The window needs to be manipulated to near bone for better calculi visualization. Attention is paid to secondary signs: in kidney: hydronephrosis, increase in renal size, decrease in renal attenuation, perinephric stranding; in ureter: dilatation, tissue rim sign, periureteric stranding, ureterovesical junction edema.[68]

Diagnostic Utility

A prospective study in 50 children compared US (without color Doppler) and CT performed within less than 8 hours of each other for suspected urolithiasis.[69] Calculation based on renal units, with CT as reference, had the following results for US: sensitivity 62%, specificity 98%, positive and predictive values 97% and 74%, respectively. Although more calculi were detected on CT, further evaluation revealed that "the difference in

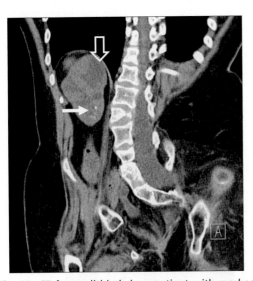

Fig. 11. CT for urolithiasis in a patient with marked thoracolumbar scoliosis with equivocal US demonstrating small stones (*solid arrow*) in the lower pole of the right kidney, pelvicaliectasis, and cortical thinning (*open arrow*).

usefulness between the 2 tests may not be clinically significant." The recommendation was to keep CT as a second imaging option after US in children suspected of urolithiasis.[69]

CT ANGIOGRAPHY

A contrast CT is used with the appropriate contrast bolus timing to depict the renal vasculature.

Indications

Renovascular hypertension and traumatic renovascular injury and other less common renovascular disorders.[5,70]

Procedure

For optimal power injection of the contrast, a suitable size of peripheral IV catheter is necessary (neonate, 24 G; infant, 22/24 G; >1 year, 20/22 G). The IV access is first tested with saline at the same flow rate planned for contrast injection. Contrast agents with high iodine concentration are preferred, particularly in infants, as the maximum contrast level is relatively small. The contrast is administered at a size-adjusted highest rate, followed by a saline chaser. Automated bolus tracking allows the optimal method for triggering the contrast injection. The scan extends from the supraceliac aorta to the upper external iliac arteries. A CT urography may be necessary in the setting of trauma. An additional postcontrast scan is performed with 5-minute delay, allowing the depiction of the urinary tract. Alternatively, a split-bolus technique may be used, injecting one-third to one-half of the contrast volume beforehand and the other two-thirds to one-half for an arterial phase scan. This allows a combination of an arterial and a urographic phase in one single acquisition. The postprocessing is important and includes 3D volume renderings and 2D thin-slab maximum-intensity projections (MIPs).[5,71–73]

Assessment

In renovascular hypertension, the focus is on morphologic changes of the renal arteries (stenoses, aneurysms, beadings) and secondary signs (poststenotic dilatation, collateral formation, focal parenchymal perfusion defects, asymmetric nephrogram, parenchymal scarring) (**Fig. 13**).[71] First-order and second-order branches of the renal arteries are usually well depicted on renal CT angiography (CTA). Intraparenchymal renal arterial changes may be difficult to visualize. If no extraparenchymal stenosis is detected and the CTAs cannot adequately demonstrate intraparenchymal arteries, a digital subtraction angiography (DSA) may be necessary for definite diagnosis. In trauma cases, the search is for renal parenchymal lesions, vascular damage, or ureteral/bladder injury. Focal or globally reduced or absent renal perfusion, perirenal fluid collection, and contrast extravasation are important imaging findings of sequela of trauma.

Diagnostic Utility

Comparative studies in the pediatric population are currently lacking. A prospective comparison of CTA with DSA in adults with suspicion of renovascular hypertension found CTA to have 94% sensitivity, 93% specificity, and 71% positive and 99% negative predictive values. These results are in contrast to the multicenter study that had been conducted approximately 6 years earlier.[74] Currently, DSA is the gold standard, but this may change, depending on the multidetector CT technology advancements.[75]

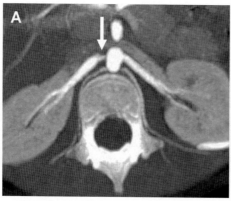 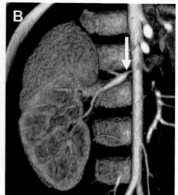

Fig. 13. CT angiography in a 3-year-old patient with hypertension and neurofibromatosis type I demonstrates a short-segment high-grade stenosis (*arrow*) of the proximal right renal artery with poststenotic dilatation in the axial MIP (*A*) and in the coronal 3D volumetric rendering (*B*). (*Courtesy of* Monica Epelman, MD.)

CT CYSTOGRAPHY

Active contrast filling of the urinary bladder, to detect extraluminal contrast, which is an indicator of rupture. Direct CT cystography entails retrograde filling of the bladder and indirect CT cystography passive antegrade filling of the bladder after IV contrast administration.

Indications

Bladder trauma with or without known pelvic fracture and hematuria[76]; workup for suspected delayed spontaneous rupture of augmented bladder.[77]

Procedure

For direct CT cystography before bladder catheterization, it is important to exclude urethral injury clinically or with retrograde urethrography. An age-appropriate Foley catheter is placed; the balloon is not inflated. A precontrast scan is performed from the diaphragm to the ischial tuberosity. A drip infusion is prepared with diluted (10%) water-soluble contrast (eg, 50 mL in 450 mL 0.9% NaCl solution).[78] The bladder is filled until the patient starts to void or the maximal bladder capacity ([age + 2] × 30, mL) is reached. Then, it is important to wait for about 5 minutes and rescan the abdomen and pelvis. If no contrast extravasation is visualized, it may be necessary to perform further delayed scan of just the pelvis. Multiplanar reformation (MPR) of the axial images in sagittal and coronal planes optimizes detection of extravasated contrast, particularly at the bladder dome. Indirect CT cystography is performed after IV contrast administration and antegrade filling, particularly in the setting of polytrauma. This includes occlusion of the Foley catheter, if present, when the patient arrives in the CT suite and a delay of 5 to 10 minutes after the IV contrast administration before rescanning the abdomen and pelvis. It is important to check if adequate distention is achieved[79]; however, the indirect cystography is much less reliable in the diagnosis of bladder rupture.

Assessment

Evaluate for extravesical contrast; may use density measurement in HU for confirmation. Contrast in lateral paravesical fossae, pericolic space, interenteric regions, Morrison pouch, and perihepatic space denote intraperitoneal bladder rupture. In extraperitoneal rupture, contrast is detected in the perivesical/prevesical space and retrorectal presacral regions.[78,80] Differentiation between intraperitoneal and extraperitoneal bladder rupture is critical, as the former is managed nonsurgically

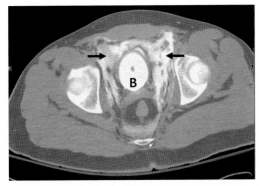

Fig. 14. CT cystography. Extraperitoneal rupture of the bladder (B) with contrast extravasation restricted to the pelvic extraperitoneal space (*arrows*), giving characteristic molar-tooth appearance.

and the latter requires emergency surgical intervention (**Figs. 14** and **15**). It is also possible to have a combined form.

Diagnostic Utility

Direct CT cystography in comparison with the surgical and clinical results in adult patients (n = 234) evaluated for bladder trauma had the following results for detecting intraperitoneal/extraperitoneal bladder rupture respectively: sensitivity 100%/92.8%, specificity 99.6%/100%, positive predictive value 85.7%/100%, NPV 100%/99.5%.[81]

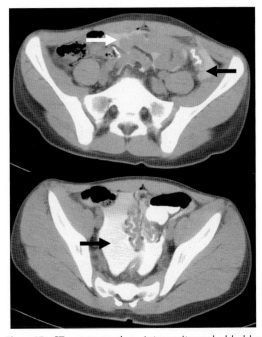

Fig. 15. CT cystography: Intraperitoneal bladder rupture with extravasated contrast diffusely outlining the bowel loops (*arrows*).

SUMMARY

The focus of pediatric uroradiologic imaging is shifting toward the use of imaging modalities that do not have radiation exposure. US is the main diagnostic imaging modality. When further evaluation is necessary, MR imaging needs to be the second choice. CT is reserved for very limited indications. These are for evaluation of possible urinary tract calculi if US proves to be inadequate and in the setting of polytrauma for assessment of blunt injuries to the urinary tract.

REFERENCES

1. Riccabona M, Avni FE, Blickman JG, et al. Imaging recommendations in paediatric uroradiology. Minutes of the ESPR uroradiology task force session on childhood obstructive uropathy, high-grade fetal hydronephrosis, childhood haematuria, and urolithiasis in childhood. ESPR Annual Congress, Edinburgh, UK, June 2008. Pediatr Radiol 2009;39:891–8.

2. Riccabona M, Avni FE, Dacher JN, et al. ESPR uroradiology task force and ESUR paediatric working group: imaging and procedural recommendations in paediatric uroradiology, part III. Minutes of the ESPR uroradiology task force minisymposium on intravenous urography, uro-CT and MR-urography in childhood. Pediatr Radiol 2010;40:1315–20.

3. Darge K. Voiding urosonography with ultrasound contrast agents for the diagnosis of vesicoureteric reflux in children. I. Procedure. Pediatr Radiol 2008;38:40–53.

4. Darge K, Anupindi SA, Jaramillo D. MR imaging of the abdomen and pelvis in infants, children, and adolescents. Radiology 2011;261:12–29.

5. Renjen P, Bellah R, Hellinger JC, et al. Advances in uroradiologic imaging in children. Radiol Clin North Am 2012;50:207–18.

6. Hiorns MP. Imaging of the urinary tract: the role of CT and MRI. Pediatr Nephrol 2011;26:59–68.

7. Boss A, Schaefer JF, Martirosian P, et al. Contrast-enhanced dynamic MR nephrography using the TurboFLASH navigator-gating technique in children. Eur Radiol 2006;16:1509–18.

8. Leyendecker JR, Barnes CE, Zagoria RJ. MR urography: techniques and clinical applications. Radiographics 2008;28:23–46.

9. Grattan-Smith JD, Little SB, Jones RA. MR urography in children: how we do it. Pediatr Radiol 2008; 38(Suppl 1):S3–17.

10. Khrichenko D, Darge K. Functional analysis in MR urography—made simple. Pediatr Radiol 2010;40: 182–99.

11. Vivier PH, Dolores M, Taylor M, et al. MR urography in children. Part 1: how we do the F0 technique. Pediatr Radiol 2010;40:732–8.

12. Jones DA, Lupton EW, George NJ. Effect of bladder filling on upper tract urodynamics in man. Br J Urol 1990;65:492–6.

13. Ergen FB, Hussain HK, Carlos RC. 3D excretory MR urography: improved image quality with intravenous saline and diuretic administration. J Magn Reson Imaging 2007;25:783–9.

14. Wakelkamp M, Gunnar A, Paintaud G. The time of maximum effect for model selection in pharmacokinetic-pharmacodynamic analysis applied to frusemide. Br J Clin Pharmacol 1998;45: 63–70.

15. Lowe J, Gray J, Henry DA, et al. Adverse reactions to frusemide in hospital inpatients. Br Med J 1979; 2(6186):360–2.

16. Healy R, Jankowski TA, Crownover B. Clinical inquiries. Which diuretics are safe and effective for patients with a sulfa allergy? J Fam Pract 2007; 56:488–90.

17. Rossleigh MA, Leighton DM, Farnsworth RH. Diuresis renography. The need for an additional view after gravity-assisted drainage. Clin Nucl Med 1993;18:210–3.

18. Kletter K, Nürnberger N. Diagnostic potential of diuresis renography: limitations by the severity of hydronephrosis and by impairment of renal function. Nucl Med Commun 1989;10:51–61.

19. Koff SA, Binkovitz L, Coley B, et al. Renal pelvis volume during diuresis in children with hydronephrosis: implications for diagnosing obstruction with diuretic renography. J Urol 2005;174:303–7.

20. Magnevist injection. Wayne, NJ: Bayer Healthcare Pharmaceuticals Inc.; 2012. Available at: http://labeling.bayerhealthcare.com/html/products/pi/MagnevistPBP_PI.pdf. Accessed on April 21, 2013.

21. Vivier PH, Dolores M, Taylor M, et al. MR urography in children. Part 2: how to use Image J MR urography processing software. Pediatr Radiol 2010; 40(5):739–46.

22. Hadjidekov G, Hadjidekova S, Tonchev Z, et al. Assessing renal function in children with hydronephrosis—additional feature of MR urography. Radiol Oncol 2011;45:248–58.

23. Rohrschneider WK, Haufe S, Wiesel M, et al. Functional and morphologic evaluation of congenital urinary tract dilatation by using combined static-dynamic MR urography: findings in kidneys with a single collecting system. Radiology 2002;224: 683–94.

24. Grattan-Smith JD, Perez-Bayfield MR, Jones RA, et al. MR imaging of kidneys: functional evaluation using F-15 perfusion imaging. Pediatr Radiol 2003; 33:293–304.

25. McDaniel BB, Jones RA, Scherz H, et al. Dynamic contrast-enhanced MR urography in the evaluation of pediatric hydronephrosis: part 2, anatomic and

functional assessment of ureteropelvic junction obstruction. Am J Roentgenol 2005;185:1608–14.

26. Jones RA, Easley K, Little SB, et al. Dynamic contrast-enhanced MR urography in the evaluation of pediatric hydronephrosis: part I, functional assessment. AJR Am J Roentgenol 2005;185: 1598–607.

27. Jones RA, Schmotzer B, Little SB, et al. MRU post-processing. Pediatr Radiol 2008;38(Suppl 1):S18–27.

28. Jones RA, Votaw JR, Salman K, et al. Magnetic resonance imaging evaluation of renal structure and function related to disease: technical review of image acquisition, postprocessing, and mathematical modeling steps. J Magn Reson Imaging 2011;33:1270–83.

29. Rutland MD. A single-injection technique for subtraction of blood background in 1311-hippuran renograms. Br J Radiol 1979;52:134–7.

30. Patlak CS, Blasberg RG, Fenstermacher JD. Graphical evaluation of blood-to-brain transfer constants from multiple time uptake data. J Cereb Blood Flow Metab 1983;3:1–7.

31. Peters AM. Graphical analysis of dynamic data: the Patlak-Rutland plot. Nucl Med Commun 1994;15: 669–72.

32. Grenier N, Mendichovszky I, de Senneville BD, et al. Measurement of glomerular filtration rate with magnetic resonance imaging: principles, limitations, and expectations. Semin Nucl Med 2008; 38:47–55.

33. Gylys-Morin VM, Minevich E, Tackett LD, et al. Magnetic resonance imaging of the dysplastic renal moiety and ectopic ureter. J Urol 2000;164: 2034–9.

34. Heidemeier A, Kirchhoff-Moradpour A, Staatz G, et al. Ectopic ureter with urinary dribbling in childhood—a diagnostic challenge: our own experience and review of the literature. Radiologe 2007;47: 411–20.

35. Stunell H, McNeill G, Browne RF, et al. The imaging appearances of calyceal diverticula complicated by urolithiasis. Br J Radiol 2010;83:888–94.

36. Mullett R, Belfield JC, Vinjamuri S. Calyceal diverticulum—a mimic of different pathologies on multiple imaging modalities. J Radiol Case Rep 2012;6:10–7.

37. Furth C, Genseke P, Amthauer H, et al. Evaluation of functional MR-urography in complex obstructive uropathy of infants: comparison to the conventional diagnostic algorithm—a pilot study. Klin Padiatr 2012;224:296–302.

38. Perez-Brayfield MR, Kirsch AJ, Jones RA, et al. A prospective study comparing ultrasound, nuclear scintigraphy and dynamic contrast enhanced magnetic resonance imaging in the evaluation of hydronephrosis. J Urol 2003;170:1330–4.

39. Zhang J, Tehrani YM, Wang L, et al. Renal masses: characterization with diffusion-weighted MR imaging—a preliminary experience. Radiology 2008;247:458–64.

40. Razek AA, Farouk A, Mousa A, et al. Role of diffusion-weighted magnetic resonance imaging in characterization of renal tumors. J Comput Assist Tomogr 2011;35:332–6.

41. Rheinheimer S, Stieltjes B, Schneider F, et al. Investigation of renal lesions by diffusion-weighted magnetic resonance imaging applying intravoxel incoherent motion-derived parameters—initial experience. Eur J Radiol 2012;81:e310–6.

42. Schenk JP, Waag KL, Graf N, et al. 3D-visualization by MRI for surgical planning of Wilms tumors. Rofo 2004;176:1447–52 [in German].

43. Günther P, Tröger J, Graf N, et al. MR volumetric analysis of the course of nephroblastomatosis under chemotherapy in childhood. Pediatr Radiol 2004;34(8):660–4.

44. Rohrschneider WK, Weirich A, Rieden K, et al. US, CT and MR imaging characteristics of nephroblastomatosis. Pediatr Radiol 1998;28:435–43.

45. Hoffer FA. Magnetic resonance imaging of abdominal masses in the pediatric patient. Semin Ultrasound CT MR 2005;26:212–23.

46. Siegel MJ, Chung EM. Wilms' tumor and other pediatric renal masses. Magn Reson Imaging Clin N Am 2008;16:479–97.

47. Finelli A, Babyn P, Lorie GA, et al. The use of magnetic resonance imaging in the diagnosis and follow-up of pediatric pelvic rhabdomyosarcoma. J Urol 2000;163:1952–3.

48. Fletcher BD, Kaste SC. Magnetic resonance imaging for diagnosis and follow-up of genitourinary, pelvic, and perineal rhabdomyosarcoma. Urol Radiol 1992;14:263–72.

49. Raza SA, Jhaveri KS. MR imaging of urinary bladder carcinoma and beyond. Radiol Clin North Am 2012;50:1085–110.

50. Green DA, Durand M, Gumpeni N, et al. Role of magnetic resonance imaging in bladder cancer: current status and emerging techniques. BJU Int 2012;110:1463–70.

51. Verma S, Rajesh A, Prasad SR, et al. Urinary bladder cancer: role of MR imaging. Radiographics 2012;32:371–87.

52. Brenner DJ. Estimating cancer risks from pediatric CT: going from the qualitative to the quantitative. Pediatr Radiol 2002;32:228–30.

53. Goske MJ, Applegate KE, Boylan J, et al. The Image Gently campaign: working together to change practice. AJR Am J Roentgenol 2008; 190:273–4.

54. Strauss KJ, Goske MJ, Kaste SC, et al. Image gently: ten steps you can take to optimize image quality and lower CT dose for paediatric patients. AJR Am J Roentgenol 2010;194: 868–73.

55. Goske MJ, Phillips RR, Mandel K, et al. Image gently: a web-based practice quality improvement program in CT safety for children. AJR Am J Roentgenol 2010;194:1177–82.

56. Maudgil DD, McHugh K. The role of computed tomography in modern paediatric uroradiology. Eur J Radiol 2002;43:129–38.

57. Damasio MB, Darge K, Riccabona M. Multi-detector CT in the paediatric urinary tract. Eur J Radiol 2013. [Epub ahead of print].

58. Sorantin E, Weissensteiner S, Hasenburger G, et al. CT in children—dose protection and general considerations when planning a CT in a child. Eur J Radiol 2012. http://dx.doi.org/10.1016/j.ejrad.2011.11.041.

59. Fenton SJ, Hansen KW, Meyers RL, et al. CT scan and the pediatric trauma patient—are we overdoing it? J Pediatr Surg 2004;39:1877–81.

60. Pietrera P, Badachi Y, Liard A, et al. Ultrasound for initial evaluation of post-traumatic renal lesions in children. J Radiol 2001;82:833–8.

61. Scaife ER, Rollins MD. Managing radiation risk in the evaluation of the pediatric trauma patient. Semin Pediatr Surg 2010;19:252–6.

62. Chow LC, Kwan SW, Olcott EW, et al. Split-bolus MDCT urography with synchronous nephrographic and excretory phase enhancement. AJR Am J Roentgenol 2007;189:314–22.

63. Ruess L, Sivit CJ, Eichelberger MR, et al. Blunt abdominal trauma in children: impact of CT on operative and non-operative management. AJR Am J Roentgenol 1997;169:1011–4.

64. Levine J, Neitlich J, Smith RC. The value of prone scanning to distinguish ureterovesical junction stones from ureteral stones that have passed into the bladder: leave no stone unturned. AJR Am J Roentgenol 1999;172:977–81.

65. Jin DH, Lamberton GR, Broome DR, et al. Renal stone detection using unenhanced multidetector row computerized tomography—does section width matter? J Urol 2009;181:2767–73.

66. Berkenblit R, Hoenig D, Lerer D, et al. Comparison of 0.625-mm source computed tomographic images versus 5-mm thick reconstructed images in the evaluation for renal calculi in at-risk patients. J Endourol 2012. http://dx.doi.org/10.1089/end.2012.0157.

67. Karmazyn B, Frush DP, Applegate KE. CT with a computer-simulated dose reduction technique for detection of pediatric nephroureterolithiasis: comparison of standard and reduced radiation doses. AJR Am J Roentgenol 2009;192:143–9.

68. Strouse PJ, Bates DG, Bloom DA, et al. Non-contrast thin-section helical CT of urinary tract calculi in children. Pediatr Radiol 2002;32:326–32.

69. Passerotti C, Chow JS, Silva A, et al. Ultrasound versus computerized tomography for evaluating urolithiasis. J Urol 2009;82:1829–34.

70. Riccabona M, Lobo ML, Papadopoulou F, et al. ESPR uroradiology task force and ESUR paediatric working group: imaging recommendations in paediatric uroradiology, part IV: minutes of the ESPR uroradiology task force mini-symposium on imaging in childhood renal hypertension and imaging of renal trauma in children. Pediatr Radiol 2011;41:939–44.

71. Kurian J, Epelman M, Darge K, et al. The role of CT angiography in the evaluation of pediatric renovascular hypertension. Pediatr Radiol 2012. http://dx.doi.org/10.1007/s00247-012-2567-z.

72. Frush DP. Pediatric abdominal CT angiography. Pediatr Radiol 2008;38(Suppl 2):S259–66.

73. Rountas C, Vlychou M, Vassiou K, et al. Imaging modalities for renal artery stenosis in suspected renovascular hypertension: prospective intraindividual comparison of color Doppler US, CT angiography, GD-enhanced MR angiography, and digital subtraction angiography. Ren Fail 2007;29:295–302.

74. Vasbinder GB, Nelemans PJ, Kessels AG, et al. Accuracy of computed tomographic angiography and magnetic resonance angiography for diagnosing renal artery stenosis. Ann Intern Med 2004;141:674–82.

75. Roebuck D. Childhood hypertension: what does the radiologist contribute? Pediatr Radiol 2008;38(Suppl 3):S501–7.

76. Sivit CJ. Imaging children with abdominal trauma. AJR Am J Roentgenol 2009;192:1179–89.

77. Glass RB, Rushton HG. Delayed spontaneous rupture of augmented bladder in children: diagnosis with sonography and CT. AJR Am J Roentgenol 1992;158:833–5.

78. Vaccaro JP, Brody JM. CT Cystography in the evaluation of major bladder trauma. Radiographics 2000;20:1373–81.

79. Mee SL, McAninch JW, Federle MP. Computerized tomography in bladder rupture: diagnostic limitations. J Urol 1986;137:207–9.

80. Sivit CJ, Cutting JP, Eichelberger MR. CT diagnosis and localization of rupture of the bladder in children with blunt abdominal trauma: significance of contrast material extravasation in the pelvis. AJR Am J Roentgenol 1995;164:1243–6.

81. Chan DP, Abujudeh HH, Cushing GL, et al. CT cystography with multiplanar reformation for suspected bladder rupture: experience in 234 cases. AJR Am J Roentgenol 2006;187:1296–302.

Pediatric Hepatobiliary Magnetic Resonance Imaging

Vy Thao Tran, MD[a], Shreyas Vasanawala, MD, PhD[b],*

KEYWORDS

- Magnetic resonance imaging • Pediatric patients • Hepatobiliary • Liver • Sequences • Protocol

KEY POINTS

- MR imaging is an effective and noninvasive modality for the evaluation of hepatobiliary tumors, congenital biliary ductal plate malformations, posttransplant complications, fibrosis, steatosis, and infection in pediatric patients.
- Various MR sequences and contrast agents can be used in pediatric hepatobiliary imaging and radiologists should familiarize themselves with both basic and new emerging MR applications.

INTRODUCTION

Pediatric liver and biliary tract imaging assessment is rapidly advancing and evolving. MR imaging is the modality of choice for detection and characterization of hepatobiliary disorders in pediatric patients at the authors' institution, virtually replacing CT and endoscopic retrograde cholangiopancreatography (ERCP). The overarching goal of this article is to provide an up-to-date review of hepatobiliary MR imaging in pediatric patients, including anatomy, indications, and imaging goals and protocols. This article also discusses some of the common MR features of pediatric liver pathologic conditions, including tumors, congenital biliary ductal plate malformations, trauma, and infection.

ANATOMY

Located beneath the diaphragm, the liver occupies the right upper abdomen, typically extends across the midline, and is the largest intraabdominal organ. Cross-sectional imaging should focus on dividing the liver into segmental anatomy based on Couinaud system. In the Couinaud system, the right and left hepatic lobe are divided by the middle hepatic vein. The superior and inferior segments of the liver are divided by the horizontal plane of the portal vein. The caudate lobe is segment I. Segments II to IV are in the left lobe and segments V to VIII are in the right lobe. The right hepatic vein divides the right lobe into anterior segments (V and VIII) and posterior segments (VI and VII). The superior segments (VII and VIII) are separated from the inferior segments (V and VI) by the horizontal plane of the right portal vein. The left hepatic vein divides the left hepatic lobe into the medial (IVa and IVb) and lateral segments (II and III). Segments II and IVa are superior to segment III and IVb with the horizontal plane of the left portal vein serving as a divider.[1]

INDICATIONS AND IMAGING GOALS

MR imaging is an effective modality for numerous hepatobiliary conditions, including pediatric and adult hepatic tumors.[2–4] MR imaging protocols can be tailored to address specific clinical queries (ie, tumor characterization, staging, resectability, biliary tract anomalies, or vascular assessment).

Disclosures: Research support from GE Healthcare.
[a] Department of Radiology, Lucile Packard Children's Hospital, Stanford University, 725 Welch Road Room 1667, Palo Alto, CA 94304, USA; [b] Department of Radiology, Lucile Packard Children's Hospital, Stanford University, 725 Welch Road, Room 1679, Palo Alto, CA 94304, USA
* Corresponding author.
E-mail address: vasanawala@stanford.edu

radiologic.theclinics.com

Pediatric MR imaging tumor characterization relies on T2 hyperintensity and contrast enhancement characteristics.[2] Delineation of lymph node involvement, vascular invasion, or biliary tract extension is crucial for determining the resectability and staging of hepatobiliary malignancies. For instance, the use of the PRETEXT staging system (Pre Treatment Extent of Disease Staging System for malignant primary liver tumors of childhood) in hepatoblastoma dictates features that must be delineated by imaging. The PRETEXT number is derived by subtracting the highest number of contiguous liver sections that are not involved by tumor from four. Additional criteria in the PRETEXT system include caudate lobe involvement, extrahepatic abdominal disease, tumor focality, distant metastases, lymph node metastases, portal vein, hepatic vein, or inferior vena cava involvement

(**Fig. 1**).[5] The same imaging principles help stage and risk stratify other malignant hepatic tumors. **Table 1** outlines key features of common benign and malignant pediatric liver tumors.

MR imaging is also useful for evaluation of the biliary tree.[6,7] Indications for biliary tract imaging include pancreatitis, cholelithiasis, sclerosing cholangitis,[8,9] ductal plate malformations, choledochal cysts,[10–13] and liver transplant biliary complications. Goals for MR imaging evaluation of the biliary tract include anatomic assessment for congenital anomalies, stones, strictures, inflammation, and evaluation of obstruction. Additionally, in a transplant patient, assessment of vascular anatomy and possible vascular complications, or infectious processes that a posttransplant patient is at increased risk for is often necessary (**Figs. 2–8**).

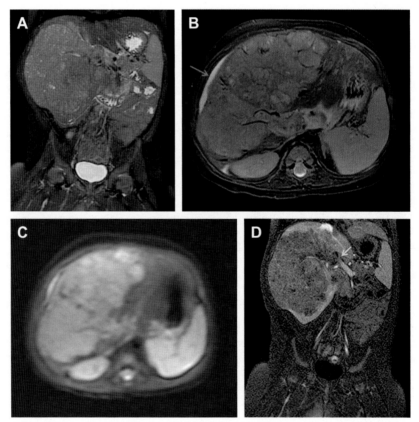

Fig. 1. Hepatoblastoma in a 7-month-old girl. (*A*) Volumetric T2-weighted coronal MR image provides high resolution (320 × 224 matrix over 28 cm field of view [FOV] with 1 mm slice thickness) to clearly demonstrate the large, heterogeneous hepatic mass involving all segment of the visualized hepatic lobes. (*B*) Volumetric data allows for multiplanar reformatting. Shown is an axial reformat from data set in 1a, comparable to conventional T2-weighted imaging. Note the perihepatic fluid collection (*red arrow*) concerning for tumor rupture. (*C*) Axial diffusion-weighted MR image of the liver demonstrates bright signal within the tumor. (*D*) Postcontrast coronal T1 postcontrast fat-saturated image (288 × 288 matrix over 26 FOV with 2 mm slice thickness) obtained during the portal venous phase demonstrates tumor thrombus (*yellow arrow*) extending into the portal vein. This is a PRETEXT stage 4P hepatoblastoma.

Table 1
Common MR imaging and clinical features of pediatric liver tumors

Tumor	T1	T2	Arterial Phase Signal	Portal Venous Phase	Other Features
Hepatoblastoma	Low	High	Heterogenous	Low	Calcification, necrosis, hemorrhage, and septa can alter signal Assess vascular invasion Most common malignant hepatic tumor in children under 3 y
HCC	Low	High	High	Low	Most common hepatic malignancy in adolescents Usually underlying liver disease Assess vascular invasion
Fibrolamellar HCC	Low	High, low scar	High	Low, central scar	Nonenhancing central scar, calcifications in 40%
Undifferentiated Embryonal Sarcoma	Low	High	Low	Low	Usually large, heterogenous, and right lobe more common than left
Biliary Rhabdomyosarcoma	Low	High	Low	Low	Rare Typically younger than age 5 y, jaundice, and some intraductal mass
Metastasis	Low	High	None or irregular rim	Low	Usually Wilms, neuroblastoma, lymphoma, or leukemia
Dysplastic Nodule	Low or high	Low	Low or high	Low or high	Seek enhancing T2 bright nodule within a nodule indicating developing HCC
Infantile Hemangioma	Low	High	Peripheral nodular	Centripetal enhancement	Most common benign pediatric liver tumor
Focal Nodular Hyperplasia	Same or low	High, higher scar	Uniformly high except scar	Usually isointense	Second-most common benign pediatric liver tumor High signal on hepatobiliary phase gadoxetate-enhanced imaging
Mesenchymal Hamartoma	Low	High	Low cysts but septa or stomal components can enhance	Low cysts, enhancing septa	Multicystic heterogenous mass with septa in children younger than 5 y
Hepatocellular Adenoma	Heterogenous	High	High	Low to isointense	Rare Associated with glycogen storage diseases, diabetes, anabolic steroids, and oral contraceptives Propensity to bleed

Abbreviation: HCC, hepatocellular carcinoma.

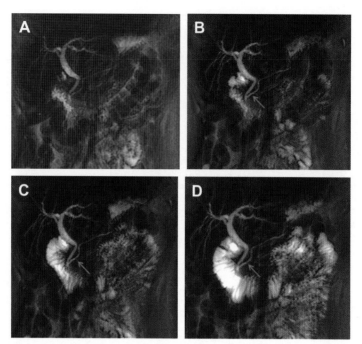

Fig. 2. Fifteen-year-old girl after cholecystostomy with persistent abdominal pain. MRCP with secretin stimulation was requested for additional evaluation. (*A–D*) Sequential coronal single-shot fast spin echo (SSFSE) T2-weighted MR images obtained every 30 seconds after the administration of secretin triggered at the end of the respiratory cycle. These MR images demonstrate minimal intrahepatic and extrahepatic biliary ductal dilatation due to reservoir effect in a patient after cholecystectomy. There is a robust exocrine response to secretin with progressive filling of the duodenum due to an increase in pancreatic secretions and the pancreatic duct (*red arrow*) becomes more prominent. No area of stricturing, beading, or side-branch ectasia is noted along the pancreatic duct. This MRCP avoided an unnecessary ERCP in this pediatric patient.

Finally, MR imaging is superb for the evaluation of diffuse hepatic disease, including hepatic fibrosis, steatosis,[14–16] and iron deposition. Quantitative evaluation of hepatic fibrosis can be obtained using elastography,[17] whereas qualitative evaluation can be gained with T2-weighted imaging and delayed contrast enhancement.[18] The degree of hepatic steatosis can be assessed by using spectroscopic methods.[19] Multiecho gradient echo imaging can be used for evaluation of steatosis and iron deposition (**Fig. 9**).[16,20]

PATIENT PREPARATION

Proper patient preparation is essential to achieving optimal hepatobiliary imaging with MR imaging. Initial patient preparation begins with evaluating the need for anesthesia or sedation. Typically, children under age six who are unable to perform a 20-second breath hold require anesthesia or sedation. The breath-hold requirement can be sacrificed when performing Magnetic Resonance Cholangiopancreatography (MRCP) (see later discussion) and in facilities with a distracting MR imaging-compatible goggle system. Pediatric

patients should take nothing by mouth 4 hours before the examination. This will help ensure the gallbladder is distended and minimize artifacts from bowel. Adequate peripheral venous access is necessary to power inject contrast and optimally evaluate the hepatobiliary vasculature. Finally, a respiratory monitoring belt or pillow should be carefully placed once the patient is comfortably situated on the MR table. Although this can be a difficult and time-consuming task in young children, its presence drastically improves image quality.

HARDWARE REQUIREMENTS

Currently, literature is scarce regarding 3 T field strength abdominal imaging in children.[21,22] The authors' experience suggests that most children (excluding those with large body habitus or large volume ascites) will benefit from the higher signal-to-noise ratio (SNR) of the 3 T MR imaging scanner. MR imaging at 3 T potentially offers twofold SNR increase over 1.5 T MR imaging. The marked improvement in MR image quality of the 3 T MR imaging scanner in children younger than 8 years of age is noteworthy. Eight

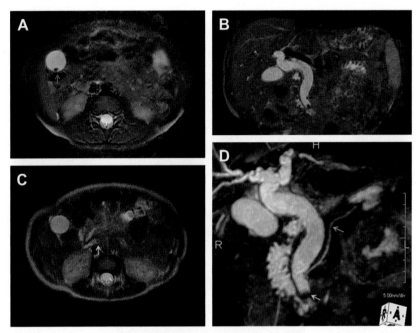

Fig. 3. Twenty-month-old girl who presented with abdominal pain, vomiting, and elevated liver transaminases, alkaline phosphatase, and gamma-glutamyl transferase. Previous ultrasound obtained at an outside hospital demonstrated gallstones and dilation of the common bile duct. MRCP was requested to evaluate for a distal obstructing stone that was presumed on a clinical basis; however, it was not delineated by ultrasound. (*A*) Axial T2-weighted MR image (320 × 256 matrix and 24 cm FOV) demonstrates small hypointense gallstone (*red arrow*) in the gallbladder. (*B*) Volumetric T2-weighted MR image exquisitely demonstrates the dilated common bile duct. Note is made of relatively low TE of 90 ms, which retains signal in liver parenchyma and kidneys permitting their evaluation. (*C*) Axial SSFSE MR image which can be used for patients with difficulty maintaining breath hold, clearly demonstrates a hypointense filling defect (*yellow arrow*) seen in the distal common bile duct. Single-shot MR imaging is complementary to volumetric T2 imaging but with lower SNR and thicker slices (4 mm); however, it typically allows for motion-free images. (*D*) 3D maximum intensity projection image clearly demonstrates marked biliary ductal dilatation and a stone (*yellow arrow*) lodged in the distal common bile duct just proximal to the ampulla. Note the main pancreatic duct (*blue arrow*), which is not dilated.

to 32 channel-phased array surface coils are now standard for hepatobiliary imaging in pediatric patients. Cardiac arrays are optimal for most children except very large patients who may require a torso array.

IMAGING PROTOCOLS

Table 2 outlines suggested protocols with summarized descriptions. Matrix, field of view, and slice thickness are parameters that should be adjusted based on patient size and are, therefore, not included. The choice of MR sequences varies based on how cooperative each patient is. Volumetric T2-weighted sequences are suboptimal in situations in which regular breathing cannot be achieved because they are susceptible to motion artifact. In semicooperative patients (those who can breath-hold but may not breathe regularly), two-dimensional (2D) T2-weighted breath-hold sequences can be used. Parallel imaging with fewer slices per acquisition can be used in this situation. Additionally, 2D spoiled gradient echo (SPGR) is an excellent alternative to three-dimensional (3D) SPGR when decreasing motion artifact is necessary. In cases where breath hold is unattainable, fast inversion recovery motion-insensitive or 2D SPGR with an inversion pulse to provide enhanced T1-weighting can be used.

Localizers

Hepatobiliary imaging at 1.5 T includes three-plane single-shot fast spin echo with low bandwidth (20 kHz) and repetition time (TR). Diagnostic single-shot images can be obtained by adjusting the matrix (320 × 256), slice thickness (4–5 mm), and echo time (TE; 80 ms) with images acquired using respiratory triggering.[23] At 3 T, localizers may be more efficiently achieved with balanced steady state imaging to conserve specific absorption rate, especially in small patients, if diagnostic

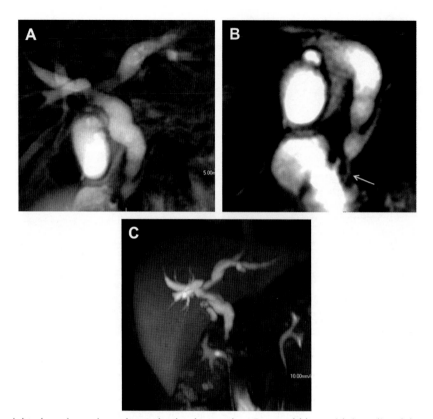

Fig. 4. T2-weighted maximum intensity projection images in a 5-year-old boy with jaundice. (*A*) Type 4a chole-dochal cyst (also sometimes referred to as Type I with intrahepatic involvement) is demonstrated with both intra-hepatic and extrahepatic biliary ductal dilatation. (*B*) Coned in T2-weighted maximum intensity projection demonstrates anomalous pancreaticobiliary pancreatic ductal union (*yellow arrow*), which is thought to be one of the predisposing factors to choledochal cyst formation. Given that the common bile duct and pancreatic duct are seen uniting greater than 15 mm before the insertion into the duodenal ampulla, this is an example of anomalous biliary pancreatic ductal union. (*C*) Delayed hepatobiliary phase imaging after the administration of Gd-EOB-DTPA clearly demonstrates the homogenous hepatocyte uptake within the parenchyma as well as 50% biliary and 50% renal excretion of the contrast.

single-shot images are not required. All localizer sequences should use parallel imaging.

Conventional T2 Imaging

Conventional T2-weighted imaging can be performed with fast spin echo in coronal and axial planes using respiratory-triggered or navigated sequences.[24,25] To maximize tissue characterization with high SNR, conventional T2-weighted imaging should be performed without parallel imaging. Typical TEs are 80 to 90 ms at 1.5 T and 70 to 80 ms at 3 T. To improve SNR, fast recovery may be used. Given the mixed opinions in the current literature about the ability of single-shot images with T2-weighting to provide an alternative to lengthier conventional T2-weighted imaging,[26] conventional T2-weighted imaging remains in the abdominal MR imaging protocol.

Volumetric T2 Imaging

Volumetric T2-weighted sequences have previously been described for musculoskeletal or neurologic imaging.[27–30] It is similar to fast spin echo in which a 90° excitation is required. However, this excitation is a slab rather than a slice. To maintain signal uniformity despite the long train (typically 60–100 echoes), the excitation in a volumetric T2-weighted sequence is followed by a train of refocusing pulses, with variation of the flip angle. The flip angle variation is automatically set by the various vendors.

Advantages of volumetric imaging include thin slices (1–2 mm) and the capability to reformat in multiple planes (see **Fig. 1**). It is necessary to use parallel imaging to maintain a reasonable scan time of 4 to 5 minutes. To minimize T2 decay-related blurring, a high bandwidth (eg, 62 kHz) should be used in addition to respiratory triggering

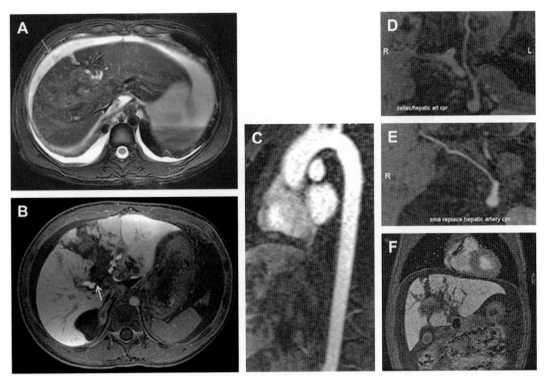

Fig. 5. Seven-year-old boy who was involved in a motor vehicle accident. Patient was clinically stabilized by an outside hospital and was transferred with known hemoperitoneum, hepatic laceration, and question of a thoracic aortic pseudoaneurysm on the outside CT. MR imaging was requested to evaluate if there was a component of biliary ductal injury and for further assessment of arterial anatomy. Given the two clinical questions to be answered, the patient was scanned using both gadofosveset trisodium and gadoxetate disodium as contrast agents. (*A*) Axial T2-weighted image (320 × 224 Matrix and 26 cm FOV) demonstrates bilateral pleural effusions and free intraperitoneal fluid (*blue arrow*) with a hepatic laceration (*red arrow*) seen extending along the anterior segment of the right hepatic lobe. (*B*) Gadoxetate disodium was used to provide functional information regarding the possibility of biliary ductal injury in the setting of trauma. MR image obtained 15 minutes after injection of contrast demonstrates hepatobiliary clearance and an active bile leak (*yellow arrow*). (*C*) Gadofosveset trisodium was given due to its prolonged intravascular phase which reduces the challenge of obtaining a correctly timed acquisition. Curved planar reformat image demonstrated a normal contour to the thoracic aorta without MR evidence for aneurysm. (*D, E*) Curved planar reformatted images demonstrate the left hepatic artery arising from the celiac axis and a replaced right hepatic artery arising separately off the superior mesenteric artery. (*F*) Portal venous phase coronal MR image demonstrates the extensive Grade 5 liver laceration.

or navigation. Typically, a TE of 70 to 90 ms allows appropriate anatomic delineation and good assessment of the bile ducts on individual slices. Use of a high TE (>500 ms) with dedicated MRCP evaluation enables excellent maximum intensity reformation of the biliary tree and pancreatic duct (see **Figs. 3** and **4**).

Single-Shot Imaging

Volumetric imaging often clearly demonstrates the bile ducts[31]; however, suboptimal image quality may occur in patients with irregular breathing or uncontrolled motion. In the case of irregular breathing, the technologist can manually trigger each slice by observing the respiratory belt tracing. Parallel imaging can be used to further reduce acquisition time per slice in single-shot imaging thus reducing motion artifacts. Methods include k-space–based (eg, generalized autocalibrating partially parallel acquisition [GRAPPA] or image domain–based (eg, sensitivity encoding parallel imaging [SENSE]) approaches. In cases in which the acquisition is short and SNR is low, more efficient image domain–based approaches may be desirable. However, care must be taken to ensure large enough field of view to avoid residual aliasing artifacts at the image center. Single-shot imaging is thus complementary[32] to volumetric imaging and a reasonable assessment of the biliary tree can be obtained in even the most challenging patients (see **Figs. 2** and **3**).

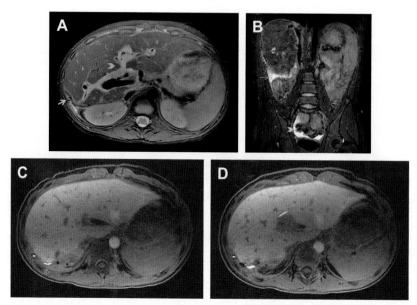

Fig. 6. Eleven-year-old boy after cut-edge hepatic transplant with persistent bilious output from Jackson-Pratt drain. MR imaging was requested to assess the site of a persistent bile leak. (*A*) Axial T2-weighted MR image (320 × 224 matrix and 28 cm FOV) demonstrates a scattered amount of hyperintense fluid adjacent to the porta hepatis (*green arrowhead*) and along the right lateral aspect of the liver where there is presence of a Jackson-Pratt drain (*yellow arrow*). (*B*) Volumetric T2-weighted MR image demonstrates a trace amount of fluid (*red arrow*) along the lateral aspect of the liver just inferior to the Jackson-Pratt drain. Additional fluid (*yellow arrowhead*) is seen inferiorly within the pelvis. (*C, D*) Axial water-specific T1-weighted high-resolution MR images (320 × 420 matrix and 32 cm FOV) after gadoxetate disodium obtained during the hepatobiliary phase demonstrate an active biliary leak (*blue arrows*) at the cut edge of the liver.

T1-Weighted Imaging

Traditionally, spin echo imaging has been used. However, recent trends in adult body imaging and personal practice have minimized use of this lengthy approach. Although exceptional images are occasionally acquired with unrivaled SNR, frequently image quality is degraded by respiratory ghosts despite use of respiratory compensation schemes.

As an alternative, dual echo imaging (SPGR with in-phase and opposed-phase echoes) or in-and-opposed phase gradient-echo (GRE) imaging can be used. Dual-echo imaging has the disadvantage of lower SNR, but offers the advantage of volumetric imaging with high resolution, sequence acquisition in a single breath hold, and more T1-weighting. Data from a single acquisition can be processed to yield four image sets: in-phase, opposed-phase, water, and fat. Representative parameters include high bandwidth (100 kHz), 4 mm slice thickness, and 12° to 15° flip angle.

Dynamic Contrast-Enhanced MR Imaging

Several contrast agents are now available that allow enhancement assessment to be tailored to specific imaging goals. Predominantly renally

excreted gadolinium agents continue to be the preferred agent for hepatic tumor characterization given the sparse literature on pediatric tumor evaluation with other gadolinium agents. The high relaxivity and longer intravascular residence time of gadobenate dimeglumine is advantageous for evaluation of vascular structures. Gadobenate dimeglumine has approximately 5% hepatobiliary elimination, which has been reported to aid in distinguishing focal nodular hyperplasia (FNH) and hepatic adenoma. Gadofosveset trisodium, a Food and Drug Administration–approved blood-pool gadolinium contrast agent for the assessment of aortoiliac disease in adults, may also be useful in pediatric vascular assessment (see **Fig. 5**). Finally, gadoxetate disodium (Gd-EOB-DTPA) is advantageous as an off-label use for biliary evaluation[33–37] given the 50% hepatobiliary excretion in the setting of normal renal and hepatic function. Gd-EOB-DTPA provides a functional and anatomic MRCP examination (see **Figs.4–6**). Single-dose Gd-EOB-DTPA has one-quarter the gadolinium of standard agents (0.025 mmol/kg), but its higher T1 relaxivity allows for adequate first-pass hepatic imaging. A single-dose administration at 1 mL/sec followed by a saline flush is acceptable for all agents. For doses less than

Dynamic gadolinium studies can be performed using a fat-suppressed 3D SPGR sequence (minimum TR, 15° flip angle, 62 kHz bandwidth). The matrix and number of slices can be adjusted to make the scan time match the patient's ability to breath-hold. If the patient is unable to breath-hold, a 30-second scan time with quiet breathing can be used. Following contrast administration, a series of three phases are acquired in rapid succession followed by delayed imaging at 3 minutes.

The technique for dynamic gadolinium studies depends on the imaging goal: vascular analysis versus tumor characterization. To optimize tumor characterization, a scan delay should be set to ensure the center of k-space is acquired at 30 seconds after half the contrast is administered: scan delay = 30 seconds − (scan duration/2) + (bolus duration/2).

As a typical example, using a 30-second scan and a 10 mL bolus infused at 1 mL/sec, the scan delay is 30 − (30/2) + (10/2) = 20 seconds. This assumes sequential, not centric, k-space encoding (**Figs. 10** and **12**).

With vascular assessment, a timing run can be performed with fluoroscopic triggering and centric k-space acquisition. Alternatively, sequential k-space acquisition and calculation of the scan delay can be performed by substituting the time to abdominal aortic peak enhancement for 30 seconds in the above equation.

TE also varies depending on the imaging goal. The minimum full TE should be selected for tumor characterization to maximize SNR. The minimum TE (ie, a fractional echo) should be used in vascular assessment to minimize artifact from flow-related spin dephasing and to minimize scan time.

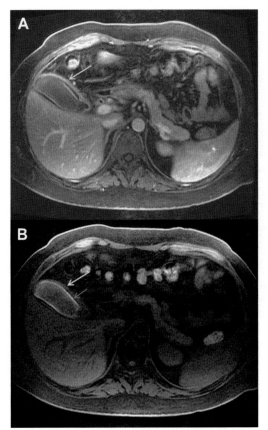

Fig. 7. Sixteen-year-old boy after liver transplant who presented with abdominal pain. (*A*) Axial T1-weighted MR image with fat saturation demonstrates marked gallbladder wall thickening with high T1 signal (*yellow arrow*) in the wall concerning for hemorrhage. Additionally, there is pericholecystic fluid (*red arrow*). (*B*) Axial T2-weighted MR image with fat saturation with a yellow arrow indicating the gallbladder wall is isointense to hypointense, concerning for subacute blood product, and the blue arrow demonstrating the hyperintense fluid. Hemorrhagic cholecystitis was confirmed at surgery.

10 mL, dilution with saline to a volume of 10 mL eases handling. Delayed images obtained between 15 and 20 minutes demonstrate hepatocyte uptake and biliary as well as renal clearance (see **Fig. 4**). Gd-EOB-DTPA has been shown to improve the detection of metastasis, better demonstrate the relationship of tumors relative to the biliary tree, and help differentiate FNH from liver metastasis, particularly in children who have been treated for a primary tumor in which there is an increased incidence of FNH. Additionally, Gd-EOB-DTPA can be used to evaluate biliary variants, including ductal plate malformations, postoperative complications, or biliary trauma (see **Figs. 4–6**).[38,39]

Noncontrast MR Angiography

Contrast-enhanced MR angiography has been the primary method for vascular assessment. However, in patients with renal insufficiency, this technique may have limited use. Also, because intravenous contrast can only be administered once, there is little room for error. Any injection-scan timing mismatch, patient motion or additional artifact during the examination cannot be rectified. Therefore, MR imaging reliability for vascular assessment is markedly improved using noncontrast-enhanced techniques.

Noncontrast-enhanced techniques based on balanced-steady state approaches have become useful for abdominal vascular evaluation, especially renal artery stenosis, whereas time-of-flight–based approaches produce limited image quality in the abdomen.[40] A variation of this

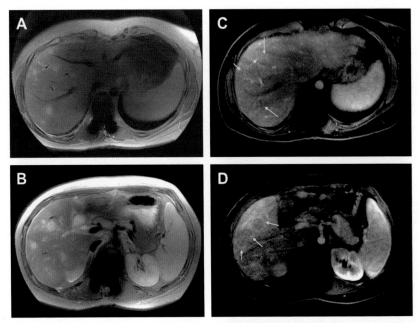

Fig. 8. Sixteen-year-old girl after orthotopic heart transplant on immunosuppressive therapy who presented with fever; a skin lesion on her forehead; and fluctuant, tender, periauricular lymphadenopathy. MR imaging was performed as part of the fever evaluation. (*A, B*) Axial T2-weighted MR images (320 × 320 matrix with 32 cm FOV) demonstrate multiple hyperintense circumscribed rounded masses. These were pathologic test–proven Bartonella abscesses. Note the loss of signal in the midline from the patient's spinal fusion. (*C, D*) Postcontrast T1-weighted water-specific images (288 × 224 matrix with 36 cm FOV) demonstrate multiple peripherally enhancing and central hypointense abscesses (*yellow arrows*).

method uses a respiratory-triggered inversion pulse covering the imaged volume and an area inferior to it followed by a balanced steady state echo train.[41] This is similar to the balanced steady state echo train used in noncontrast-enhanced coronary artery imaging, but cardiac gating is not used. With this technique, an MR angiography is produced because the blood flowing from superior to the inverted region is bright. Pitfalls similar to time-of-flight–based techniques can occur, including flow-related dephasing, slow-flow–related signal dropout, and intrinsic high T1 signal. Non-contrast MR angiography, however, provides an excellent complement to contrast-enhanced MR angiography.

Iron Quantification

There are several methods to quantify hepatic iron based on T2 signal and a composite of signals, including proton density, T2, T2*, and T1 (see http://www.radio.univ-rennes1.fr/Sources/EN/Hemo.html by Y. Gandon). However, the most common quantification method for hepatic iron is based on T2*measurement alone. Although T2* can be performed on any scanner, it is typically performed on 1.5 T as the T2* value depends on field strength. Additionally, most of the literature on calibration of iron concentration is based on T2* at 1.5 T.

T2* can be obtained by performing multiple gradient echo sequences at different TE values using a fixed TR. TE values should typically range from 1 ms to 20 ms. Prescanning should not be performed between sequences because the transmit and receiver gains could change. A region of interest in the same area of the liver on each series of images can be drawn. Mean signal at each TE is established and will demonstrate an exponential decay relationship (signal = $Ae^{-R_2^* \, TE} + B$, where $R2^* = 1/T2^*$). Various readily available software packages and programs can determine R_2^* and hence T_2^* using logarithms and linear regression.

Until recently, the process for determining T2* was quite lengthy. A breath-hold was required for each TE and regression performed, which is disruptive to patient throughput and workflow. Multiecho gradient echo serves as a reasonable alternative. A series of gradient echoes are obtained at various TEs after each excitation allowing for 2D acquisition of a single slice of the liver or a 3D volume acquisition. Regardless, the acquisition is a single breath-hold that serves to avoid slice misregistration issues, is easier on the patient,

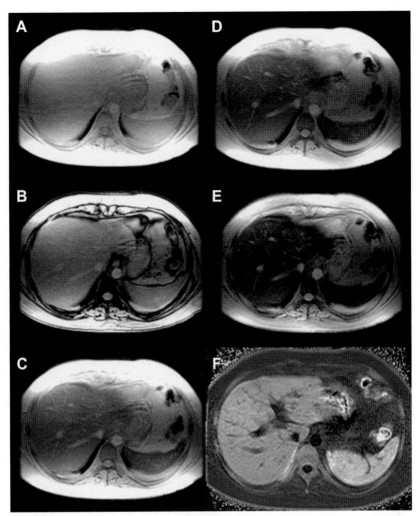

Fig. 9. Iron overload in a 16-year-old boy with acute lymphoblastic leukemia after stem cell transplant. (*A–E*) Sequential TE images demonstrate progressive decrease in hepatic signal consistent with T2* decay. The signal is fit to exponential decay to yield R2*. (*F*) R2* parametric map demonstrates mild to moderate hepatic iron deposition. Additionally noted is splenic iron deposition.

and facilitates workflow. When coupled with an image reconstruction algorithm that performs a fit to determine R_2^*,[41] image maps are obtained (see **Fig. 9**).

Determining pediatric hepatic iron deposition can be challenging given the wide range of T2* values that are acquired in practice. Obtaining accurate T2* over such a wide range can be difficult. T2* can be overestimated in a patient with severe iron deposition when a long train of echoes or long echo spacing is used. This is because rapid signal decay results in images dominated by noise. Conversely, poor estimation of T2* may occur when a series of echoes with short TEs is used to address the situation of mild iron deposition because the minimal signal decay precludes good exponential fitting. Therefore, the longest

TE used to determine T_2^* should be based in part on the expected T_2^*. By acquiring two datasets, one with long TEs and the other with short TEs, the appropriate set could be used.

MR Elastography

A wide variety of underlying conditions result in hepatic fibrosis, including infectious, autoimmune, drug-related, genetic, and metabolic disorders. Early intervention can slow or halt the progression of hepatic fibrosis. Although liver biopsy remains the gold standard for the definitive diagnosis, it is prone to sampling error, is costly, and places the patient at risk for procedural complications, including bleeding and infection. MR elastography has recently emerged as a noninvasive alternative

Table 2
Suggested MR protocols for hepatobiliary imaging

Pulse Sequences	Scan Time	Indication		
		Tumors	MRCP	Transplant
Localizer (1.5 T: SSFSE, HASTE 3T: FIESTA True FISP)	20 s–3 min	X	X	X
FSE T2	3–4 min	X	X	X
Volumetric T2 (CUBE SPACE, VISTA)	4–5 min	Optional	X	X
Single-shot (SSFSE, HASTE)	2–3 min	—	X	X
Dual Echo	30 s	X	X	X
Noncontrast MR angiography	4–5 min	—	—	X
SPGR (LAVA, VIBE, THRIVE)	30 s	Full echo	Optional	Partial echo

Abbreviations: FIESTA, fast imaging employing steady state acquisition; FISP, fast imaging with steady state precession; FSE, fast spin echo; HASTE, half-fourier acquisition single shot turbo spin echo; SPGR, spoiled gradient echo; SSFSE, single-shot fast spin echo; CUBE, SPACE, and VISTA are Single Slab 3 Dimensional Fast Spin Echo Sequences from various vendors. LAVA, VIBE, and THRIVE are 3 Dimensional Spoiled Gradient Sequences (SPGR) from various vendors.

for the evaluation of hepatic inflammation and fibrosis because it provides a more global assessment of the hepatic parenchyma. As much as 20% of the liver volume can be assessed based on the number of slices imaged and the liver size.[42] MR elastography has also been shown to be accurate in the staging of liver fibrosis in adults when compared with liver biopsy and pathologic grading.[43] MR elastography is based on the principle that infiltrative processes and tumors alter the mechanical properties of soft tissues and typically result in increased firmness. With vibrational stress, transmission of energy in the form of a shear wave will penetrate deeper into tissues with fibrosis, whereas softer tissues will dissipate that energy. Dynamic MR elastography uses harmonic motion that is introduced into the body through an external vibration system. Using phase contrast MR pulse sequences, the motion is imaged by measuring tissue displacement or

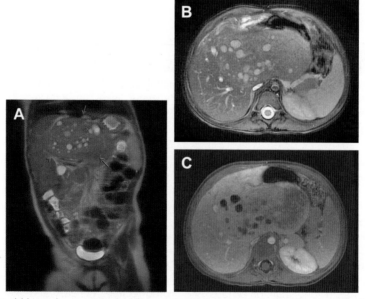

Fig. 10. Three-year-old boy who presented with an enlarging abdominal mass. No elevation in Alpha Fetal Protein (AFP) was present. (*A, B*) Conventional T2-weighted MR coronal and axial MR images demonstrate a large solid and cystic mass (*red arrows*) seen spanning the right and left hepatic lobes. (*C*) Postcontrast T1-weighted MR image with fat saturation timed to optimize tumor characterization sets a scan delay so that the center of k-space is acquired 30 seconds after half the contrast is administered. Note the clear enhancement of the solid portions of the mass and nonenhancement of the cysts. Additionally, there is decreased enhancement along the left aspect of the tumor, potentially reflecting an underlying microcystic component. Surgical pathology confirmed the diagnosis of mesenchymal hamartoma, a benign tumor.

velocity. Using an inversion algorithm, data can then generate elastograms that reflect the mechanical properties of the tissue. Limited pediatric MR elastography data is currently available, and protocols provided have been altered and modified from adult MR elastography scan methods developed by Ehman and colleagues[43] at the Mayo Clinic. A suggested MR elastography protocol adapted from Serai and colleagues[44] and Yin and colleagues[45] for the pediatric patient includes a fast gradient echo sequence that is synchronized with the vibrational input in the axial plane through the widest portion of the liver beneath the heart during end expiration. Recommended parameters include a TR of 50 ms, TE of 20 ms, flip angle of 25°, slice thickness of 10 mm, GAP of 1 mm, and 32 kHz bandwidth. A total of four slices are obtained with a parallel imaging acceleration factor of two, and four time points are evenly sampled over one period of motion. Typically four 15-second breath holds at end expiration is needed. MR elastography can be incorporated with a diagnostic MR liver examination, with only about 10 minutes of additional setup and table time. Scans must be performed with at least 4 hours of nothing per mouth because the increase in portal venous blood flow after eating has been shown to transiently increase hepatic stiffness in patients with liver disease but not in normal patients.[46] Technical issues unique to the pediatric patient include use of a child life specialist who uses a vibrating passive driver simulator before the MR elastography to help children prepare for the sensation they will feel during the scanning, decreasing the driver power that emits the vibration by 20% in all pediatric patients and by 50% in patients less than 2 years of age, and placement of a towel between the driver and the child to help improve mechanical coupling and minimize any theoretical risk of mechanical or thermal injury to the child.[42,44]

Although no normal pediatric liver MR elastography database has been established for mild,

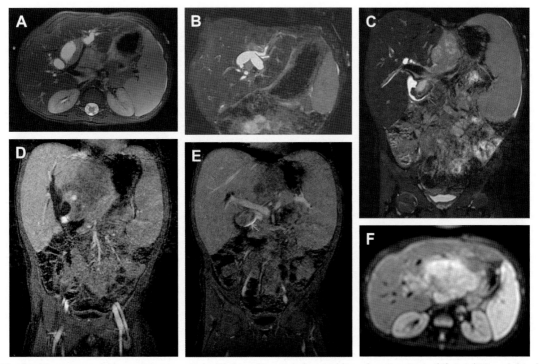

Fig. 11. Three-year-old boy who presented with jaundice and elevated liver function tests. (A) Axial T2-weighted MR image with fat saturation (320 × 224 matrix with 24 cm FOV) demonstrates dilated central biliary ducts with associated hyperintense soft tissue surrounding the central biliary tree and porta hepatis. (B, C) Coronal volumetric fast spine echo T2-weighted images (320 × 320 matrix with 28 cm FOV) demonstrate a polypoid mass (*red arrow*) projecting centrally within the common bile duct. Splenomegaly and a trace amount of perisplenic fluid are also present. (D, E) Postcontrast T1-weighted MR images with fat saturation demonstrate an ill-defined hypointense solid mass involving the porta hepatis and left hepatic lobe; however, with some solid enhancing soft tissue component (*blue arrow*) extending into the common bile duct. (F) Axial diffusion-weighted MR image demonstrates marked bright signal within the tumor. Surgical pathologic result was consistent with a biliary rhabdomyosarcoma.

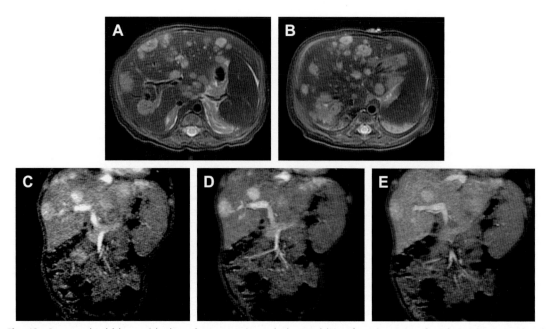

Fig. 12. One-week old boy with thrombocytopenia and elevated liver function tests. (*A, B*) Axial T2-weighted MR images demonstrate multiple homogenous hyperintense rounded masses within the liver. No substantial perilesional edema is noted. No architectural distortion is noted to the hepatic parenchyma. (*C–E*) Sequential coronal postcontrast T1-weighted images clearly demonstrate avid arterial enhancement with persistent retention of the contrast within the hepatic masses. No evidence of substantial washout of contrast is noted on subsequent portal venous phase images. MR imaging findings are pathognomonic for multiple infantile or congenital hemangiomas, which is currently the preferred term. This was previously referred to as a congenital hemangioendothelioma.

moderate, or severe fibrosis in children, normal pediatric controls have been found to have ultrasound transient elastography (UTE) measurements similar to adult patients.[47] Prospective studies still need to be performed comparing MR elastography with percutaneous biopsy in the pediatric patient before it can be completely accepted as a replacement for hepatic biopsy. However, the use of MR elastography to help target biopsy by creating visual maps, follow posttreatment changes of known cases of hepatic fibrosis, and aid in identifying early prefibrotic hepatic changes to prompt biopsy seems promising.

Diffusion-Weighted Imaging

Diffusion-weighted imaging (DWI) is an additional imaging tool to aid in evaluation of hepatic lesions, particularly malignant tumors and pyogenic abscesses (see **Figs. 1** and **11**).[48] However, there is a lack of literature on DWI use in the pediatric population. DWI sequences are obtained quickly, ranging from 1 to 5 minutes. Additionally, DWI sequences may provide further diagnostic information in patients with contraindications to intravenous contrast administration, such as those in renal failure. Well performed DWI sequences are complementary to T2-weighted sequences (see **Fig. 11**), especially in cases in which T2-weighted images are less than optimal. However, pitfalls in DWI interpretation can occur due to difficulty in accurately comparing studies that are performed using different imaging protocols.[49] An advantage of DWI is its relatively fast acquisition resulting in motion-free degradation. Disadvantages include low resolution and susceptibility-related image distortion, which can be minimized by using parallel imaging. Recent research suggests that DWI and apparent diffusion coefficient (ADC) maps are helpful in discerning malignant from benign pediatric tumors with a cut-off ADC value of 1.29×10^{-3} mm²/s as being statistically significant. Tumors less than this value are worrisome for malignancy.[50]

SUMMARY

MR imaging techniques and protocols continue to progress and advance in hepatobiliary imaging in pediatric patients. MR imaging provides radiologists with a nonradiative, noninvasive, and reliable modality to aid clinicians in the accurate diagnosis and follow-up of various hepatic and biliary disorders in the pediatric population. An up-to-date knowledge of proper MR imaging techniques and clear understanding of characteristic MR imaging appearance of these hepatobiliary disorders in pediatric patients hold great potential for optimal patient care.

REFERENCES

1. Couinaud V. The paracaval segments of the liver. J Hepatobiliary Pancreat Surg 1994;2:145–51.

2. Finn JP, Hall-Craggs MA, Dicks-Mireaux C, et al. Primary malignant liver tumors in childhood: assessment of resectability with high-field MR and comparison with CT. Pediatr Radiol 1990;21: 34–8.

3. Semelka RC, Shoenut JP, Kroeker MA, et al. Focal liver disease: comparison of dynamic contrast-enhanced CT and T2-weighted fat-suppressed, FLASH, and dynamic gadolinium-enhanced MR imaging at 1.5 T. Radiology 1992; 184:687–94.

4. Weinreb JC, Cohen JM, Armstrong E, et al. Imaging the pediatric liver: MRI and CT. AJR Am J Roentgenol 1986;147:785–90.

5. Roebuck DJ, Aronson D, Clapuyt P, et al. 2005 PRETEXT: a revised staging system for primary malignant liver tumours of childhood developed by the SIOPEL group. Pediatr Radiol 2007;37: 123–32 [quiz: 249–50].

6. Arcement CM, Meza MP, Arumanla S, et al. MRCP in the evaluation of pancreaticobiliary disease in children. Pediatr Radiol 2001;31:92–7.

7. Delaney L, Applegate KE, Karmazyn B, et al. MR cholangiopancreatography in children: feasibility, safety, and initial experience. Pediatr Radiol 2008; 38:64–75.

8. Chavhan GB, Roberts E, Moineddin R, et al. Primary sclerosing cholangitis in children: utility of magnetic resonance cholangiopancreatography. Pediatr Radiol 2008;38:868–73.

9. Ferrara C, Valeri G, Salvolini L, et al. Magnetic resonance cholangiopancreatography in primary sclerosing cholangitis in children. Pediatr Radiol 2002;32:413–7.

10. Hamada Y, Tanano A, Takada K, et al. Magnetic resonance cholangiopancreatography on postoperative work-up in children with choledochal cysts. Pediatr Surg Int 2004;20:43–6.

11. Irie H, Honda H, Jimi M, et al. Value of MR cholangiopancreatography in evaluating choledochal cysts. AJR Am J Roentgenol 1998;171:1381–5.

12. Kim MJ, Han SJ, Yoon CS, et al. Using MR cholangiopancreatography to reveal anomalous pancreaticobiliary ductal union in infants and children with choledochal cysts. AJR Am J Roentgenol 2002; 179:209–14.

13. Krause D, Cercueil JP, Dranssart M, et al. MRI for evaluating congenital bile duct abnormalities. J Comput Assist Tomogr 2002;26:541–52.

14. Fishbein M, Castro F, Cheruku S, et al. Hepatic MRI for fat quantitation: its relationship to fat morphology, diagnosis, and ultrasound. J Clin Gastroenterol 2005;39:619–25.

15. Fishbein MH, Gardner KG, Potter CJ, et al. Introduction of fast MR imaging in the assessment of hepatic steatosis. Magn Reson Imaging 1997;15: 287–93.

16. Qayyum A, Goh JS, Kakar S, et al. Accuracy of liver fat quantification at MR imaging: comparison of out-of-phase gradient-echo and fat-saturated fast spin-echo techniques–initial experience. Radiology 2005;237:507–11.

17. Yin M, Talwalkar JA, Glaser KJ, et al. Assessment of hepatic fibrosis with magnetic resonance elastography. Clin Gastroenterol Hepatol 2007;5: 1207–1213.e2.

18. Fujita T, Ito K, Honjo K, et al. Hepatic parenchymal enhancement in the cirrhotic liver: evaluation by triple-phase dynamic MRI. Abdom Imaging 2002; 27:29–33.

19. Lee JK, Dixon WT, Ling D, et al. Fatty infiltration of the liver: demonstration by proton spectroscopic imaging. Preliminary observations. Radiology 1984;153:195–201.

20. Wood JC, Enriquez C, Ghugre N, et al. MRI R2 and R2* mapping accurately estimates hepatic iron concentration in transfusion-dependent thalassemia and sickle cell disease patients. Blood 2005;106:1460–5.

21. Dagia C, Ditchfield M. 3T MRI in paediatrics: challenges and clinical applications. Eur J Radiol 2008; 68:309–19.

22. Schindera ST, Merkle EM, Dale BM, et al. Abdominal magnetic resonance imaging at 3.0 T what is the ultimate gain in signal-to-noise ratio? Acad Radiol 2006;13:1236–43.

23. Runge VM, Clanton JA, Partain CL, et al. Respiratory gating in magnetic resonance imaging at 0.5 Tesla. Radiology 1984;151:521–3.

24. Kim BS, Kim JH, Choi GM, et al. Comparison of three free-breathing T2-weighted MRI sequences in the evaluation of focal liver lesions. AJR Am J Roentgenol 2008;190:W19–27.

25. Klessen C, Asbach P, Kroencke TJ, et al. Magnetic resonance imaging of the upper abdomen using a free-breathing T2-weighted turbo spin echo sequence with navigator triggered prospective acquisition correction. J Magn Reson Imaging 2005;21: 576–82.

26. Lee SS, Byun JH, Hong HS, et al. Image quality and focal lesion detection on T2-weighted MR imaging of the liver: comparison of two high-resolution free-breathing imaging techniques with

two breath-hold imaging techniques. J Magn Reson Imaging 2007;26:323–30.

27. Busse RF, Hariharan H, Vu A, et al. Fast spin echo sequences with very long echo trains: design of variable refocusing flip angle schedules and generation of clinical T2 contrast. Magn Reson Med 2006;55:1030–7.

28. Hennig J, Weigel M, Scheffler K. Multiecho sequences with variable refocusing flip angles: optimization of signal behavior using smooth transitions between pseudo steady states (TRAPS). Magn Reson Med 2003;49:527–35.

29. Kijowski R, Davis KW, Woods MA, et al. Knee joint: comprehensive assessment with 3D isotropic resolution fast spin-echo MR imaging–diagnostic performance compared with that of conventional MR imaging at 3.0 T. Radiology 2009;252:486–95.

30. Mugler J, Brookeman J. Three-dimensional T2-weighted imaging of the brain using very long spin-echo trains. In: International Society of Magnetic Resonance in Medicine 8th Meeting. Denver, Colorado April 3–7, 2000. p. 687.

31. Nandalur KR, Hussain HK, Weadock WJ, et al. Possible biliary disease: diagnostic performance of high-spatial-resolution isotropic 3D T2-weighted MRCP. Radiology 2008;249:883–90.

32. Miyazaki T, Yamashita Y, Tang Y, et al. Single-shot MR cholangiopancreatography of neonates, infants, and young children. AJR Am J Roentgenol 1998;170:33–7.

33. Carlos RC, Branam JD, Dong Q, et al. Biliary imaging with Gd-EOB-DTPA: is a 20-minute delay sufficient? Acad Radiol 2002;9:1322–5.

34. Koelblinger C, Schima W, Weber M, et al. Gadoxate-enhanced T 1-weighted MR cholangiography: comparison of 1.5 T and 3.0 T. Rofo 2009;181:587–92.

35. Lee NK, Kim S, Lee JW, et al. Biliary MR imaging with Gd-EOB-DTPA and its clinical applications. Radiographics 2009;29:1707–24.

36. Seale MK, Catalano OA, Saini S, et al. Hepatobiliary-specific MR contrast agents: role in imaging the liver and biliary tree. Radiographics 2009;29:1725–48.

37. Takao H, Akai H, Tajima T, et al. MR imaging of the biliary tract with Gd-EOB-DTPA: effect of liver function on signal intensity. Eur J Radiol 2011;77(2):325–9.

38. Meyers A, Towbin A, Serai S, et al. Characterization of pediatric liver lesions with gadoxetate disodium. Pediatr Radiol 2011;41:1183–97.

39. Tamrazi A, Vasanawal S. Functional hepatobiliary MR imaging in children. Pediatr Radiol 2011;41:1250–8.

40. Maki JH, Wilson GJ, Eubank WB, et al. Steady-state free precession MRA of the renal arteries: breath-hold and navigator-gated techniques vs. CE-MRA. J Magn Reson Imaging 2007;26:966–73.

41. Katoh M, Buecker A, Stuber M, et al. Free-breathing renal MR angiography with steady-state free-precession (SSFP) and slab-selective spin inversion: initial results. Kidney Int 2004;66:1272–8.

42. Binkovitz LA, El-Youssef M, Glaser KJ, et al. Pediatric MR elastography of hepatic fibrosis: principles, technique and early clinical experience. Pediatr Radiol 2012;42:402–9.

43. Ehman R, Glaser K, Manduca A. Review of MR elastography applications and recent developments. J Magn Reson Imaging 2012;36:757–74.

44. Serai S, Towbin A, Podberesky DJ. Pediatric liver MR elastography. Dig Dis Sci 2012;57:2713–9.

45. Yin M, Chen J, Glaser K, et al. Assessment of hepatic fibrosis with magnetic resonance elastography. Clin Gastroenterol Hepatol 2007;5:1207–13.

46. Yin M, Talwakar JA, Glaser K, et al. Dynamic postprandial hepatic stiffness augmentation assessed with MR elastography in patients with chronic liver disease. AJR Am J Roentgenol 2007;197:64–70.

47. Nobili V, Vizzutti F, Arena U, et al. Accuracy and reproducibility or transient elastography for the diagnosis of fibrosis in pediatric nonalcoholic steatohepatitis. Hepatology 2008;48:442–8.

48. Namasivayam S, Martin DR, Saini S. Imaging of liver metastases: MRI. Cancer Imaging 2007;7:2–9.

49. Koh DM, Collins DJ. Diffusion-weighted MRI in the body: applications and challenges in oncology. AJR Am J Roentgenol 2007;188:1622–35.

50. Gawande R, Daldrup-Link H, Gonzalez G. Role of diffusion-weighted imaging in differentiating benign and malignant pediatric abdominal tumors. Pediatr Radiol, in press.

Multidetector Computed Tomographic and Magnetic Resonance Enterography in Children: State of the Art

Matthew R. Hammer, MD[a],*, Daniel J. Podberesky, MD[b], Jonathan R. Dillman, MD[a]

KEYWORDS

- Computed tomographic enterography • Magnetic resonance enterography • Bowel imaging
- Inflammatory bowel disease • Crohn disease • Ulcerative colitis • Children • Pediatric

KEY POINTS

- Multidetector computed tomographic and magnetic resonance imaging (CT and MR enterography, respectively) allow for detailed imaging of the bowel and mesentery in children.
- CT enterography excellently depicts the pediatric bowel, even when adhering to "as low as reasonably achievable" and "image gently" principles.
- CT and MR enterography can identify and characterize many inflammatory and noninflammatory abnormalities affecting the bowel and mesentery, directly influencing the medical and surgical management of pediatric patients.
- MR enterography has several advantages over CT enterography in the pediatric population, including superior contrast resolution and lack of ionizing radiation.
- MR enterography is often considered the study of choice when evaluating pediatric inflammatory bowel disease, particularly at follow-up after the diagnosis has been established.

INTRODUCTION

Advances in computed tomographic (CT) and magnetic resonance (MR) imaging techniques have revolutionized assessment of the pediatric abdomen and pelvis over the past decade (Box 1). For example, state-of the-art multidetector CT enterography allows for imaging of the entire pediatric small bowel and colon with radiation doses similar to or less than those used for traditional bowel-imaging techniques, such as small bowel-follow-through (SBFT) examinations.[1,2]

Recent MR imaging hardware and software advances now allow for rapid acquisition of high-quality images that superbly depict various abdominopelvic structures, including peristalsing bowel.[3] As a result, MR enterography has become a first-line imaging examination for evaluating bowel abnormality in many pediatric radiology practices.[4–7] Cross-sectional enterographic techniques, including both CT and MR enterography, can evaluate for a wide variety of abnormalities affecting the bowel and mesentery, including both inflammatory

[a] Section of Pediatric Radiology, Department of Radiology, C.S. Mott Children's Hospital, University of Michigan Health System, 1540 East Hospital Drive, Room 3-220, Ann Arbor, MI 48109-4252, USA; [b] Department of Radiology, Cincinnati Children's Hospital Medical Center, University of Cincinnati College of Medicine, 3333 Burnet Avenue, MLC 5031, Cincinnati, OH 45229, USA
* Corresponding author.
E-mail address: hammerm@med.umich.edu

Radiol Clin N Am 51 (2013) 615–636
http://dx.doi.org/10.1016/j.rcl.2013.04.001
0033-8389/13/$ – see front matter © 2013 Elsevier Inc. All rights reserved.

Box 1
What the referring physician needs to know

- CT and MR enterography superbly depict the pediatric bowel, allowing for evaluation of the bowel lumen, bowel wall, and adjacent soft-tissue structures

- CT and MR enterography are appropriate first-line imaging tests for evaluation of IBD in children, although MR enterography may be preferred because of its superior contrast resolution and lack of ionizing radiation despite less availability

- Using state-of-the-art iterative image reconstruction techniques and low kVp imaging, low-dose CT enterography is possible (<1–2 mSv) while maintaining image quality

- CT and MR enterography superbly depict bowel-wall inflammation in IBD as well as various abdominopelvic IBD-related complications and extraintestinal manifestations

- CT and MR enterography can satisfactorily evaluate various non-IBD abnormalities affecting the bowel, such as other inflammatory conditions, ischemia, obstruction, congenital anomalies, polyps, and masses

and noninflammatory conditions. In recent years, the advent and refinement of these imaging methods has caused fundamental paradigm shifts in the diagnosis and management (medical and surgical) of pediatric patients with suspected or known abnormalities affecting the bowel or adjacent soft tissues, especially in the setting of inflammatory bowel disease (IBD). The purpose of this article is to provide a contemporary review of CT and MR enterography in the pediatric population, including state-of-the-art techniques and clinical applications. A range of bowel abnormalities is illustrated, with an emphasis on IBD and its various abdominopelvic manifestations.

CURRENT ROLE OF CT AND MR ENTEROGRAPHY

Cross-sectional enterography is usually performed in the pediatric population to evaluate suspected or known IBD. The term IBD typically refers to 3 specific entities: Crohn disease (CD), ulcerative colitis (UC), and indeterminate colitis. CD is characterized by relapsing, remitting transmural granulomatous inflammation of the bowel wall, sometimes with discontinuous ("skip") segments of involved intestine. Inflammation may involve any portion of the gastrointestinal tract from the mouth to the anus. The inflammation of UC is generally more superficial and is typically limited to the rectum and colon, although small bowel manifestations can be noted, including "backwash ileitis."[8] The diagnosis of IBD will be made during the pediatric period in up to 30% of affected individuals.[9,10] Approximately 600,000 individuals are affected by CD in North America, with a prevalence of 5 to 16 cases per 100,000 children.[9,11] Based on recent studies, the incidence of pediatric CD appears to be increasing.[12,13] Whereas many children present with typical clinical findings of IBD, such as weight loss, gastrointestinal tract bleeding, diarrhea, and abdominal pain, some present with other nonspecific signs and symptoms that can delay diagnosis. Such nonspecific or atypical presentations can include failure to thrive, poor longitudinal growth or weight gain, unexplained anemia, arthropathy, elevated blood inflammatory markers, and a variety of skin disorders.[9,14,15]

Classically the initial diagnosis and monitoring of pediatric IBD activity and associated complications have relied on a combination of clinical assessment, optical endoscopy, and fluoroscopic imaging examinations. While CT and MR enterography in many ways provide information complementary to that of these traditional methods of assessment, these newly developed diagnostic techniques also provide additional data. The sensitivities and specificities of CT and MR enterography for detecting the presence of CD are excellent for noninvasive tests, approaching or greater than 90% in both children and adults[5,6,16–20]; based on several studies, these imaging modalities deliver increased diagnostic yield over both capsule endoscopy and SBFT examinations.[21–24] CT and MR enterography allow direct visualization of the bowel lumen, bowel wall, and adjacent soft tissues by a single test, which permits detailed assessment of disease activity and increased discovery of IBD complications such as abscesses, penetrating tracts (intra-abdominal/perianal sinus tracts and fistulas), and a variety of hepatopancreaticobiliary abnormalities.[10,25]

CT and MR enterography can also clearly depict countless other non-IBD bowel and mesenteric abnormalities in children, including:

- Other inflammatory conditions (eg, infectious enteritis and colitis, graft vs host disease [GVHD])
- Bowel (mesenteric) ischemia (including vasculitis)
- Bowel obstruction due to multiple causes
- Congenital anomalies (eg, enteric duplication cysts, Meckel diverticula)

- Benign and malignant polyps/masses
- Intestinal bleeding sources

IMAGING TECHNIQUES AND PROTOCOLS
CT Enterography

CT enterography is a first-line imaging study for evaluating pediatric patients with suspected or known CD based on American College of Radiology (ACR) appropriateness criteria,[26] particularly at the time of initial diagnosis.

Advantages of CT enterography in comparison with MR enterography include:

- Superior spatial resolution
- Less susceptibility to motion artifacts, including bowel peristalsis
- Shorter examination time
- Lesser need for sedation/general anesthesia
- Greater availability (particularly at nondedicated children's hospitals)
- Increased radiologist comfort and interpreting experience
- Lower cost
- Increased safety in patients with pacemakers/implanted MR-sensitive devices

The primary disadvantage of CT enterography in comparison with MR enterography is its use of ionizing radiation. Many pediatric IBD patients require repetitive imaging to assess disease activity and known or suspected complications.[27] When compared with adult IBD patients, children are likely more susceptible to the potentially harmful effects of ionizing radiation, owing to their longer expected life spans for adverse effects to manifest and because they have a considerably larger number of dividing cells in the body.[28,29] Recent efforts to increase awareness of the potentially harmful effects of ionizing radiation, including the possibility of radiation-induced cancers,[28–30] have decreased pediatric use of CT based on at least one recent study,[31] including CT enterography at C.S. Mott Children's Hospital. However, newly developed CT iterative image reconstruction algorithms are making possible CT examinations in adults and children at significantly reduced doses.[32–35] While it remains reasonable to limit repeated CT imaging in pediatric IBD patients and use MR enterography for follow-up imaging,[27,29,36] when possible, it is conceivable that use of CT enterography could increase in the near future, as estimated effective doses routinely approach less than 1 to 2 mSv with preserved image quality. In a recent review of pediatric IBD imaging in children, Duigenan and Gee[37] concluded that CT enterography can serve as a primary imaging modality for diagnosing suspected IBD and for differentiating CD from UC.

Low-attenuation oral contrast materials are required for CT enterography.[1,38,39] Commonly used contrast materials include low-density barium sulfate (VoLumen; Bracco Imaging, Princeton, NJ) and water, which increase the conspicuity of mucosal postcontrast hyperenhancement and distend bowel loops to improve the assessment of wall thickness. Numerous other oral contrast materials have been described for pediatric and adult CT enterography, but are less often used. CT enteroclysis is possible in children,[40] but is only very rarely performed because of the invasiveness of the procedure, which includes placement of a nasojejunal tube.

Intravenous low-osmolality iodinated contrast material is administered for CT enterography examinations, preferably using a power injector and 22-gauge or larger peripheral catheter. At the C.S. Mott Children's Hospital, 2 mL/kg of iopamidol (Isovue-370; Bracco Imaging, Princeton, NJ) is administered for routine pediatric CT enterography examinations, up to a maximum 125 mL. Single-phase enteric (about 40 seconds) or portal venous (about 60–70 seconds) phase CT enterography yields satisfactory results in both children and adults while minimizing radiation exposure.[41] Antiperistaltic agents, such as glucagon, are not necessary for CT enterography, as imaging is very rapid when using current-generation multidetector CT scanners, and motion artifacts attributable to bowel peristalsis are rarely encountered.

CT enterography images are typically acquired from the level of the diaphragm through the perianal region using submillimeter collimation to obtain an isotropic volumetric data set, thus allowing the creation of 2-dimensional (2D) multiplanar reformatted images in any plane as well as 3-dimensional (3D) reconstructions. From the source data, thicker reconstructed 2.5-5 mm axial images (often with 1.25–2.5 mm section overlap) also can be generated for primary review. The submillimeter axial source images are available for problem-solving purposes and to create additional reformations/reconstructions, as needed. Isotropic reformatted images are typically of diagnostic quality, and help identify the presence of disease as well as determine the extent.[42,43]

A multidetector CT scanner (16–64-slice or greater) with iterative image reconstruction capability is ideal for maximizing image quality while minimizing radiation dose.[44,45] At the C.S. Mott Children's Hospital where model-based iterative image reconstruction is used, tube current (mA) is established using automatic exposure control and a noise index of 40–50, while low tube potentials (kVp = 80–100) are used to lower radiation dose and increase image contrast. A recent study by Kaza and colleagues[46] demonstrated that low-kVp CT enterography imaging in smaller adult patients provides a significant dose reduction while maintaining image quality. The authors expect this observation to hold true for the pediatric population.

MR Enterography

MR enterography is also a first-line imaging study of choice for evaluating pediatric patients with CD based on ACR appropriateness criteria,[26] particularly when evaluating known disease.

Advantages of MR enterography in comparison with CT enterography include:

- Lack of ionizing radiation, which allows for:
  - Dynamic postcontrast imaging
  - Assessment of areas of luminal narrowing over an extended period of time to confirm the presence of a stricture
  - Repeat imaging if a series is of limited diagnostic quality
- Superior contrast resolution
- Availability of cine imaging techniques
- Availability of qualitative and quantitative functional techniques, such as diffusion-weighted (DW) imaging
- Lower frequency of adverse reactions of intravenous contrast material[47]

Multiple studies have validated MR enterography against CT enterography, endoscopy, and/or histology in children and adults, in some instances showing advantages for MR enterography in detecting inflammation and complications.[17,48–50] Gee and colleagues[5] concluded that "MR enterography can substitute for CT as the first-line imaging modality in pediatric patients with CD, based on its ability to detect intestinal pathologic abnormalities in both small and large bowel as well as extraintestinal disease manifestations."

Although MR enterography has several advantages over CT enterography, it has one primary disadvantage. Many younger children cannot tolerate MR enterography owing to the duration of the examination and an inability to remain motionless within the scanner. In the authors' experience, a substantial percentage of children younger than 10 years cannot undergo routine MR enterography while awake. At present, most pediatric institutions do not perform MR enterography examinations in sedated or anesthetized children. However, at C.S. Mott Children's Hospital MR enterography examinations are commonly performed in younger children using general anesthesia, and at Cincinnati Children's Hospital they are also infrequently performed using general anesthesia on a case-by-case basis. Following endotracheal tube placement and balloon inflation, oral contrast material is delivered into the stomach or proximal small bowel through a nasogastric or nasojejunal tube using a weight-based algorithm. The patient is then kept asleep for 45 to 60 minutes before imaging, to allow distal passage of contrast material in the bowel.

Multiple pediatric MR enterography protocols have been described in the literature, most of which rely on a variety of axial and coronal precontrast and postcontrast pulse sequences acquired after the administration of oral contrast material. Biphasic (T1-weighted hypointense and T2-weighted hyperintense) oral contrast agents are generally preferred, such as VoLumen and water. Similarly to CT enterography, oral contrast materials distend bowel loops, minimizing artifactual bowel-wall thickening and improving visualization of mucosal postcontrast hyperenhancement. MR enteroclysis has been described, although this technique is rarely used in children, and some studies have shown comparable results for MR enterography following a standard preparation of oral contrast material.[51,52]

Antiperistaltic medications, such as intravenous or intramuscular glucagon, can be used to reduce bowel peristalsis and improve image quality. At C.S. Mott Children's Hospital, glucagon is administered immediately before postcontrast imaging using a weight-based algorithm. When administered intravenously, glucagon should be injected slowly to minimize patient nausea and emesis. A recent study by Dillman and colleagues[53] showed that intravenous glucagon improves bowel-wall visualization in most children undergoing MR enterography, although nearly 50% experience transient nausea during or immediately after injection.

Diagnostic quality pediatric MR enterography can be performed on both 1.5-T and 3-T MR scanners. Although 3-T imaging has a few drawbacks, such as more pronounced susceptibility artifact, standing wave artifacts, and less homogeneous fat saturation, it may be preferred in children because it provides greater image signal and spatial resolution, as well as allowing for faster imaging. Dagia and colleagues[54] demonstrated the feasibility of pediatric 3-T MR enterography for the evaluation of CD. The C.S. Mott Children's Hospital routine clinical pediatric 3-T MR enterography protocol is presented in **Table 1**.

Each MR enterography pulse sequence permits evaluation of certain findings while offering particular benefits and drawbacks. Single-shot fast spin-echo (SSFSE) images provide an excellent

Table 1
Pediatric MR enterography pulse sequences and key parameters at 3 T

Sequence	Plane	Fat Saturation (Yes/No)	Flip Angle (°)	Echo Time (ms)	Repetition Time (ms)	Slice Thickness (mm)	NSA	Respiratory-Triggered vs Breath-Held
Single-shot fast spin-echo	Coronal and axial	No	90	80	Shortest	5	1	RT
T2-weighted fast spin-echo	Axial	Yes	90	80	1700	5	2	RT
Diffusion-weighted[a] (echo planar imaging, single-shot)	Axial	Yes	90	Shortest	Shortest	5	3	RT
Dynamic pre- and postcontrast T1-weighted 3D SPGR[b]	Coronal	Yes	10	Shortest	Shortest	4	1	BH
Delayed postcontrast T1-weighted 3D SPGR[b]	Coronal and axial	Yes	10	Shortest	Shortest	3–4	1	BH

"Shortest" echo time and/or repetition time set to be the shortest allowed by scanner.

Abbreviations: 3D SPGR, 3-dimensional spoiled-gradient recalled echo; BH, breath-held; NSA, number of signal averages; RT, respiratory-triggered.

[a] Diffusion-weighted imaging b-values = 0, 150, and 750 s/mm^2.
[b] T1-weighted 3D SPGR images have 50% section overlap.

anatomic overview while being resistant to motion and susceptibility artifacts. 2D balanced steady-state free precession (b-SSFP) imaging also allows for assessment of anatomy and is commonly used for cine imaging, although this sequence can be sensitive to banding and susceptibility artifacts. T2-weighted fat-saturated pulse sequences excellently depict inflammation, edema, and fluid as areas of signal hyperintensity, and areas of hyperenhancement on postcontrast imaging (0.1 mmol/kg of gadolinium-based contrast material, up to 20 mL) suggest the presence of inflammation and/or hyperemia. DW imaging, which is gaining popularity in pediatric abdominal MR imaging, assists with identifying segments of bowel affected by IBD.[55–57] This pulse sequence also aids in the detection of lymph nodes, intra-abdominal and perianal abscesses, and penetrating complications.[10,58]

SPECTRUM OF UNDERLYING PATHOLOGY AND IMAGING FINDINGS
Inflammatory Bowel Disease

MR and CT enterography both depict the inflammatory findings of IBD with a high degree of accuracy when compared with other imaging modalities as well as endoscopy and histology. In addition, cross-sectional enterography can assist in making a precise diagnosis in IBD. In the setting of indeterminate colitis (as established

by endoscopy and histology), the pattern of bowel inflammation by imaging can sometimes suggest a specific diagnosis. For example, notable small bowel inflammation in addition to proctocolitis suggests CD, as does the presence of noncontiguous "skip" segments of small and/or large bowel inflammation. Conversely, the presence of isolated contiguous proctocolitis is more suggestive of UC, although CD can have this imaging appearance. The presence of certain disease-related complications, such as fistulas, abscesses, and perianal disease, is also highly suggestive of CD.

Bowel-wall findings

The wall of noninflamed small bowel and colon segments normally appears thin and smooth at CT and MR enterography, measuring less than 3 mm in maximum thickness. On T2-weighted MR enterography images, normal bowel wall is generally of intermediate signal intensity, whereas normal bowel is not well seen or appears minimally hyperintense on DW imaging. Normal bowel wall typically mildly homogeneously enhances without a layered appearance on postcontrast CT and MR enterography.[25,59]

Bowel-wall thickening is usually present in CD and UC, and is most pronounced when inflammation is active (**Figs. 1–3**). In CD, bowel-wall thickening may be concentric or eccentric, with luminal surfaces sometimes appearing nodular or

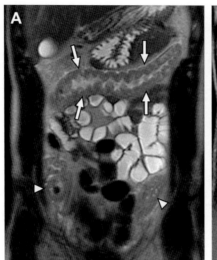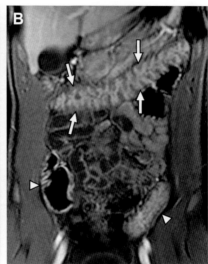

Fig. 1. A 16-year-old boy with known ulcerative colitis (UC) and worsening bloody diarrhea. (*A*) Coronal single-shot fast spin-echo (SSFSE) image demonstrates marked circumferential wall thickening and "thumb printing" involving the transverse colon (*arrows*) as well as partially visualized wall thickening of the cecum and sigmoid colon (*arrowheads*). (*B*) Coronal postcontrast T1-weighted 3-dimensional (3D) spoiled-gradient recalled echo (SPGR) fat-saturated image shows corresponding mucosal and submucosal hyperenhancement of the transverse colon (*arrows*) and cecum and sigmoid colon (*arrowheads*), consistent with active inflammation.

irregular owing to deep ulcers and pseudopolyps. Bowel-wall thickening is usually concentric in UC in the authors' experience. "Thumb printing" of the colon may be observed in severe UC inflammatory flares as a result of marked submucosal edema (see **Fig. 1**), whereas the colon can appear featureless ("lead pipe" colon) in long-standing UC. Underdistended normal bowel loops may appear falsely thickened owing to an inadequate preparation of oral contrast material, and in this setting other bowel-wall and mesenteric inflammatory findings are absent. An advantage of MR enterography is that bowel loops that are initially underdistended can be evaluated at multiple time points over the course of the examination to assess whether apparent wall thickening eventually resolves.

Bowel-wall signal characteristics are also helpful when evaluating IBD at MR enterography. For example, T2-weighted signal hyperintensity within the bowel wall suggests the presence of edema and active inflammation. Conversely, unusually low T2-weighted signal within the bowel wall may indicate the presence of fibrosis, a finding that can lead to eventual bowel obstruction.[60–62] However, the detection of bowel-wall fibrosis by MR and CT enterography remains difficult, as active inflammation and fibrosis commonly coexist.[63]

Postcontrast hyperenhancement is probably the most sensitive and specific indicator of active bowel-wall inflammation at CT and MR enterography. Findings suggestive of moderate to severe

active bowel-wall inflammation include avid postcontrast hyperenhancement or striated/stratified (target-like) appearance of the bowel wall (with the inner wall or mucosa/submucosa and the serosa hyperenhancing) (see **Figs. 1–5**).[59,64–66] It is interesting that although UC is generally considered to be a superficial process involving the inner bowel wall, in the authors' experience apparent transmural postcontrast hyperenhancement is commonly observed at CT and MR enterography. Striated appearance of the bowel wall caused by deposition of submucosal fat (which appears hypointense on fat-saturated pulse sequences) has been described in individuals with long-standing IBD but is very rarely seen in children, and has also been reported in a variety of other conditions, including in normal patients.[64,67] Impeded bowel-wall diffusion on DW imaging recently has been shown to be an imaging biomarker of bowel-wall inflammation in children and adults with CD, and may be an alternative to postcontrast imaging, particularly when gadolinium-based contrast agents are contraindicated or intravenous access cannot be obtained.[56,57,68]

CT and MR enterography also excellently depict the caliber of small bowel and colon. In CD and (much less commonly) UC, persistent inflammation with attempted healing over time can lead to deposition of fibrous tissue in the bowel wall. Bowel-wall fibrosis can cause fixed luminal narrowing with obstructive symptoms (fibrostenotic disease). In

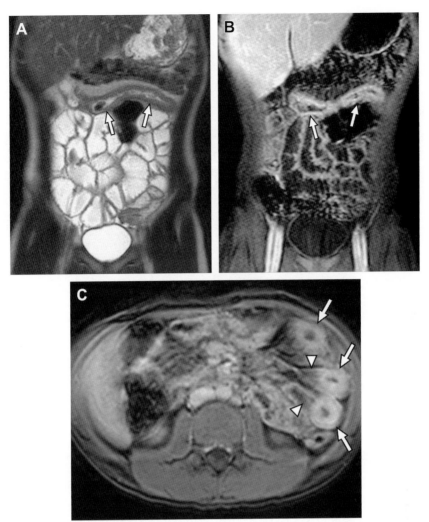

Fig. 2. An 11-year-old boy with Crohn disease (CD). (*A*) Coronal SSFSE image shows marked wall thickening of the jejunum (*arrows*) with adjacent mesenteric fibrofatty proliferation. (*B, C*) Coronal and axial postcontrast T1-weighted 3D SPGR fat-saturated images show jejunal wall thickening and hyperenhancement (*arrows*), consistent with active inflammation. Engorged mesenteric vessels are seen on the axial image (*arrowheads*).

CD, strictures can also be either purely inflammatory or contain a mixture of inflammation and fibrosis. Symptomatic strictures usually appear as areas of moderate or severe luminal narrowing (which persist over time at MR enterography) with upstream bowel dilatation (see **Fig. 3**). Postcontrast imaging and DW imaging are useful for establishing the presence of inflammation within a stricture, although superimposed fibrosis is challenging to identify. Strictures that persist after resolution of bowel-wall inflammation are likely mostly fibrotic. Recently published studies have shown that magnetization transfer MR imaging and ultrasound elasticity imaging may be able to discriminate bowel-wall fibrosis from inflammation, even when superimposed.[55,69–71] Distinguishing

inflammatory from fibrotic strictures is important, as fibrosis is often considered irreversible and requires endoscopic or surgical intervention.[72]

Mesenteric findings
Inflammatory changes in IBD frequently extend beyond the bowel to involve perienteric and pericolic soft tissues, including the small bowel and colonic mesenteries. An increased number of prominent and/or enlarged hyperenhancing typically reactive lymph nodes is often seen adjacent to inflamed bowel segments (including the rectum) in both CD and UC. Normal mesenteric lymph nodes are usually well defined, only mildly enhance, and measure less than about 5 mm in the short axis.[72]

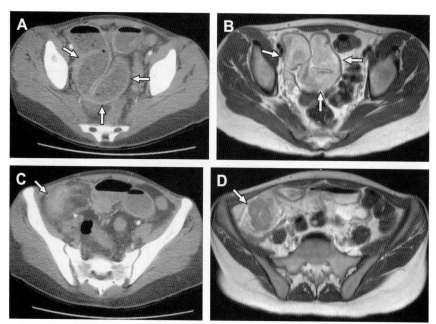

Fig. 3. A 16-year-old girl with CD and increasing abdominal pain and emesis. (*A, B*) Axial CT enterography and SSFSE MR enterography images show a dilated loop of distal ileum in the pelvis filled with fecal material (*arrows*) (small bowel feces sign). Finding is suspicious for more distal bowel obstruction. (*C, D*) Slightly more cephalad images show marked thickening and luminal narrowing of the terminal ileum (*arrow*) with adjacent mesenteric stranding, consistent with an inflammatory stricture. Note that the possibility of superimposed fibrosis in the stricture cannot be excluded by either CT or MR enterography.

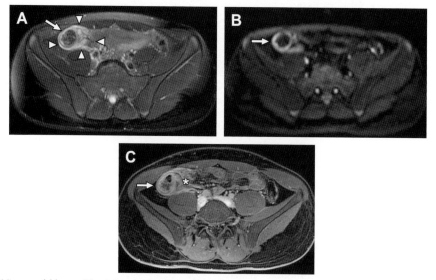

Fig. 4. An 11-year-old boy with abdominal pain and previously undiagnosed CD. (*A*) Axial T2-weighted fast spin-echo (FSE) image with fat saturation shows distal ileal circumferential bowel-wall thickening (*arrow*) with surrounding soft-tissue signal hyperintensity (*arrowheads*) attributable to a combination of mesenteric inflammation, edema, and fluid. Fecal material distending the lumen of the ileum (small bowel feces sign) is due to more distal small bowel obstruction. (*B*) Axial diffusion-weighted image demonstrates impeded (restricted) diffusion of water within the distal ileum, presumably because of inflammation (*arrow*). (*C*) Axial postcontrast T1-weighted 3D SPGR fat-saturated image shows transmural hyperenhancement of the distal ileum (*arrow*) as well as extensive enhancement of the adjacent small bowel mesentery (*asterisk*), consistent with active inflammation.

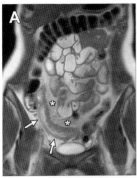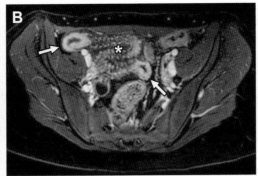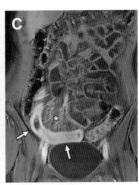

Fig. 5. A 16-year-old girl with CD and rising inflammatory markers. (*A*) Coronal SSFSE image shows circumferential wall thickening (*arrows*) of the terminal ileum. Increased fibrofatty material in the right lower quadrant small bowel mesentery (*asterisks*), so-called creeping fat, suggests long-standing terminal ileitis. (*B, C*) Axial and coronal postcontrast T1-weighted 3D SPGR fat-saturated images show transmural distal and terminal ileal wall thickening and hyperenhancement (*arrows*) as well as marked engorgement of adjacent mesenteric vessels (*asterisk*) (comb sign), consistent with active inflammation.

Increased T2-weighted signal intensity and enhancement within the mesentery and perienteric/pericolic soft tissues at MR enterography, or fat stranding at CT enterography, is commonly observed in active CD and UC, and may result from inflammation, edema, and/or fluid (see **Figs. 3 and 4**). Thin linear hyperenhancing structures located adjacent to affected bowel segments are due to engorged vasa recta vessels, sometimes referred to as the comb sign, and indicate active inflammation (see **Figs. 2 and 5**).[25,73] Over time, inflammation also can lead to deposition of fibrofatty material next to bowel segments affected by CD and UC. This finding, sometimes referred to as creeping fat, is commonly seen in the right lower quadrant adjacent to inflamed terminal ileum, and can cause separation of bowel loops at radiography (see **Figs. 2 and 5**).

Mesenteric and perienteric/pericolic areas of linear signal abnormality at MR enterography or altered attenuation at CT enterography arising from the serosal surface of the bowel wall suggest the presence of penetrating disease.[1,10] Penetrating disease is almost always due to CD and is very rarely present in UC. Penetrating tracts are considered sinuses when blind-ending and fistulas when they communicate with another epithelialized surface. Enteroenteric, enterocolic, enterocutaneous, enteroappendiceal, and perianal fistulas are regularly encountered by the authors in pediatric CD patients. Gastrocolic, enterovesicular, colovesicular, and anoscrotal fistulas are also seen, although these are less common (**Fig. 6**). Fistulas can be simple, appearing as a linear, hyperenhancing tract between 2 structures, or complex, appearing as multiple tracts (sometimes stellate in appearance) communicating between multiple

structures.[7,10] These tracts demonstrate variable signal intensity on T2-weighted MR enterography imaging, as they can contain any combination of fluid, gas, and bowel contents. The possibility of a fistula should also be investigated when a bowel loop appears to be tethered to an adjacent structure (**Fig. 7**).

Although intraperitoneal free fluid can be seen in both CD and UC, focal fluid collections are typically associated with CD. Complex yet poorly organized inflammatory fluid collections are sometimes referred to as phlegmons, whereas organized fluid collections that have a discrete wall are abscesses (**Fig. 8**).[10,74] The presence of an intra-abdominal or perianal peripherally enhancing fluid collection containing gas (nondependent foci of low signal that demonstrate susceptibility artifact at MR enterography or air attenuation at CT enterography) is highly indicative of an abscess. Phlegmons and abscesses usually arise from infected sinus tracts or fistulas.

Cutaneous findings

Cutaneous involvement by IBD almost always occurs in the setting of CD. In children, cutaneous granulomatous inflammation caused by CD may be diagnosed before bowel involvement.[75,76] Skin involvement can be contiguous with the gastrointestinal tract, or separated from the gastrointestinal tract by intervening normal skin. Although cutaneous CD can occur anywhere, it most often affects the perianal and perineal (scrotum in boys and labia in girls) regions.[14,76,77] Perianal abnormalities are common in pediatric CD, occurring in 13% to 49% of affected children.[78,79] Cutaneous CD manifestations that can

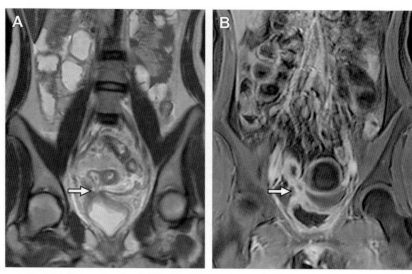

Fig. 6. A 16-year-old girl with previously undiagnosed CD and recurrent urinary tract infections. (*A*) Coronal SSFSE image demonstrates abnormal linear signal between inflamed terminal ileum and urinary bladder with associated tethering (*arrow*). The urinary bladder wall appears asymmetrically thickened. (*B*) Coronal postcontrast T1-weighted 3D SPGR fat-saturated image confirms the presence of a fistula (*arrow*). The terminal ileum and urinary bladder walls are abnormally thickened and hyperenhance because of active inflammation.

be detected by imaging include uncomplicated skin inflammation, fistulas, and abscesses.

Although CT enterography can detect cutaneous CD manifestations in some pediatric patients, MR imaging generally is more sensitive because of its inherent superior contrast resolution. Dedicated high-resolution, small field-of-view imaging is ideal for identifying and characterizing perianal and

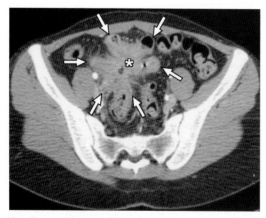

Fig. 7. An 18-year-old male patient with CD and increasing abdominal pain. Axial CT enterography image demonstrates multiple tethered, inseparable loops of small bowel and colon with associated wall thickening and abnormal postcontrast hyperenhancement (*arrows*). Abnormal bowel loops have a stellate appearance (*asterisk*), consistent with complex fistulous disease including multiple interloop fistulas.

perineal cutaneous inflammation, fistulas, and abscesses,[3,80] although standard MR enterography pulse sequences can often identify these abnormalities.[10] At MR enterography, perianal and perineal uncomplicated cutaneous granulomatous inflammation presents as skin and subcutaneous tissue thickening with associated T2-weighted signal hyperintensity and postcontrast hyperenhancement, mimicking infectious cellulitis (**Fig. 9**).[10,14,76,77] Perianal fistulas, when active, are typically hyperintense on T2-weighted imaging, may contain fluid signal, and hyperenhance on postcontrast imaging (**Fig. 10**). Low signal foci within fistulas that demonstrate "blooming" on gradient-recalled echo sequences suggest the presence of gas. Perianal fistulas arise from the anal canal, and may be transsphincteric (traversing the anal sphincter mechanism) or intersphincteric (coursing between the layers of the anal sphincter). A recent study by Horsthuis and colleagues[75] showed that dynamic contrast-enhanced MR imaging can characterize perianal CD activity in adults. Perianal abscesses arise from superinfected perianal fistulas, and appear as focal fluid collections within or adjacent to the anal sphincter mechanism that are hyperintense on T2-weighted imaging and demonstrate peripheral postcontrast hyperenhancement.[10]

Hepatopancreaticobiliary findings
Numerous abnormalities of the liver, bile ducts, and pancreas are associated with CD and UC.

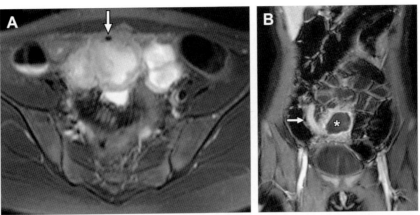

Fig. 8. A 14-year-old girl with chronic abdominal pain and previously undiagnosed CD. (*A*) Axial T2-weighted FSE fat-saturated image shows a bilobed, thick-walled fluid collection containing gas (*arrow*) in the lower abdomen. (*B*) Coronal postcontrast T1-weighted 3D SPGR fat-saturated image shows hyperenhancement of the terminal ileum with circumferential wall thickening and luminal narrowing (*arrow*), consistent with a stricture containing active inflammation. The adjacent fluid collection peripherally enhances, consistent with an abscess (*asterisk*).

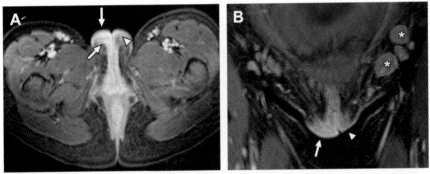

Fig. 9. An 11-year-old girl with CD and vulvar skin thickening and erythema on physical examination. (*A*) Axial postcontrast T1-weighted 3D SPGR fat-saturated image shows abnormal enhancement of the labia, greater on the right (*arrows*) than on the left (*arrowhead*). Skin biopsy confirmed extraintestinal cutaneous vulvar CD. (*B*) Coronal postcontrast image using same pulse sequence shows similar findings, including abnormal labial thickening and hyperenhancement on the right (*arrow*) and left (*arrowhead*). Enlarged left inguinal lymph nodes (*asterisks*) are likely reactive.

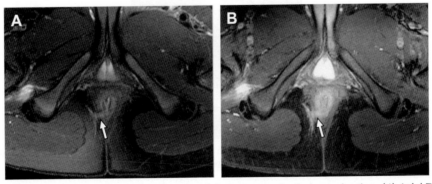

Fig. 10. A 17-year-old with history of CD and perianal drainage on physical examination. (*A*) Axial T2-weighted FSE image with fat saturation shows a linear, hyperintense tract (*arrow*) arising from the 7 o'clock position of the anal canal and extending laterally through both the internal and external sphincters, consistent with transsphincteric perianal fistula. (*B*) Axial postcontrast T1-weighted 3D SPGR fat-saturated image shows enhancement of this tract (*arrow*), likely caused by associated inflammation.

Sclerosing cholangitis, an inflammatory condition affecting the biliary tree that can lead to cirrhosis, is present in up to 5% of UC patients, with approximately 70% to 80% of patients with sclerosing cholangitis having UC.[81,82] This condition less commonly affects CD patients, although these patients are also at higher risk than the general population. Biliary dilatation at MR or CT enterography in the setting of IBD should be considered suspicious for sclerosing cholangitis and should prompt further evaluation, such as MR cholangiopancreatography (**Fig. 11**). Autoimmune cholangitis, an immunoglobulin G4 (IgG4)-mediated process, can have an appearance similar to that of sclerosing cholangitis, but is corticosteroid responsive.[82] IBD patients also are at increased risk for hepatic abscesses, owing to the spread of bacteria from the bowel or mesentery through the portal venous system to the liver.[82]

Cholelithiasis occurs with increased frequency in pediatric and adult CD patients with terminal ileitis or who are status post ileocecectomy due to disruption of normal bile salt enterohepatic circulation. Although gallstones are difficult to visualize at CT enterography unless they are calcified or contain gas, they can be readily identified at MR enterography, appearing as hypointense filling defects within the gallbladder on T2-weighted pulse sequences (**Fig. 12**).[10]

Pancreatitis can also be observed in IBD; causes include IgG4-mediated autoimmune pancreatitis and pancreatitis as a complication of medical therapy (such as azathioprine).[82,83] Acute pancreatitis can be detected by both CT and MR enterography, presenting as focal or diffuse glandular enlargement. Focal or diffuse pancreatic parenchymal signal hyperintensity with associated peripancreatic edema or fluid is noted on T2-weighted MR enterography images (**Fig. 13**). Findings suggestive of autoimmune pancreatitis at CT and MR enterography include delayed pancreatic parenchymal enhancement due to glandular

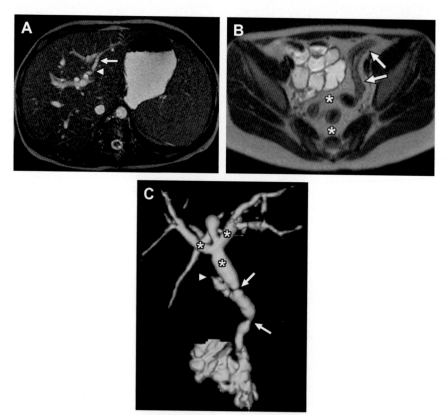

Fig. 11. A 13-year-old girl with ulcerative colitis and sclerosing cholangitis. (*A*) Axial 2-dimensional (2D) balanced steady-state free precession (b-SSFP) image demonstrates intrahepatic biliary dilation (*arrow*) and irregularity (*arrowhead*). (*B*) Axial SSFSE image through the pelvis shows rectosigmoid wall thickening (*arrows*) with adjacent fibrofatty proliferation (*asterisks*), consistent with long-standing proctocolitis. (*C*) 3D volume-rendered MR cholangiopancreatography image (follow-up examination) reveals multiple extrahepatic biliary strictures (*arrows*) and central biliary dilatation (*asterisks*), consistent with sclerosing cholangitis. The gallbladder is surgically absent (*arrowhead* indicates cystic duct stump). There is anomalous branching of intrahepatic bile ducts, with the right posterior duct draining into the central left bile duct.

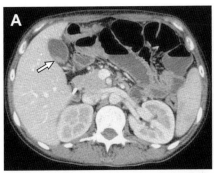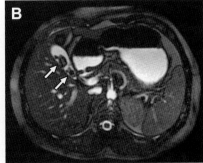

Fig. 12. An 18-year-old female patient with CD with prior ileocecectomy. (*A*) Axial CT enterography image reveals subtle focal high attenuation (*arrow*) within the gallbladder lumen caused by cholelithiasis. (*B*) Axial 2D b-SSFP image shows multiple low-signal foci (*arrows*) within the gallbladder lumen, consistent with gallstones.

fibrosis, rim-like peripheral signal abnormality or altered attenuation, and narrowing of the common bile duct in the region of the pancreatic head.[84,85]

Sacroiliitis

Both CD and UC are associated with inflammatory arthritis, particularly in patients with HLA-B27 major histocompatibility complex.[15] Peeters and colleagues[15] demonstrated that up to 27% of CD patients have radiographic evidence of sacroiliitis. At CT enterography, findings include articular erosions, subchondral sclerosis, and eventual joint fusion (ankylosis) (**Fig. 14**).[1] At MR enterography, findings include intra-articular T2-weighted signal hyperintensity because of the presence of synovitis and fluid, periarticular bone marrow edema, and postcontrast hyperenhancement. Bollow and colleagues[86] showed that contrast-enhanced MR imaging is useful for detecting sacroiliitis in children, with greater sensitivity than radiography.

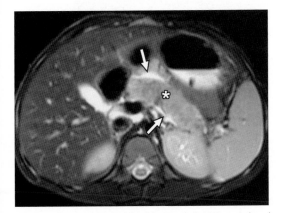

Fig. 13. A 9-year-old girl with CD. Axial T2-weighted FSE image with fat saturation shows diffuse enlargement of the pancreas (*asterisk*) with heterogeneously increased parenchymal signal intensity and peripancreatic fluid (*arrows*), consistent with acute pancreatitis.

Cross-sectional enterography beyond IBD

In the authors' experience, both CT and MR enterography have proved valuable for evaluating children with other bowel and mesenteric abnormalities, including non-IBD inflammatory conditions, ischemia, obstruction, congenital anomalies, and benign and malignant polyps and masses.

Infection

Infectious enteritis and colitis do not generally require CT or MR enterography for diagnosis in children. However, these diagnoses can sometimes be suggested based on the presence of inflammatory changes on the bowel wall, such as thickening, in the appropriate clinical setting. Cross-sectional enterography may be particularly useful for evaluating suspected or known unusual bowel infections, such as tuberculous enteritis. Numerous intra-abdominal infections, including tuberculosis and histoplasmosis, can have an appearance similar to that of CD, presenting with ileocecal bowel-wall thickening and intra-abdominal lymph node enlargement.[87]

Graft versus host disease

GVHD affects the small and large bowel of children who have undergone bone marrow transplantation, and can be an acute or chronic process. Donor T cells can attack the mucosa of the intestines, causing the bowel to appear thickened, featureless (ribbon-like), and hyperenhancing at both CT and MR enterography (**Fig. 15**).[88] Other common findings in GVHD include mesenteric stranding/edema, vasa recta engorgement, and ascites.[89]

Bowel ischemia (including vasculitis)

Ischemic bowel is rare in children and may be due to a state of low blood flow (shock), arterial or venous vascular occlusion, vascular compromise caused by bowel obstruction (eg, intussusception

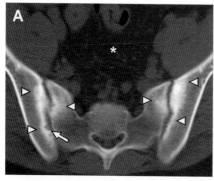
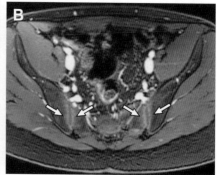

Fig. 14. (A) A 17-year-old girl with UC. Axial CT enterography image using a bone window/level setting shows subchondral sclerosis along both sacroiliac joints (*arrowheads*) with visible erosive changes on the right (*arrow*). Fibrofatty proliferation in the pelvis (*asterisk*) is related to long-standing rectosigmoid inflammation. (B) A 17-year-old boy with CD. Axial postcontrast T1-weighted 3D SPGR fat-saturated image shows symmetric enhancement along both sacroiliac joints (*arrows*), suspicious for sacroiliitis.

or volvulus), and vasculitis. Imaging findings of ischemic or infarcted bowel at CT and MR enterography include bowel-wall thickening, luminal dilatation, and postcontrast hypoenhancement.[90] The presence of pneumatosis and portal venous gas suggest severe ischemia or bowel infarction.

Henoch-Schonlein purpura (HSP) is a common vasculitis that affects the bowel of children, and is associated with abdominal pain and a characteristic rash.[91,92] Bowel-wall thickening in HSP may be due to ischemia and/or intramural hemorrhage. Small bowel intussusceptions are common in HSP, and frank bowel obstruction can occur.[93] Other vasculitides, such as Behçet disease and radiation-induced enteritis, can have a similar imaging appearance, often presenting with bowel-wall thickening (**Fig. 16**). Over time, radiation-induced enteritis can be complicated by obstructions caused by strictures and adhesions.[87]

Bowel obstruction

Both CT and MR enterography can detect the presence of bowel obstruction.[91] In the authors' experience, numerous causes of non-IBD bowel obstruction can be identified and characterized by cross-sectional enterography, including hernias, intussusceptions, malrotation with volvulus, superior mesenteric artery syndrome, intramural hemorrhage, and neoplasms (**Figs. 17** and **18**). Obstructions resulting from common inflammatory conditions, such as appendicitis, can also be readily identified. CT and MR enterography

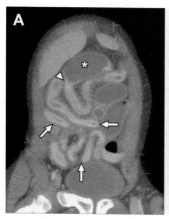
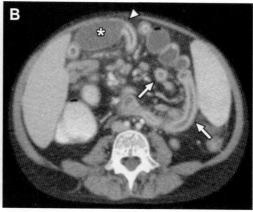

Fig. 15. A 5-year-old girl with history of acute leukemia status post bone marrow transplant complicated by severe graft versus host disease. (A) Coronal reformatted CT enterography image shows numerous loops of thickened, ribbon-like small bowel with mucosal hyperenhancement (*arrows*). A site of focal stricture (*arrowhead*) with proximal luminal dilation (*asterisk*) is noted. (B) Axial image from same study demonstrates similar appearance of the bowel (*arrows*) with a site of stricture (*arrowhead*) and upstream dilation (*asterisk*). Note that hyperattenuating contrast material in the colon was from prior small bowel follow-through examination.

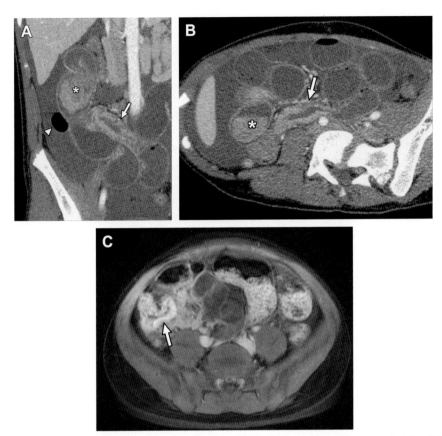

Fig. 16. (*A, B*) A 12-year-old boy with acute abdominal pain and rash caused by Henoch-Schonlein purpura. Coronal-oblique and axial-oblique reformatted CT enterography images show focally thickened, hyperenhancing distal ileum (*arrow*) that is narrowed and associated with proximal small bowel dilatation suggestive of obstruction. Intraluminal hemorrhage (*asterisk*) was present as was a focus of adjacent free air (*arrowhead*). Surgical resection of the terminal ileum confirmed the presence of vasculitis and perforation. (*C*) An 8-year-old girl with known Behçet disease with periumbilical abdominal pain and vomiting. Axial postcontrast T1-weighted 3D SPGR fat-saturated image shows wall thickening and hyperenhancement of the terminal ileum and cecum (*arrow*), consistent with active inflammation likely as a result of known vasculitis.

findings suggestive of bowel obstruction include proximally dilated fluid-filled bowel loops with de-compressed, more distal bowel loops. The exact site of bowel obstruction is often identified as an abrupt change in luminal caliber. If the point of transition appears angulated or tethered, adhesive disease should be considered.[87]

Congenital anomalies of the bowel

CT and MR enterography can detect a variety of congenital anomalies affecting the bowel, including Meckel diverticula and enteric duplication cysts. Meckel diverticula are blind-ending remnants of the omphalomesenteric duct that arise from the antimesenteric surface of the mid to distal ileum. Most are asymptomatic, although common pediatric presentations include painless bleeding in the gastrointestinal tract, diverticulitis, and obstruction (due to intussusception or internal

hernia from an omphalomesenteric band).[91,94,95] Though often difficult to prospectively detect at CT and MR enterography, the possibility of a Meckel diverticulum should be strongly entertained in children with painless bleeding in the gastrointestinal tract. Meckel diverticulitis may both clinically and radiologically mimic acute appendicitis (**Fig. 19**).[95] Bowel obstructions caused by Meckel diverticula can be easily detected, although an underlying Meckel diverticulum or omphalomesenteric band may not be discovered until surgery.

Congenital bowel duplication cysts commonly arise from the ileum or ileocecal valve, but can occur anywhere along the gastrointestinal tract. Most are diagnosed in children younger than 2 years.[96] Both CT and MR enterography can suggest the diagnosis of duplication cyst based on a lesion's relationship with the bowel wall and

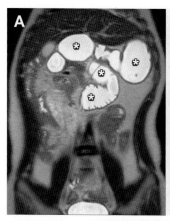
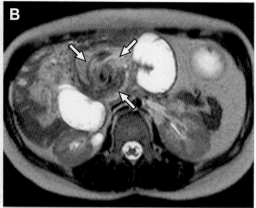

Fig. 17. An 11-year-old girl with trisomy 21 and intermittent abdominal pain of 3 weeks' duration. (*A*) Coronal SSFSE image shows fluid-filled, dilated stomach, duodenum, and very proximal jejunum (*asterisks*) with more distal decompressed small bowel loops and colon. Findings are consistent with small bowel obstruction. (*B*) Axial SSFSE image shows abnormal swirling of the superior mesenteric artery and vein (*arrows*), consistent with the diagnosis of malrotation with midgut volvulus.

cystic nature (**Fig. 20**).[97] Though commonly asymptomatic, duplication cysts can serve as a lead point for intussusception and present with obstructive symptoms.[91] Most duplication cysts do not communicate with the bowel lumen.

Bowel polyps and masses

A variety of bowel masses and polyps may be detected in children using CT and MR enterography. Some polyps, such as colonic juvenile polyps, commonly present with painless bleeding in the lower gastrointestinal tract, whereas others, such as hamartomatous polyps in Peutz-Jeghers syndrome, can present with intermittent abdominal pain attributable to intussusceptions. At MR enterography, juvenile polyps appear as 1- to 3-cm pedunculated masses within the colon that contain numerous tiny cystic spaces on SSFSE and other forms of T2-weighted imaging (**Fig. 21**). These polyps also enhance on postcontrast imaging.

Peutz-Jeghers polyps are frequently multiple and may affect the stomach, small bowel, or colon. In the authors' experience, these polyps are usually best appreciated by MR enterography on SSFSE

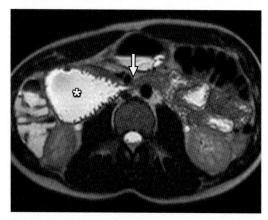

Fig. 18. A 19-year-old male patient with recurrent abdominal pain, nausea, and emesis. Axial SSFSE image shows marked dilatation of the duodenum (*asterisk*) to the level of the aortomesenteric interval (*arrow*), with the duodenum narrowed and likely partially obstructed as it passes between the superior mesenteric artery and abdominal aorta. Given the clinical history, findings are suspicious for superior mesenteric artery syndrome.

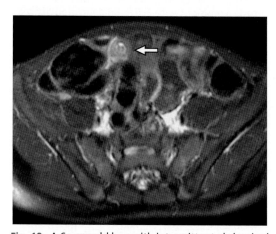

Fig. 19. A 6-year-old boy with intermittent abdominal pain and hematochezia. Axial T2-weighted FSE image with fat saturation shows an apparent focally thickened bowel loop (*arrow*) in the anterior right lower quadrant with intramural edema and adjacent inflammatory changes. Surgery and histopathology confirmed the diagnosis of Meckel diverticulum.

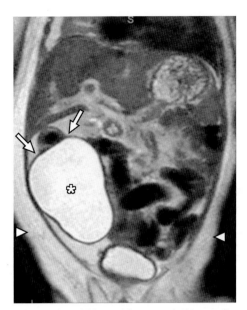

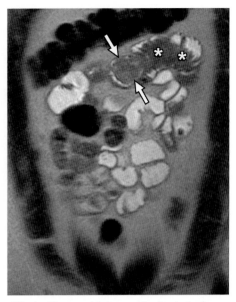

Fig. 20. A 9-day-old boy with congenital heart disease and cystic intra-abdominal mass at ultrasonography. Coronal SSFSE image shows a large homogeneously hyperintense cystic lesion (*asterisk*) in the right hemi-abdomen measuring 4 × 4 × 6 cm, inseparable from the ascending colon (*arrows*), surgically confirmed to represent a colonic duplication cyst. Diffuse body-wall thickening (*arrowheads*) is due to subcutaneous edema related to the patient's heart condition.

Fig. 22. A 13-year-old boy with Peutz-Jeghers syndrome and sudden abdominal pain. Coronal SSFSE image shows a 3-cm filling defect (*arrows*) in the proximal jejunum caused by a polyp. The patient's abdominal pain is due to an associated jejunojejunal intussusception (*asterisks*).

and b-SSFP pulse sequences as hypointense filling defects within the bowel lumen. These lesions also generally hyperenhance and may restrict diffusion. Small bowel intussusceptions are commonly noted in association with these polyps (**Fig. 22**). Gupta and colleagues[98] showed that MR enterography can be used successfully to perform polyp surveillance in patients with

Peutz-Jeghers syndrome. An excellent preparation of oral contrast material is essential to optimize polyp detection.

CT and MR enterography can also be used to diagnose suspected and unsuspected bowel neoplasms in the setting of abdominal pain and gastrointestinal bleeding. At CT and MR enterography, adenocarcinomas of the small and large bowel typically present as either eccentric or concentric bowel-wall thickening with abrupt margins ("shouldering") and associated postcontrast

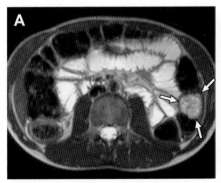

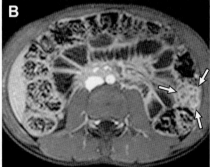

Fig. 21. A 9-year-old boy with hematochezia caused by colonic juvenile polyp. (*A*) Axial SSFSE image through the midabdomen shows a predominantly hyperintense 2.5-cm mass in the descending colon (*arrows*). Numerous tiny cystic spaces are present within the mass. (*B*) Axial postcontrast T1-weighted 3D SPGR fat-saturated image shows that the mass (*arrows*) heterogeneously enhances. The mass is difficult to distinguish from adjacent fecal material on this pulse sequence.

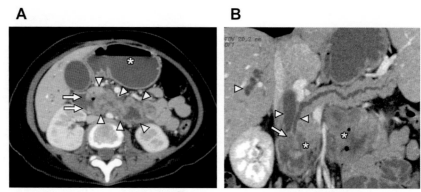

A **B**

Fig. 23. A 16-year-old girl with Lynch syndrome, abdominal pain, and weight loss. (*A*) Axial CT enterography image shows a large, nodular, ulcerating enhancing soft-tissue mass involving the transverse duodenum (*arrowheads*) with abrupt margins proximally (*arrows*). The stomach is distended with an air-fluid level (*asterisk*) because of partial obstruction. (*B*) Coronal-oblique reformatted image confirms that the mass (*asterisks*) is causing obstruction of the ampulla of Vater (*arrow*), with resulting double-duct sign (dilation of the main pancreatic duct and intra-/extrahepatic bile ducts [*arrowheads*]).

enhancement (**Figs. 23** and **24**). Large masses may contain areas of ulceration or necrosis, and adjacent mesenteric or omental fat stranding is suggestive of extramural spread of tumor. When a bowel mass is identified, images should be reviewed for local extension as well as lymphatic and hematogenous metastases.

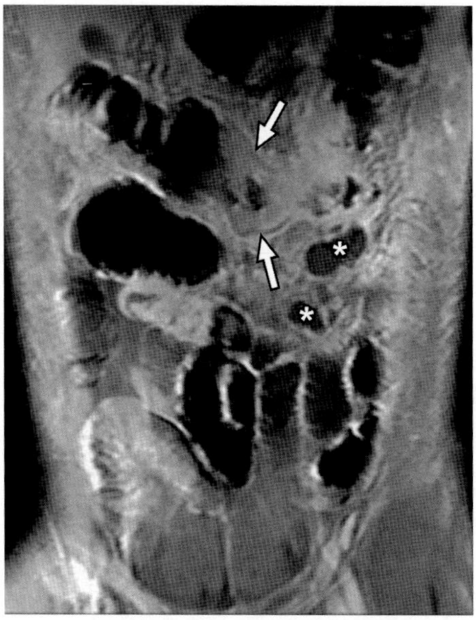

SUMMARY

Computed tomography and MR imaging have transformed imaging of the pediatric abdomen over the past decade, including assessment of the bowel. CT enterography can be now performed in just a few seconds with a radiation dose similar to or less than that used for SBFT examinations. MR enterography allows for high-quality images of the bowel while adhering to "as low as reasonably achievable" and "image gently" principles. Today cross-sectional enterographic examinations are the first-line diagnostic tests for the noninvasive assessment of IBD as well as many other conditions affecting the bowel and mesentery, and they are having a substantial impact on the care of pediatric patients, influencing both medical and surgical management. Using essentially any modern CT or MR imaging scanner, protocols for imaging of the bowel that generate high-quality diagnostic examinations in pediatric patients of all ages can be easily created.

Fig. 24. A 17-year-old boy with abdominal pain and fever of 4 days' duration caused by perforated adenocarcinoma of the colon. Coronal postcontrast T1-weighted 3D SPGR fat-saturated image shows an enhancing annular mass (*arrows*) affecting the transverse colon with well-demarcated "shoulders." Peripherally enhancing fluid collections (*asterisks*) within the greater omentum are due to abscesses from tumor rupture.

REFERENCES

1. Dillman JR, Adler J, Zimmermann EM, et al. CT enterography of pediatric Crohn disease. Pediatr Radiol 2010;40(1):97–105.
2. Gaca AM, Jaffe TA, Delaney S, et al. Radiation doses from small-bowel follow-through and abdomen/pelvis MDCT in pediatric Crohn disease. Pediatr Radiol 2008;38(3):285–91.

3. Darge K, Anupindi SA, Jaramillo D. MR imaging of the abdomen and pelvis in infants, children, and adolescents. Radiology 2011;261(1):12–29.

4. Absah I, Bruining DH, Matsumoto JM, et al. MR enterography in pediatric inflammatory bowel disease: retrospective assessment of patient tolerance, image quality, and initial performance estimates. AJR Am J Roentgenol 2012;199(3): W367–75.

5. Gee MS, Nimkin K, Hsu M, et al. Prospective evaluation of MR enterography as the primary imaging modality for pediatric Crohn disease assessment. AJR Am J Roentgenol 2011;197(1):224–31.

6. Wallihan DB, Towbin AJ, Denson LA, et al. Inflammatory bowel disease in children and adolescents: assessing the diagnostic performance and interreader agreement of magnetic resonance enterography compared to histopathology. Acad Radiol 2012;19(7):819–26.

7. Toma P, Granata C, Magnano G, et al. CT and MRI of paediatric Crohn disease. Pediatr Radiol 2007; 37(11):1083–92.

8. Rubenstein J, Sherif A, Appelman H, et al. Ulcerative colitis associated enteritis: is ulcerative colitis always confined to the colon? J Clin Gastroenterol 2004;38(1):46–51.

9. Diefenbach KA, Breuer CK. Pediatric inflammatory bowel disease. World J Gastroenterol 2006;12(20): 3204–12.

10. Smith EA, Dillman JR, Adler J, et al. MR enterography of extraluminal manifestations of inflammatory bowel disease in children and adolescents: moving beyond the bowel wall. AJR Am J Roentgenol 2012;198(1):W38–45.

11. Hyams JS. Crohn's disease in children. Pediatr Clin North Am 1996;43(1):255–77.

12. Heyman MB, Kirschner BS, Gold BD, et al. Children with early-onset inflammatory bowel disease (IBD): analysis of a pediatric IBD consortium registry. J Pediatr 2005;146(1):35–40.

13. Malaty HM, Fan X, Opekun AR, et al. Rising incidence of inflammatory bowel disease among children: a 12-year study. J Pediatr Gastroenterol Nutr 2010;50(1):27–31.

14. Pinna AL, Atzori L, Ferreli C, et al. Cutaneous Crohn disease in a child. Pediatr Dermatol 2006; 23(1):49–52.

15. Peeters H, Vander Cruyssen B, Mielants H, et al. Clinical and genetic factors associated with sacroiliitis in Crohn's disease. J Gastroenterol Hepatol 2008;23(1):132–7.

16. Dillman JR, Ladino-Torres MF, Adler J, et al. Comparison of MR enterography and histopathology in the evaluation of pediatric Crohn disease. Pediatr Radiol 2011;41(12):1552–8.

17. Siddiki HA, Fidler JL, Fletcher JG, et al. Prospective comparison of state-of-the-art MR enterography and CT enterography in small-bowel Crohn's disease. AJR Am J Roentgenol 2009; 193(1):113–21.

18. Borthne AS, Abdelnoor M, Rugtveit J, et al. Bowel magnetic resonance imaging of pediatric patients with oral mannitol MRI compared to endoscopy and intestinal ultrasound. Eur Radiol 2006;16(1): 207–14.

19. Horsthuis K, de Ridder L, Smets AM, et al. Magnetic resonance enterography for suspected inflammatory bowel disease in a pediatric population. J Pediatr Gastroenterol Nutr 2010; 51(5):603–9.

20. Casciani E, Masselli G, Di Nardo G, et al. MR enterography versus capsule endoscopy in paediatric patients with suspected Crohn's disease. Eur Radiol 2011;21(4):823–31.

21. Hara AK, Leighton JA, Heigh RI, et al. Crohn disease of the small bowel: preliminary comparison among CT enterography, capsule endoscopy, small-bowel follow-through, and ileoscopy. Radiology 2006;238(1):128–34.

22. Hara AK, Swartz PG. CT enterography of Crohn's disease. Abdom Imaging 2009;34(3):289–95.

23. Jamieson DH, Shipman PJ, Israel DM, et al. Comparison of multidetector CT and barium studies of the small bowel: inflammatory bowel disease in children. AJR Am J Roentgenol 2003;180(5): 1211–6.

24. Wold PB, Fletcher JG, Johnson CD, et al. Assessment of small bowel Crohn disease: noninvasive peroral CT enterography compared with other imaging methods and endoscopy—feasibility study. Radiology 2003;229(1):275–81.

25. Chalian M, Ozturk A, Oliva-Hemker M, et al. MR enterography findings of inflammatory bowel disease in pediatric patients. AJR Am J Roentgenol 2011; 196(6):W810–6.

26. Huprich JE, Rosen MP, Fidler JL, et al. ACR Appropriateness Criteria on Crohn's disease. J Am Coll Radiol 2010;7(2):94–102.

27. Sauer CG, Kugathasan S, Martin DR, et al. Medical radiation exposure in children with inflammatory bowel disease estimates high cumulative doses. Inflamm Bowel Dis 2011;17(11):2326–32.

28. Brenner DJ, Hall EJ. Computed tomography—an increasing source of radiation exposure. N Engl J Med 2007;357(22):2277–84.

29. Brenner DJ. Should computed tomography be the modality of choice for imaging Crohn's disease in children? The radiation risk perspective. Gut 2008;57(11):1489–90.

30. Goske MJ, Applegate KE, Boylan J, et al. The 'Image Gently' campaign: increasing CT radiation dose awareness through a national education and awareness program. Pediatr Radiol 2008;38(3): 265–9.

31. Townsend BA, Callahan MJ, Zurakowski D, et al. Has pediatric CT at children's hospitals reached its peak? AJR Am J Roentgenol 2010;194(5):1194–6.

32. Lee SH, Kim MJ, Yoon CS, et al. Radiation dose reduction with the adaptive statistical iterative reconstruction (ASIR) technique for chest CT in children: an intra-individual comparison. Eur J Radiol 2012;81(9):e938–43.

33. Mieville FA, Berteloot L, Grandjean A, et al. Model-based iterative reconstruction in pediatric chest CT: assessment of image quality in a prospective study of children with cystic fibrosis. Pediatr Radiol 2013;43(5):558–67.

34. Singh S, Kalra MK, Hsieh J, et al. Abdominal CT: comparison of adaptive statistical iterative and filtered back projection reconstruction techniques. Radiology 2010;257(2):373–83.

35. Singh S, Kalra MK, Shenoy-Bhangle AS, et al. Radiation dose reduction with hybrid iterative reconstruction for pediatric CT. Radiology 2012;263(2):537–46.

36. Guimaraes LS, Fidler JL, Fletcher JG, et al. Assessment of appropriateness of indications for CT enterography in younger patients. Inflamm Bowel Dis 2010;16(2):226–32.

37. Duigenan S, Gee MS. Imaging of pediatric patients with inflammatory bowel disease. AJR Am J Roentgenol 2012;199(4):907–15.

38. Applegate KE, Maglinte DD. Imaging of the bowel in children: new imaging techniques. Pediatr Radiol 2008;38(Suppl 2):S272–4.

39. Elsayes KM, Al-Hawary MM, Jagdish J, et al. CT enterography: principles, trends, and interpretation of findings. Radiographics 2010;30(7):1955–70.

40. Brown S, Applegate KE, Sandrasegaran K, et al. Fluoroscopic and CT enteroclysis in children: initial experience, technical feasibility, and utility. Pediatr Radiol 2008;38(5):497–510.

41. Vandenbroucke F, Mortele KJ, Tatli S, et al. Noninvasive multidetector computed tomography enterography in patients with small-bowel Crohn's disease: is a 40-second delay better than 70 seconds? Acta Radiol 2007;48(10):1052–60.

42. Sandrasegaran K, Rydberg J, Akisik F, et al. Isotropic CT examination of abdomen and pelvis diagnostic quality of reformat. Acad Radiol 2006; 13(11):1338–43.

43. Raptopoulos V, Schwartz RK, McNicholas MM, et al. Multiplanar helical CT enterography in patients with Crohn's disease. AJR Am J Roentgenol 1997;169(6):1545–50.

44. Lee SJ, Park SH, Kim AY, et al. A prospective comparison of standard-dose CT enterography and 50% reduced-dose CT enterography with and without noise reduction for evaluating Crohn disease. AJR Am J Roentgenol 2011;197(1):50–7.

45. Kambadakone AR, Chaudhary NA, Desai GS, et al. Low-dose MDCT and CT enterography of patients with Crohn disease: feasibility of adaptive statistical iterative reconstruction. AJR Am J Roentgenol 2011;196(6):W743–52.

46. Kaza RK, Platt JF, Al-Hawary MM, et al. CT enterography at 80 kVp with adaptive statistical iterative reconstruction versus at 120 kVp with standard reconstruction: image quality, diagnostic adequacy, and dose reduction. AJR Am J Roentgenol 2012;198(5):1084–92.

47. Dillman JR, Ellis JH, Cohan RH, et al. Frequency and severity of acute allergic-like reactions to gadolinium-containing i.v. contrast media in children and adults. AJR Am J Roentgenol 2007; 189(6):1533–8.

48. Lee SS, Kim AY, Yang SK, et al. Crohn disease of the small bowel: comparison of CT enterography, MR enterography, and small-bowel follow-through as diagnostic techniques. Radiology 2009;251(3):751–61.

49. Low RN, Francis IR, Politoske D, et al. Crohn's disease evaluation: comparison of contrast-enhanced MR imaging and single-phase helical CT scanning. J Magn Reson Imaging 2000;11(2):127–35.

50. Fiorino G, Bonifacio C, Peyrin-Biroulet L, et al. Prospective comparison of computed tomography enterography and magnetic resonance enterography for assessment of disease activity and complications in ileocolonic Crohn's disease. Inflamm Bowel Dis 2011;17(5):1073–80.

51. Negaard A, Paulsen V, Sandvik L, et al. A prospective randomized comparison between two MRI studies of the small bowel in Crohn's disease, the oral contrast method and MR enteroclysis. Eur Radiol 2007;17(9):2294–301.

52. Schreyer AG, Geissler A, Albrich H, et al. Abdominal MRI after enteroclysis or with oral contrast in patients with suspected or proven Crohn's disease. Clin Gastroenterol Hepatol 2004;2(6):491–7.

53. Dillman JR, Smith EA, Khalatbari S, et al. Intravenous glucagon use in pediatric MR enterography: effect on image quality, length of examination, and patient tolerance. AJR Am J Roentgenol, in press.

54. Dagia C, Ditchfield M, Kean M, et al. Feasibility of 3-T MRI for the evaluation of Crohn disease in children. Pediatr Radiol 2010;40(10):1615–24.

55. Al-Hawary M, Zimmermann EM. A new look at Crohn's disease: novel imaging techniques. Curr Opin Gastroenterol 2012;28(4):334–40.

56. Oto A, Zhu F, Kulkarni K, et al. Evaluation of diffusion-weighted MR imaging for detection of bowel inflammation in patients with Crohn's disease. Acad Radiol 2009;16(5):597–603.

57. Oto A, Kayhan A, Williams JT, et al. Active Crohn's disease in the small bowel: evaluation by diffusion weighted imaging and quantitative dynamic contrast enhanced MR imaging. J Magn Reson Imaging 2011;33(3):615–24.

58. Oto A, Schmid-Tannwald C, Agrawal G, et al. Diffusion-weighted MR imaging of abdominopelvic abscesses. Emerg Radiol 2011;18(6):515–24.

59. Leyendecker JR, Bloomfeld RS, DiSantis DJ, et al. MR enterography in the management of patients with Crohn disease. Radiographics 2009;29(6): 1827–46.

60. Maccioni F, Viscido A, Broglia L, et al. Evaluation of Crohn disease activity with magnetic resonance imaging. Abdom Imaging 2000;25(3):219–28.

61. Maccioni F, Bruni A, Viscido A, et al. MR imaging in patients with Crohn disease: value of T2- versus T1-weighted gadolinium-enhanced MR sequences with use of an oral superparamagnetic contrast agent. Radiology 2006;238(2):517–30.

62. Maccioni F, Staltari I, Pino AR, et al. Value of T2-weighted magnetic resonance imaging in the assessment of wall inflammation and fibrosis in Crohn's disease. Abdom Imaging 2012;37(6):944–57.

63. Adler J, Punglia DR, Dillman JR, et al. Computed tomography enterography findings correlate with tissue inflammation, not fibrosis in resected small bowel Crohn's disease. Inflamm Bowel Dis 2012; 18(5):849–56.

64. Fidler JL, Guimaraes L, Einstein DM. MR imaging of the small bowel. Radiographics 2009;29(6): 1811–25.

65. Fidler J. MR imaging of the small bowel. Radiol Clin North Am 2007;45(2):317–31.

66. Del Vescovo R, Sansoni I, Caviglia R, et al. Dynamic contrast enhanced magnetic resonance imaging of the terminal ileum: differentiation of activity of Crohn's disease. Abdom Imaging 2008;33(4): 417–24.

67. Harisinghani MG, Wittenberg J, Lee W, et al. Bowel wall fat halo sign in patients without intestinal disease. AJR Am J Roentgenol 2003;181(3):781–4.

68. Neubauer H, Pabst T, Dick A, et al. Small-bowel MRI in children and young adults with Crohn disease: retrospective head-to-head comparison of contrast-enhanced and diffusion-weighted MRI. Pediatr Radiol 2013;43(1):103–14.

69. Adler J, Swanson SD, Schmiedlin-Ren P, et al. Magnetization transfer helps detect intestinal fibrosis in an animal model of Crohn disease. Radiology 2011;259(1):127–35.

70. Dillman JR, Stidham RW, Higgins PD, et al. Elastography-derived shear wave velocity helps distinguish acutely inflamed from fibrotic bowel in a crohn disease animal model. Radiology 2013. [Epub ahead of print].

71. Stidham RW, Xu J, Johnson LA, et al. Ultrasound elasticity imaging for detecting intestinal fibrosis and inflammation in rats and humans with Crohn's disease. Gastroenterology 2011;141(3):819–826.e1.

72. Lawrance IC, Welman CJ, Shipman P, et al. Correlation of MRI-determined small bowel Crohn's disease categories with medical response and surgical pathology. World J Gastroenterol 2009; 15(27):3367–75.

73. Lee SS, Ha HK, Yang SK, et al. CT of prominent pericolic or perienteric vasculature in patients with Crohn's disease: correlation with clinical disease activity and findings on barium studies. AJR Am J Roentgenol 2002;179(4):1029–36.

74. Yamaguchi A, Matsui T, Sakurai T, et al. The clinical characteristics and outcome of intraabdominal abscess in Crohn's disease. J Gastroenterol 2004; 39(5):441–8.

75. Horsthuis K, Lavini C, Bipat S, et al. Perianal Crohn disease: evaluation of dynamic contrast-enhanced MR imaging as an indicator of disease activity. Radiology 2009;251(2):380–7.

76. Pai D, Dillman JR, Mahani MG, et al. MRI of vulvar Crohn disease. Pediatr Radiol 2011;41(4):537–41.

77. Corbett SL, Walsh CM, Spitzer RF, et al. Vulvar inflammation as the only clinical manifestation of Crohn disease in an 8-year-old girl. Pediatrics 2010;125(6):e1518–22.

78. Markowitz J, Daum F, Aiges H, et al. Perianal disease in children and adolescents with Crohn's disease. Gastroenterology 1984;86(5 Pt 1):829–33.

79. Tolia V. Perianal Crohn's disease in children and adolescents. Am J Gastroenterol 1996;91(5):922–6.

80. O'Malley RB, Al-Hawary MM, Kaza RK, et al. Rectal imaging: part 2, perianal fistula evaluation on pelvic MRI—what the radiologist needs to know. AJR Am J Roentgenol 2012;199(1):W43–53.

81. Bernstein CN, Blanchard JF, Rawsthorne P, et al. The prevalence of extraintestinal diseases in inflammatory bowel disease: a population-based study. Am J Gastroenterol 2001;96(4):1116–22.

82. Navaneethan U, Shen B. Hepatopancreatobiliary manifestations and complications associated with inflammatory bowel disease. Inflamm Bowel Dis 2010;16(9):1598–619.

83. Riello L, Talbotec C, Garnier-Lengline H, et al. Tolerance and efficacy of azathioprine in pediatric Crohn's disease. Inflamm Bowel Dis 2011;17(10): 2138–43.

84. Vlachou PA, Khalili K, Jang HJ, et al. IgG4-related sclerosing disease: autoimmune pancreatitis and extrapancreatic manifestations. Radiographics 2011;31(5):1379–402.

85. Ravi K, Chari ST, Vege SS, et al. Inflammatory bowel disease in the setting of autoimmune pancreatitis. Inflamm Bowel Dis 2009;15(9):1326–30.

86. Bollow M, Braun J, Biedermann T, et al. Use of contrast-enhanced MR imaging to detect sacroiliitis in children. Skeletal Radiol 1998;27(11):606–16.

87. Amzallag-Bellenger E, Oudjit A, Ruiz A, et al. Effectiveness of MR enterography for the assessment of small-bowel diseases beyond Crohn disease. Radiographics 2012;32(5):1423–44.

88. Mentzel HJ, Kentouche K, Kosmehl H, et al. US and MRI of gastrointestinal graft-versus-host disease. Pediatr Radiol 2002;32(3):195–8.

89. Kalantari BN, Mortele KJ, Cantisani V, et al. CT features with pathologic correlation of acute gastrointestinal graft-versus-host disease after bone marrow transplantation in adults. AJR Am J Roentgenol 2003;181(6):1621–5.

90. Aidlen J, Anupindi SA, Jaramillo D, et al. Malrotation with midgut volvulus: CT findings of bowel infarction. Pediatr Radiol 2005;35(5):529–31.

91. Hryhorczuk AL, Lee EY. Imaging evaluation of bowel obstruction in children: updates in imaging techniques and review of imaging findings. Semin Roentgenol 2012;47(2):159–70.

92. Mills JA, Michel BA, Bloch DA, et al. The American College of Rheumatology 1990 criteria for the classification of Henoch-Schonlein purpura. Arthritis Rheum 1990;33(8):1114–21.

93. Chang WL, Yang YH, Lin YT, et al. Gastrointestinal manifestations in Henoch-Schonlein purpura: a review of 261 patients. Acta Paediatr 2004;93(11):1427–31.

94. Park JJ, Wolff BG, Tollefson MK, et al. Meckel diverticulum: the Mayo Clinic experience with 1476 patients (1950-2002). Ann Surg 2005;241(3):529–33.

95. Hegde S, Dillman JR, Gadepalli S, et al. MR enterography of perforated acute Meckel diverticulitis. Pediatr Radiol 2012;42(2):257–62.

96. Ildstad ST, Tollerud DJ, Weiss RG, et al. Duplications of the alimentary tract. Clinical characteristics, preferred treatment, and associated malformations. Ann Surg 1988;208(2):184–9.

97. Dillman JR, Neef HC, Ehrlich PF, et al. Ileal dysgenesis coexisting with multiple enteric duplication cysts in a child-MR enterography, CT, and Meckel scan appearances. Pediatr Radiol 2012;42(12):1517–22.

98. Gupta A, Postgate AJ, Burling D, et al. A prospective study of MR enterography versus capsule endoscopy for the surveillance of adult patients with Peutz-Jeghers syndrome. AJR Am J Roentgenol 2010;195(1):108–16.

Primary Lung and Large Airway Neoplasms in Children
Current Imaging Evaluation with Multidetector Computed Tomography

Behrang Amini, MD, PhD[a], Steven Y. Huang, MD[a],
Jason Tsai, MD[b], Marcelo F. Benveniste, MD[a],
Hector H. Robledo, MD[c], Edward Y. Lee, MD, MPH[d,e],*

KEYWORDS

- Multidetector computed tomography (MDCT) • Primary lung neoplasm • Primary airway neoplasm
- Radiation dose • Pediatric patients

KEY POINTS

- The relative rarity of primary neoplasms of the lung and large airway may lead to a low index of suspicion for these lesions, with subsequent delay in achieving a correct diagnosis and initiating effective treatment.
- In the case of malignant neoplasms, this delay can adversely affect prognosis by allowing progression of disease to an advanced stage.
- Multidetector computed tomography (MDCT), with its improved efficiency and diagnostic capability compared with single-detector computed tomography, offers an important noninvasive imaging modality for confirmation and further characterization of these lesions in pediatric patients.
- Clear understanding of the proper MDCT techniques and the MDCT imaging appearance of primary lung and airway neoplasms aids in accurate diagnosis and thus contributes to optimal pediatric patient care.

INTRODUCTION

Primary malignant neoplasms of the lung and large airway represent 0.2% of all malignancies in the pediatric population.[1] Such low incidence often results in a low index of suspicion for these lesions, and the correct diagnosis is often missed or delayed. Early and accurate diagnosis is particularly important in cases of malignant tumors involving the lung and large airway, because a missed or delayed diagnosis can lead to progression to advanced stages before effective treatment is initiated, adversely affecting prognosis. Benign neoplasms of the lung and large airway must also be kept in mind as mimics of more aggressive processes. Familiarity with both, therefore, is important in the effective workup and optimal management of a child who presents with a primary lung or airway neoplasm on imaging evaluation.

Financial Disclosure and Conflict of Interest Obligations: None.
[a] Department of Diagnostic Radiology, The University of Texas MD Anderson Cancer Center, 1515 Holcombe Blvd, Houston, TX 77030, USA; [b] Division of Diagnostic Imaging and Radiology, Children's National Medical Center, 111 Michigan Avenue NW, Washington, DC 20010, USA; [c] Department of Radiology, Córdoba Children's Hospital, Bajada Pucara 1900, Córdoba, CP 5000, Argentina; [d] Division of Thoracic Imaging, Department of Radiology, Boston Children's Hospital, Harvard Medical School, 300 Longwood Avenue, Boston, MA 02115, USA; [e] Magnetic Resonance Imaging, Boston Children's Hospital, Harvard Medical School, 300 Longwood Avenue, Boston, MA 02115, USA
* Corresponding author. Division of Thoracic Imaging, Department of Radiology, Boston Children's Hospital, Harvard Medical School, 300 Longwood Avenue, Boston, MA 02115.
E-mail address: Edward.Lee@childrens.harvard.edu

Computed tomography (CT) has been an important noninvasive imaging modality for confirmation and further characterization of primary lung and large airway neoplasms after radiographic assessment. In recent years, rapid advances in multidetector CT (MDCT) technology have further enhanced the diagnostic capability of CT for evaluating primary lung and large airway neoplasms encountered in pediatric patients. MDCT offers the combination of faster acquisition times, increased anatomic coverage, and decreased need for sedation, which is particularly beneficial in pediatric patients. In addition, superb-quality two-dimensional (2D) multiplanar and three-dimensional (3D) CT images generated from MDCT axial data sets have been shown to increase the diagnostic capability in evaluating large airway anomalies and abnormalities in the pediatric population.[2–5]

The overarching goal of this article is to review an imaging algorithm, up-to-date imaging techniques, and clinical applications of MDCT for evaluating benign and malignant primary neoplasms of lung and large airway in infants and children.

IMAGING ALGORITHM

The first step in imaging pediatric patients using CT, which is associated with potentially harmful ionizing radiation, is a careful assessment of the benefits of the imaging study balanced against the risks from radiation, and consideration of alternative imaging modalities. Beside CT, the 2 most commonly used alternative imaging modalities after initial radiographic evaluation are ultrasonography (US) and magnetic resonance (MR) imaging in the pediatric population. Although US can help differentiate a large pleural effusion from a mass occupying the entire hemithorax, and can characterize cystic components within a mass, it is markedly limited in assessing the airway, thoracic lymph nodes, and invasion of vital structures, the last 2 of which are essential for staging and operative planning.[6] MR imaging, although helpful for characterizing vascular anomalies of the thorax in pediatric patients, is not commonly used for assessment of airway and pulmonary parenchymal lesions.[7] Therefore, MDCT is considered the imaging modality of choice for confirmation and characterization of suspected or known large airway and lung neoplasms after initial chest radiographic assessment. After the decision is made to use CT, the overarching goal must be to obtain an examination with sufficient diagnostic quality needed for answering the specific clinical question using the lowest possible radiation dose, closely following the ALARA (as low as reasonably achievable) principle, as discussed in the next section.

IMAGING TECHNIQUES
Patient Preparation

In MDCT evaluation of the lung and airway of children, patient factors such as inability to follow instructions and motion can lead to a suboptimal or nondiagnostic study. Although MDCT has reduced the need for sedation,[8] it is still usually required for children younger than 5 years and those unable to stay still.[5] Conscious sedation is a safe and effective alternative to general anesthesia in suitable pediatric patients. It allows infants and young children to maintain a patent airway and respond appropriately to physical stimulation or verbal commands.[2]

MDCT Parameters

MDCT parameters should be optimized according to the ALARA principle, keeping radiation exposure as low as reasonably achievable. This goal can be typically achieved by varying tube current (mA) and kilovoltage peak (kVp) according to patient age or weight.[9] The recommended weight-based MDCT parameters are shown in **Table 1**. Detailed MDCT protocols can be found in the article titled "Managing Radiation Dose from Thoracic MDCT in Pediatric Patients: Background, Current Issues, and Recommendations" by MacDougall and colleagues elsewhere in this issue.

Other essential MDCT imaging parameters include fast table speeds (with scan times <1 second) and thin detector collimation, both of which vary based on the type of MDCT scanner used.[5] For obtaining high-quality multiplanar 2D or 3D reformations, a 1-mm to 2-mm reconstruction interval with approximately 50% overlap is ideal.[9] However, when very thin collimation (0.5–1.0 mm) is used, an isotropic data set is achieved, and spatial resolution is the same regardless of whether images are reviewed in the transverse, sagittal, or coronal plane, without the need for overlapping reconstruction intervals.[10]

Table 1		
Pediatric MDCT parameters by patient weight		
Weight (kg)	**Tube Current (mA)**	**Kilovoltage (kVp)**
<10	40	80
10–14	50	80
15–24	60	80
25–34	70	80
35–44	80	80
45–54	90	90
55–70	100–120	100–120

For evaluation of lung and large airway, intravenous contrast may not be necessary. However, for assessing lymphadenopathy and involvement of adjacent major vessels and chest wall from lung and large airway neoplasms, the use of intravenous contrast is helpful. The recommended dose of contrast material is typically 1.5 to 2 mL per kg of patient body weight (not to exceed 3 mL/kg or 125 mL). Intravenous contrast can be administered manually or with mechanical injection, with the choice depending on the size, location, and stability of the catheter (**Table 2**).[9] In general, mechanical injection and exact timing of the bolus are not needed for assessment of pulmonary neoplasms, as they would be for dedicated assessment of the vascular structures of the chest.

SPECTRUM OF IMAGING FINDINGS
Primary Neoplasms of the Lung

Solid lung masses in pediatric patients are typically caused by underlying inflammatory, infectious, or reactive processes.[11] Primary pulmonary neoplasms are uncommon in the pediatric patient, with most neoplasms representing metastases. Pulmonary neoplasm should be considered when a patient's clinical presentation and chest radiographic findings are incongruent, or unusual chest radiographic findings are encountered. For example, a pulmonary neoplasm should be considered when a pediatric patient's clinical presentation resembles pneumonia, but does not respond to antibiotic therapy as expected.[11]

Benign Primary Neoplasms of the Lung

Most primary neoplasms of lung are malignant; benign primary neoplasms of the lung account for only 1% to 5% of lung tumors.[12]

Table 2 Intravenous catheter size, injection rate and methods		
Intravenous Catheter Size (Gauge)	Injection Rate	Injection Methods
24	0.5–1.0 mL/s	Hand injection
24–22	1.0–2.0 mL/s	Mechanical injection
22	2.0–2.5 mL/s	Mechanical injection
20	2.5–3.5 mL/s	Mechanical injection
18	5–6 mL/s	Mechanical injection

Inflammatory myofibroblastic tumor

Inflammatory myofibroblastic tumor, formerly known as inflammatory pseudotumor and plasma cell granuloma, is the most common primary benign lung tumor in children.[13,14] It is a slow-growing benign pulmonary neoplasm with characteristics of both reactive and neoplastic components on histology.[11,15] These tumors are characterized by a spindle cell proliferation mixed with an inflammatory infiltrate of lymphocytes, plasma cells, and histiocytes.[16] Aggressive features such as local invasion, recurrence, and metastasis are rarely seen in pediatric patients with inflammatory myofibroblastic tumors.[17–22]

Most affected children are older than 5 years, and there is an equal sex distribution.[14] Inflammatory myofibroblastic tumors are usually solitary, but multiple lesions are present in approximately 5% of cases.[19,20,23–25] Although most inflammatory myofibroblastic tumors arise from the lung, they can also appear as endobronchial lesions in about 12% of cases.[26] This presentation is discussed in the section on primary neoplasms of large airways. Approximately 40% to 60% of affected patients are asymptomatic. Symptoms, which are more likely to occur with endobronchial lesions than with parenchymal lesions, include fever, cough, chest pain, hemoptysis, and pneumonitis.[14,19,23,26–29]

On chest radiograph, inflammatory myofibroblastic tumor typically presents as a solitary, well-circumscribed, peripherally located lesion with a predilection for the lower lobes (**Fig. 1**A).[23] On CT, most lesions are well marginated, with lobulated contours and heterogeneous attenuation (**Fig. 1**B). Variable amounts of calcification and degree of contrast enhancement can be seen within the tumor. The calcification pattern can be amorphous, mixed, fine flecklike, or dense.[23,30–33] On MR imaging, inflammatory myofibroblastic tumors typically have low to intermediate signal intensity on T1-weighted images and increased signal intensity on T2-weighted images.[23,34] Homogeneous delayed enhancement has been described in 1 case report.[34] The inflammatory cells in pulmonary inflammatory myofibroblastic tumor can result in increased fluorodeoxyglucose (FDG) avidity.[35–38]

Definite diagnosis of inflammatory myofibroblastic tumor solely based on transbronchial or transthoracic needle biopsies can be challenging. This is because inflammatory cells and fibrosis, key components of this tumor, can also be found in the periphery of a variety of other tumors and reactive processes, including fibrohistiocystic neoplasm, plasmacytoma, Hodgkin sclerosing lymphoma, primary lung cancers or sarcoma,

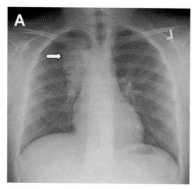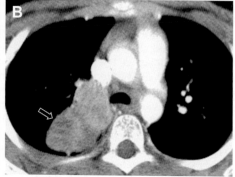

Fig. 1. Inflammatory myofibroblastic tumor in a 10-year-old boy who presented with recurrent cough. (*A*) Frontal chest radiograph shows an opacity (*arrow*) with relatively well-circumscribed borders in the medial right upper lung. (*B*) Enhanced axial CT image shows a heterogeneously enhancing mass (*arrow*) with smooth outer margins abutting the right side of mediastinum.

and mediastinal fibrosis.[20,39–44] However, frozen section specimens from surgery are usually sufficient to exclude other possible malignant and reactive processes.[41,43] Therefore, surgery is generally recommended not only for treatment but also to reach a definitive diagnosis of suspected inflammatory myofibroblastic tumor.[40,45,46] The prognosis of affected patients is excellent if complete surgical resection of tumor with clear margin can be achieved. Radiation therapy, chemotherapy, and steroids have variable success and are reserved for unresectable or multifocal tumors and patients with contraindications to surgery.[40,47,48]

Pulmonary hamartoma

Pulmonary hamartomas are benign neoplasms, and not, as their name suggests, developmental anomalies.[49] They are composed of variable amounts of cartilage, fat, connective tissue, and smooth muscle. Pulmonary hamartomas are the most common benign lung tumor across all ages and account for approximately 6% of all solitary pulmonary nodules.[50] Although the peak incidence is in the sixth decade of life, it also occurs in pediatric patients.[51] Most patients are asymptomatic, and the lesions are incidentally detected on imaging studies such as chest radiograph or CT obtained for investigating other medical conditions.

On chest radiographs, pulmonary hamartoma typically presents as a well-defined, round, or oval nodule, which frequently has lobulated contours. The lesions tend to occur peripherally and grow slowly. Larger lesions are more likely to have the characteristic popcorn calcification.[51] On CT, it is usually a well-circumscribed lesion with lobulated contours (**Fig. 2**). CT better shows fatty and calcific components of the lesion. CT

has been shown to be highly predictive for correctly detecting pulmonary hamartoma in the setting of macroscopic fat and popcorn calcifications.[52,53] However, the fat and popcorn calcifications are reported to be present in 50% and 5% to 15% of cases, respectively, and accurate diagnosis becomes challenging when neither of these elements is present.[54,55] On MR imaging, pulmonary hamartomas tend to be well-defined and lobulated lesions, with intermediate signal intensity on TI-weighted images and high signal intensity on T2-weighted images. Internal septations, when present, demonstrate marked enhancement

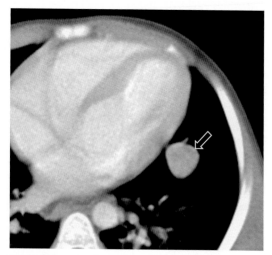

Fig. 2. Pulmonary hamartoma in a 3-year-old boy who presented with a focal lung lesion seen on chest radiograph obtained for evaluation of pneumonia. Enhanced axial CT image show a round lung lesion (*arrow*) located in the left lower lobe with areas of low attenuation, likely representing fat components. Surgical pathology confirmed the diagnosis of pulmonary hamartoma.

on postcontrast images. Foci of calcification can appear as signal voids on all MR imaging sequences. Fat within pulmonary hamartoma may not be easily shown on MR imaging.[56,57] Most lesions are not FDG-avid; however, false-positive cases have been reported.[58]

Transthoracic needle aspiration and core needle biopsy can be used to establish the definitive diagnosis, obviating surgery in cases with nonspecific imaging features. In a case series by Hamper and colleagues,[59] transthoracic needle aspiration and biopsy yielded the correct diagnosis in 12 of 14 (86%) patients with pulmonary hamartoma. In this study, cytology was diagnostic in only 5 of 14 (36%) patients, whereas histologic examination was diagnostic in 11 of 13 (85%) patients (insufficient material in 1 patient precluded histologic examination). Fine-needle aspirates of lesions are diagnostic if cartilage or fibromyxoid fragments are recognized, as opposed to epithelial cells and adipocytes, which hold no diagnostic value.[60] In a case series of 14 patients, Dunbar and Leiman[60] successfully diagnosed pulmonary hamartoma in 11 cases by transthoracic fine-needle aspiration with 22-gauge needles, but cited needle diameter as a major determinant in the proportion of cartilage and fibromyxoid elements in the aspirate. Previous reports have commented on the difficulty of sampling hard, firm, possibly calcified pulmonary hamartomas despite accurate placement and multiple passes for fine-needle biopsy.[61,62] Nevertheless, percutaneous needle aspiration and core needle biopsies have been shown to be an efficient and valuable method to achieve a definitive diagnosis in cases of uncertainty regarding the diagnosis of pulmonary hamartoma. However, some investigators prefer resection for pulmonary hamartomas with nonspecific imaging features, because of low accuracy of cytologic diagnosis.[63] Either enucleation or wedge resection has been reported to be an appropriate method of surgical resection.[64]

Pulmonary sclerosing hemangioma

Pulmonary sclerosing hemangioma of the lung, also known as pneumocytoma, is a rare benign or very low-grade malignant neoplasm of uncertain histogenesis. Originally called a hemangioma because of the prominence of angiomatoid features, it is believed to represent a neoplasm arising from primitive respiratory epithelium.[65]

Sclerosing hemangiomas are uncommon in Western populations but represent the second most common benign lung neoplasm in Asian populations.[66,67] There is a 5:1 female/male ratio. Although it predominantly affects middle-aged adults, it can also occur in adolescents. One of the 7 patients included in the original case series of Liebow and Hubbell[68] was a 15-year-old girl. Most affected patients are asymptomatic, and the lesions are typically incidental findings. Symptomatic patients with sclerosing hemangiomas usually present with hemoptysis, cough, and chest pain.[69]

Chest radiographs typically show a small (<3 cm), well-circumscribed, solitary, peripheral lesion (Fig. 3A).[70] Although most cases are solitary, approximately 4% of cases are multiple.[69] Rarely, a crescent-shaped lucency (air meniscus sign) may be seen around the periphery of the lesion, similar to that seen with invasive pulmonary aspergillosis in immunocompromised pediatric patients.[71] On CT, pulmonary sclerosing hemangioma is typically located adjacent to a pleural surface (Fig. 3B). Pulmonary sclerosing hemangiomas usually show soft tissue attenuation; however, they may also have cystic areas of low attenuation and foci of calcification. After contrast administration, pulmonary sclerosing hemangiomas markedly enhance.[70] The air meniscus sign sometimes associated with pulmonary sclerosing hemangioma is better depicted on CT. It is believed to represent areas of air-trapping surrounding the lesion, possibly resulting from peritumoral hemorrhage followed by clearance through the airway.[72,73] Lymph node metastases from pulmonary sclerosing hemangioma are rare.[69,74,75] On MR imaging, lesions can be hyperintense on both T1-weighted and T2-weighted images and have intense contrast enhancement or appear heterogeneous, with areas of hemorrhage and cystic change.[76,77] Most lesions have increased FDG avidity (Fig. 3C), which positively correlates with increasing lesion size. Lesions larger than 2 cm can be falsely interpreted as malignancy because of high FDG avidity.[78]

The preoperative diagnosis of sclerosing hemangioma is important, because a limited, but complete, surgical resection is associated with excellent prognosis.[67] A preoperative diagnosis using fine-needle aspiration is difficult, because the cytology of sclerosing hemangioma has not been fully evaluated in a large number of cases.[79] Furthermore, case reports that have used fine-needle aspiration to diagnose sclerosing hemangioma have described different cytologic features, some of which can mimic those of adenocarcinoma.[80–84] The diagnosis of sclerosing hemangioma is grounded in histology, relying on recognition of the 4 architectural patterns (papillary, solid, sclerotic, and hemorrhagic) and 2 cell types (surface and round cells).[79]

Surgical excision is the treatment of choice.[67,85] Recurrence is rare and does not seem to affect prognosis after reexcision.[86,87]

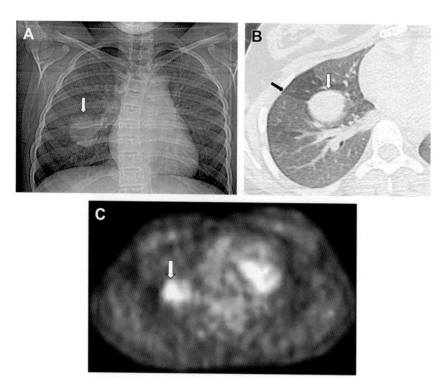

Fig. 3. Sclerosing hemangioma in an 11-year-old girl who was found to have a solitary pulmonary nodule on radiography performed for scoliosis. Core needle biopsy revealed a low-grade epithelial neoplasm, concerning for low-grade adenocarcinoma, highlighting the difficulty encountered on needle biopsy of these lesions. Surgical biopsy revealed sclerosing hemangioma. A subcarinal lymph node was positive for metastatic disease. (*A*) Scout image from chest CT reveals a well-defined mass (*arrow*) in the right midlung zone. (*B*) Noncontrast CT from PET-CT reveals a well-defined, 3.3-cm mass (*white arrow*) contacting the minor fissure (*black arrow*). The mass extended to the upper and middle lobes. No hilar or mediastinal adenopathy was identified. (*C*) [^{18}F]FDG-PET obtained as part of preoperative staging reveals an FGD-avid lesion with SUV$_{max}$ (maximum standardized uptake value) = 5.2 (*arrow*). No other FDG-avid abnormality was identified.

Malignant Primary Neoplasms of the Lungs

Most primary neoplasms of lung in pediatric patients are malignant. Pleuropulmonary blastoma (PPB) and carcinoid tumor are the 2 most common primary lung malignancies in children. Other malignant neoplasms of the lungs, such as small cell carcinoma, adenocarcinoma, and squamous cell carcinoma, are rare in pediatric patients.[11]

Pleuropulmonary blastoma

PPB is an aggressive malignant mesenchymal tumor arising from lung, and less commonly, parietal pleura.[88] It belongs to the family of dysembryonic or dysontogenetic neoplasms: tumors with pathologic features resembling those of the developing organ or tissues in which the neoplasms arise. Other tumors in this family include neuroblastoma, retinoblastoma, Wilms tumor (nephroblastoma), and hepatoblastoma.[89] PPBs are classified into 3 types based on underlying histologic features. Type I is purely cystic without a grossly detectable solid component. Cysts are lined by a benign respiratory type epithelium covering a population of primitive malignant cells. Type III is a solid tumor without an epithelial-lined cystic component. Type II has both solid and cystic areas that are identifiable on gross inspection.[90] It is believed that PPBs progress from cystic lesions (type I) to mixed cystic and solid (type II) or exclusively solid (type III) lesions through progressive overgrowth of mesenchymal cells.[90,91]

PPBs exclusively affect infants and young children, with a median age of diagnosis of 3 years.[90] The median age at diagnosis is different among the 3 types, with type I patients being the youngest (median age, 10 months), and type III patients being the oldest (median age, 44 months).[90] For unknown reasons, the tumor has a predilection for the right lung.[90] Patients with type I PPB may be asymptomatic or present with respiratory distress with or without pneumothorax. Patients with type II and III PPB often present with dyspnea, fever, cough, and chest or abdominal pain. Those with type II PPB can also present with pneumothorax.[92]

On radiographs, PPBs typically present as a peripherally located mass with or without cysts (**Fig. 4**A). There may be complete opacification of the hemithorax, with contralateral mediastinal shift if the lesion is large and solid. Pleural effusion and pneumothorax can also be concomitantly present and may result in complicated radiographic findings.[93] On CT, type I PPBs appear as cystic lesions with variable numbers of cysts (**Fig. 4**B). Cyst diameters range from 2 cm to 9 cm.[94] The cysts exert mass effect on adjacent structures and result in lobar expansion, sometimes with mediastinal shift. Concomitant pneumothorax can also be present.[94] Type II PPBs can appear as a complex mass with air-filled cavities (with or without air-fluid levels) and solid components.[95] Intralesional hemorrhage or infection can occupy the cavities and result in a more solid appearance (**Fig. 5**). Pleural effusion and mediastinal shift can also be seen if the lesion is large.[95] Type III PPBs appear as predominantly solid tumors with heterogeneous contrast enhancement. There may be associated pleural effusion, atelectasis, and mediastinal shift.[95,96] On MR imaging, the lesions with solid components (types II and III) can have heterogeneous contrast enhancement with hemorrhagic and cystic areas.[96] [18F]FDG-positron emission tomography (PET) reveals heterogeneous, predominantly peripheral, FDG avidity in type III lesions.[96]

Complete surgical resection is the treatment of choice for PPB, and reduces the risk of recurrence and metastasis. However, complete surgical resection may be hindered by the size of the tumor and involvement of vital structures. Neoadjuvant chemotherapy can help reduce tumor bulk and increase the chance of complete resection.[97,98] There is a suggestion that type I PPB is more readily resectable and may be associated with

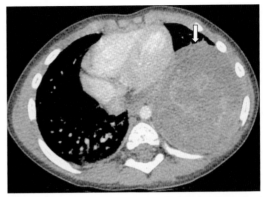

Fig. 5. PPB type II in a 3-year-old girl who presented with fever and lethargy. The patient had been treated 5 months previously for left lower lobe pneumonia complicated by abscess, which had been drained. On initial follow-up chest radiography (not shown), left lower lobe cystic lesions were seen and believed to represent postinfectious pneumatoceles. CT scan was performed, showing large complex mass (*arrow*) in the left lower lobe and no air-filled cavities. The patient subsequently underwent left lower lobectomy and was found to have a type II PPB on pathologic evaluation. The air-filled cavities normally present in a type II PPB contained hemorrhage and inflammatory debris.

a better survival outcome than either types II or III.[90] Unpublished data from the PPB Registry show improved overall survival for type I lesions compared with type II and type III lesions, but no significant difference between type II and type III lesions.[99]

Carcinoid tumors

Neuroendocrine tumors of the lung share microscopic, immunohistochemical, and molecular characteristics, including organoid nesting,

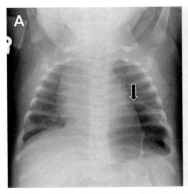
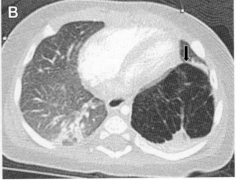

Fig. 4. PPB type I in a 4-month-old girl who presented with left chest mass. The patient subsequently underwent left lower lobe resection, which confirmed the diagnosis of PPB type I. (*A*) Frontal chest radiograph shows a cystic mass (*arrow*) in the lower left hemithorax. (*B*) On CT, a cystic lesion (*arrow*) is seen in the left lower lobe, causing mild mass effect on the heart.

palisading, a trabecular pattern, and rosettelike structures. The 4 major types of neuroendocrine tumors of the lung are typical and atypical carcinoid tumors, large cell neuroendocrine carcinoma, and small cell carcinoma. They are distinguished by mitotic activity and the presence or absence of necrosis, with mitotic activity increasing from typical to atypical carcinoid to large cell neuroendocrine carcinoma and to small cell carcinoma.[100]

Carcinoid tumors are low-grade neuroendocrine tumors, with locally aggressive behavior and low potential for metastasis. Most (85%) intrathoracic lesions arise from the lobar or mainstem bronchi, with 15% arising within the lung parenchyma.[101] In the spectrum of neuroendocrine tumors, typical carcinoid tumors are characterized by fewer than 2 mitoses per 2 mm^2 (10 high-power fields) and no necrosis, whereas atypical carcinoid tumors have 2 to 10 mitoses per 2 mm^2 or foci of necrosis. A mitotic count of 11 or more mitoses per 2 mm^2 separates atypical carcinoids from large cell neuroendocrine carcinoma and small cell carcinomas.[102]

Carcinoid tumors of the lung typically affect older children and adolescents, with a mean age of presentation of 12 years. More cases are reported in boys than girls, with a ratio of 1.4:1.[103] Patients with peripheral lesions are more likely to be asymptomatic when compared with those with central endobronchial lesions, who tend to present with respiratory tract infection, wheezing, and chest pain. Carcinoid syndrome in pediatric patients with carcinoid tumors of the lung is rare.[103]

On radiographs, carcinoid tumors of the lung typically appear as a round or ovoid opacity with well-circumscribed margins.[104] Nonspherical carcinoid tumors of the lung tend to be oriented along the axis of the nearest major bronchus or pulmonary arterial branch (parallel sign).[104,105] CT reveals a soft tissue attenuation mass with well-defined or lobulated margins (**Fig. 6**). Centrally located carcinoid tumors are more likely to have internal calcification compared with peripherally located tumors. Intense enhancement within the tumor is often seen on postcontrast CT images.[104,105]

CT-guided fine-needle aspiration is generally considered reliable for diagnosis of typical carcinoid tumors.[106] However, atypical carcinoid tumors show increased mitoses, pleomorphism, hyperchromatic nuclei, coarse chromatin, necrosis, and nuclear molding, making preoperative differentiation from carcinoma difficult solely based on specimens obtained with fine-needle aspiration.[107,108] Complete surgical resection is the treatment of choice for pulmonary carcinoid tumors and is associated with good long-term

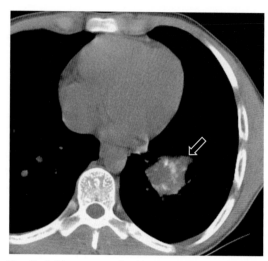

Fig. 6. Pulmonary carcinoid tumor in a 14-year-old boy who presented with cough and fever. Unenhanced axial CT image shows a round mass (*arrow*) with internal calcification located in the left lower lobe. Surgical pathology confirmed the diagnosis of typical carcinoid tumor.

survival (10-year survival rates of >90% in pediatric patients with typical carcinoid tumors).[109] Some advocate parenchyma-sparing resection (when technically feasible), as achieving similar results with a decreased morbidity and better quality of life.[109,110]

Small cell carcinoma

Small cell carcinoma of the lung is a malignant epithelial tumor that consists of small round, oval, or spindle-shaped cells with scant cytoplasm. In adults, small cell carcinoma is the most aggressive lung-cancer subtype and is strongly associated with cigarette smoking.[111] Only 2 cases of small cell carcinoma of the lung have been reported in children in the English-language literature.[112,113] These 2 patients had different clinical presentations. One, a 14-year-old boy, presented with a 10-day history of cough, hemoptysis, and fever unresponsive to oral antibiotics. The second, a 14-year-old girl, presented with a 6-month history of cough, fatigue, anorexia, and weight loss, unresponsive to antibiotics and antiasthmatic drugs. As with small cell carcinomas in adults, the tumors were located centrally in these 2 cases and resulted in postobstructive symptoms such as atelectasis and pneumonia. Because of the limited number of cases, specific imaging features of small cell carcinoma in pediatric patients have not been fully understood and established. Radiographs may show a central mass with or without postobstructive atelectasis or pneumonia, findings that are better depicted on CT (**Fig. 7**A, B).

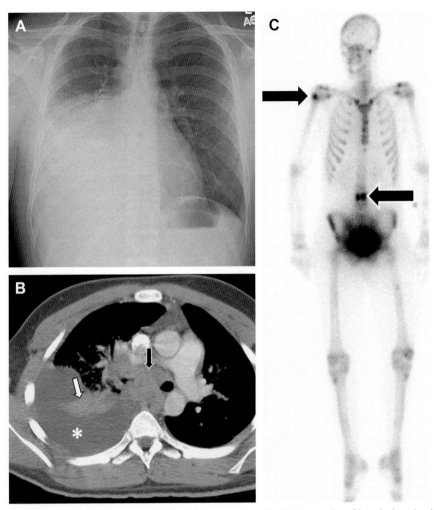

Fig. 7. Small cell carcinoma in an 18-year-old male who presented with 2 months of headaches, back, neck, and shoulder pain, as well as pneumonia only partially responsive to treatment. (*A*) Posteroanterior chest radiograph reveals opacification of most of the right hemithorax. (*B*) Enhanced axial CT image shows a large central mass (*black arrow*) with resultant right lower lobe collapse (*white arrow*) and a pleural effusion (*asterisk*). (*C*) Bone scintigraphy shows bone metastases (*arrows*) at the right humerus and lower lumbar spine. The patient died 4 months after presentation.

Malignant pleural effusion, lymphadenopathy, and distant osseous metastasis can also be seen in affected pediatric patients.

Histologic findings from core needle biopsy and cytologic features from fine-needle aspirations can both be used for diagnosis of small cell carcinoma of the lung. However, although malignant cells obtained from fine-needle aspiration can show cytoplasmic globules or the so-called paranuclear blue inclusions, considered to be characteristic of small cell carcinoma, cytology can sometimes be inaccurate.[114,115] Lymphocytes can mimic small cell carcinoma, and carcinoid tumor can be misclassified as small cell carcinoma.[116] In order to obtain an accurate diagnosis, flow cytometry or immunohistochemistry can be performed to differentiate small cell carcinoma from lymphoid infiltrates, other neuroendocrine tumors, other small round blue cell tumors, and primary or metastatic nonsmall cell carcinomas.[115]

Although small cell carcinomas tend to initially respond to chemotherapy, the local recurrence rate (between 41% and 52% at 2 years) is high in adults.[117,118] In the cases reported in children, both patients initially responded to chemotherapy, but progressed soon after (**Fig. 7**C). One patient was followed for only 7 months. The other patient had progressive disease after 2 courses of chemotherapy, and died 21 months after initial diagnosis, with brain metastases and intestinal perforation.

Adenocarcinoma and squamous cell carcinoma
Adenocarcinomas and squamous cell carcinomas are malignant epithelial neoplasms, which are common in adults. In children, most of these rare tumors are associated with congenital pulmonary airway malformations, but sporadic cases have been also reported.[119,120] Histopathologically, adenocarcinomas show glandular differentiation or mucin production, whereas squamous cell carcinomas show keratinization or intercellular bridges arising from bronchial epithelium.[121]

Adenocarcinomas of the lung in children are similar to those in adults, and have a poor prognosis.[121] A rare subtype of adenocarcinoma is fetal adenocarcinoma, also known as well-differentiated fetal adenocarcinoma, which is distinguished by epithelium that resembles fetal lung in the pseudoglandular stage.[122] Most pediatric squamous cell carcinomas reported in case series are centrally located. Affected patients with centrally located tumors tend to present with symptoms mimicking those of pneumonia, whereas those with peripherally located tumors tend to be asymptomatic.[123–130]

Imaging features of pediatric pulmonary adenocarcinomas and squamous cell carcinomas have been described in the nonradiology literature in case reports and small series, but have not been systematically investigated.[120,123–132] Radiographic and CT findings of these neoplasms range from a well-defined solitary lesion to postobstructive pneumonia. Radiographs may reveal an area of peripheral consolidation (**Fig. 8**A). CT findings range from ground-glass to more solid nodular

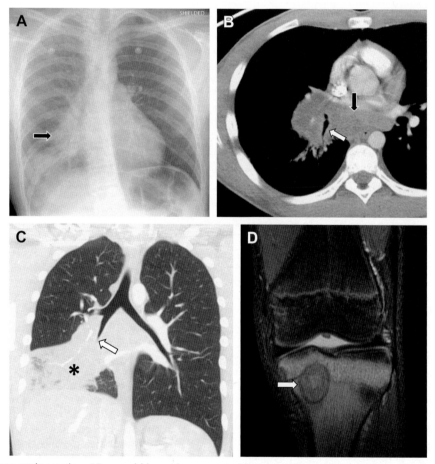

Fig. 8. Adenocarcinoma in a 15-year-old boy who presented because of knee pain and later developed cough. The patient expired 3 months after coming to medical attention. (*A*) Frontal chest radiograph shows an infrahilar opacity (*arrow*) extending to the right lower lung. The opacity did not resolve on antibiotics and chest CT was performed a few days later. (*B*) Enhanced axial CT image shows an infiltrating central soft tissue mass (*black arrow*). Also noted is adjacent airway narrowing (*white arrow*). (*C*) Coronal reformatted CT image shows narrowing (*arrow*) of the right middle and lower lobe bronchi and resultant obstructive atelectasis (*asterisk*). (*D*) Coronal fat-saturated proton-density image from MR imaging of the left knee shows a metastatic lesion (*arrow*) in the proximal tibia, with extensive surrounding marrow edemalike signal.

opacities (**Fig. 8**B, C). MR imaging may reveal a T2-hyperintense lesion in a peripheral location with variable enhancement patterns, ranging from heterogeneous to homogeneous.[133]

Because of the rarity in pediatric patients, no standardized treatment exists for these tumors, although surgical resection is attempted in children who present with resectable tumors. However, metastases are common, and prognosis is usually poor (**Fig. 8**D).

Primary Neoplasms of Large Airways

Neoplasms of the large airway are rare in the pediatric population. Unlike in adults, most primary neoplasms of the large airway in children are benign. Benign neoplasms such as subglottic hemangiomas, recurrent respiratory papillomatosis, and inflammatory myofibroblastic tumors are located in the proximal portion of the central airways, malignant neoplasms such as carcinoid tumors and mucoepidermoid carcinomas tend to be located in the distal trachea or bronchi.[134–136]

Benign Primary Neoplasms of Large Airways

Recurrent respiratory papillomatosis
Recurrent respiratory papillomatosis refers to repeated growth of multiple warts in the respiratory tract. It is believed to be caused by human papillomavirus (HPV), usually type 6 or 11, transmitted from infected mothers to their infants.[137] Recurrent respiratory papillomatosis lesions are composed of a fibrovascular core, with papillary fronds that are covered by bland, stratified squamous epithelium.[138] Although recurrent respiratory papillomatosis is rare in children, with a prevalence of 1 to 4 per 100,000 children in the United States, it is the most common neoplasm of the large airway in the pediatric population.[136,139,140]

Pediatric recurrent respiratory papillomatosis has a bimodal distribution of the age of diagnosis, with peaks at 2 and 11 years of age.[137]

Clinical symptoms in affected pediatric patients are related to the number and location of the lesions, as well as degree of airway obstruction. The classic presentation in children is persistent hoarseness or weak cry occurring between 2 and 4 years of age. However, presenting symptoms can mimic those of more commonly encountered disorders in pediatric patients, such as asthma and croup. Although severe respiratory distress caused by upper airway obstruction from recurrent respiratory papillomatosis is a rare presenting symptom, it may require tracheostomy when it occurs.[141]

On radiographs, the respiratory papillomas appear as lobulated masses or nodules in the laryngeal or subglottic region.[142,143] Although the entire large airway can be affected, recurrent respiratory papillomatosis most commonly affects the larynx. Involvement of the lower trachea, bronchi, and lung is rare. Associated postobstructive atelectasis and consolidation may be present with endobronchial lesions. Concomitant pulmonary parenchymal papillomas are present in less than 1% of affected patients and manifest as well-defined pulmonary nodules with or without cyst or cavity formation.[144] Such pulmonary parenchymal papillomas are believed to be caused by seeding of more proximal disease during endoscopic evaluation and treatment.[138,145] Although malignant transformation of laryngeal disease into squamous cell carcinoma from recurrent respiratory papillomatosis has been reported, it is rare.[146] On CT, nodular or polypoid lesions are usually present in the airway in affected patients (**Fig. 9**A). 3D MDCT virtual bronchoscopy can provide a noninvasive assessment of the tracheobronchial tree, especially in cases of

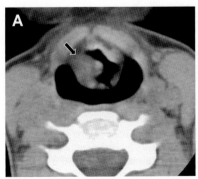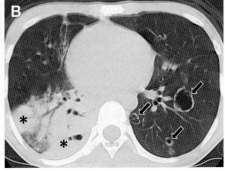

Fig. 9. Recurrent respiratory papillomatosis in a 7-year-old girl who presented with respiratory distress and hoarseness. (*A*) Axial nonenhanced CT image shows a lobular mass (*arrow*) located in the right side of the larynx. (*B*) Axial lung window CT image shows areas of consolidation (*asterisks*) and cavitary pulmonary nodules (*arrows*), likely from distal seeding of tumor.

obstructing lesions, and can reduce the risk of distal seeding that may occur during endoscopic examination (**Fig. 9**B).[147,148]

The diagnosis of recurrent respiratory papillomatosis can be made on bronchoscopy by observing the typical cauliflowerlike lesion with smooth surfaces, with later confirmation on histology. Serum antibody detection is also useful for establishing a diagnosis of HPV infection.[149] Treatment is typically endoscopic surgery with CO_2 laser excision, cryotherapy, or microdebrider treatment.[139] However, current therapies are not curative, and management includes periodic resections of papillomas to maintain the patency of the airway and preserve the patient's voice.[150] Patients with HPV11 infection and those younger than 3 years at diagnosis are more likely to have more aggressive disease.[151]

Subglottic hemangioma

Infantile hemangiomas can be located in the supraglottic area, subglottic region, trachea, or mainstem bronchi.[152] Subglottic hemangiomas are uncommon congenital benign vascular neoplasms, which account for 2% of all congenital laryngeal anomalies.[153] Most patients present before the age of 6 months (mean age at diagnosis is 3–4 months), and girls are more commonly affected than boys, with a ratio of 2:1.[154] The typical clinical presentation is often that of an infant who develops progressively worsening stridor at 4 to 6 weeks of age, with temporary relief with steroids.[155] The stridor is typically biphasic (ie, inspiratory and expiratory) in affected pediatric patients. Less common symptoms include hoarseness, cough, dysphagia, cyanosis, vomiting, and hemoptysis.[154] Approximately 15% of affected patients have cutaneous hemangiomas in the so-called beard distribution (preauricular region, chin, anterior neck, or lower lip). It has been reported that the risk of symptomatic airway involvement increases with the number of cutaneous lesions in this distribution.[156,157]

Frontal radiographs of the neck (**Fig. 10**) typically reveal asymmetric narrowing of the subglottic airway, which is contrasted with the typically symmetric narrowing seen in congenital subglottic stenosis or croup.[157] However, circumferential subglottic hemangiomas, those located at the anterior or posterior wall, or lesions causing a marked fibrotic reaction can have a more symmetric appearance and should be recognized as an important limitation of radiography.[152,158] CT typically shows a lesion along the airway wall, with intense early enhancement after contrast administration (**Fig. 11**). The latter can help differentiate hemangiomas from other causes of airway

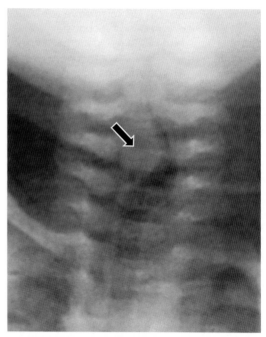

Fig. 10. Subglottic hemangioma in a 42-day-old boy who presented with biphasic stridor. Frontal radiograph of the neck shows asymmetric narrowing of the subglottic airway caused by soft tissue mass (*arrow*). Bronchoscopy confirmed the diagnosis of subglottic hemangioma.

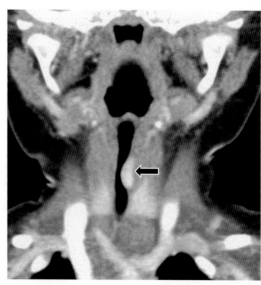

Fig. 11. Subglottic hemangioma in a 2-month old boy who presented with cough and stridor. On physical examination, the patient had a large cutaneous hemangioma on the face. Enhanced coronal CT image shows markedly enhancing subglottic mass (*arrow*) arising from the left side of the subglottic wall. Bronchoscopy confirmed the diagnosis of subglottic hemangioma. (*Courtesy of* Ricardo Restrepo, MD.)

narrowing in infants, such as tracheomalacia, laryngeal papilloma, granuloma, mucocele, cysts, lymphangioma, or acquired subglottic stenosis after infection or intubation.[152]

Definitive diagnosis of subglottic hemangioma is made with bronchoscopy. Management has typically been placement of a tracheotomy, with removal between 1 and 2 years of age, after involution of the lesion. However, children with mild to moderate symptoms can be treated with systemic steroids. Alternatives to tracheotomy include intralesional steroid administration, laser ablation, microdebrider resection, and open surgical resection.[159] In general, prognosis of pediatric patients with subglottic hemangioma is good with prompt diagnosis and appropriate treatment.[160]

Inflammatory myofibroblastic tumor

As described earlier, inflammatory myofibroblastic tumor has characteristics of both reactive and neoplastic lesions[11,15] and can appear as an endobronchial lesion in 12% of cases.[26] Affected patients typically present with cough, wheezing, chest pain, or hemoptysis.[161–165]

Small inflammatory myofibroblastic tumors within the airway can lead to normal radiographs. However, larger lesions can present with secondary signs of airway obstruction, such as segmental or lobar atelectasis or collapse (**Fig. 12A**).[162,163,165] CT is more sensitive than radiographs for detecting the lesion and characterizing the size, location, and transmural extension (**Fig. 12B**).[161,165] Variable degrees of enhancement can be seen within the tumor after administration of contrast. The degree of contrast enhancement in an inflammatory myofibroblastic tumor of the

bronchus is typically less than that seen in a carcinoid tumor located within the large airway (see next section).

Surgical resection is the current management of choice for inflammatory myofibroblastic tumor of the large airway.[162]

Malignant Primary Neoplasms of Large Airways

Carcinoid tumor

Carcinoid tumors are low-grade neuroendocrine tumors with locally aggressive behavior and low potential for metastasis. As noted earlier, most carcinoid tumors arise from the large airway, particularly the lobar and mainstem bronchi.[101] These bronchial carcinoids account for 10% to 20% of all primary lung tumors in pediatric patients.[11,13,103] As endobronchial lesions, carcinoid tumors often cause obstructive symptoms such as unilateral wheezing. However, affected patients can also present with symptoms related to respiratory tract infection, chest pain, or rarely carcinoid syndrome.[103,166]

The most common radiographic finding of large airway involvement of carcinoid tumors is postobstructive segmental or lobar atelectasis or collapse (**Fig. 13A**). Other less common radiographic findings include a well-defined perihilar opacity or focal obstructive hyperinflation.[167] On CT, carcinoid tumor of the large airway typically presents as a well-defined soft tissue attenuation mass with well-defined, lobulated margins (**Fig. 13B–F**). Central tumors are more likely to have internal calcification compared with peripheral tumors. Intense enhancement within the tumor is usually observed on postcontrast CT images.[104,105]

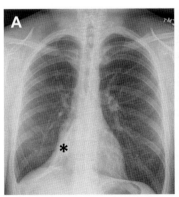
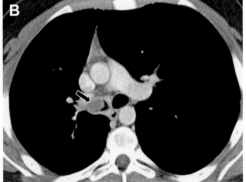

Fig. 12. Inflammatory myofibroblastic tumor of the bronchus in a 17-year-old male who presented with acute onset of hemoptysis. Surgical pathology confirmed the diagnosis of inflammatory myofibroblastic tumor. (*A*) Frontal chest radiograph shows a triangular opacity (*asterisk*) abutting the medial right lower lobe and associated right lower lobe atelectasis. (*B*) Enhanced axial CT image shows a minimally enhancing endobronchial mass (*arrow*) located in the proximal right mainstem bronchus.

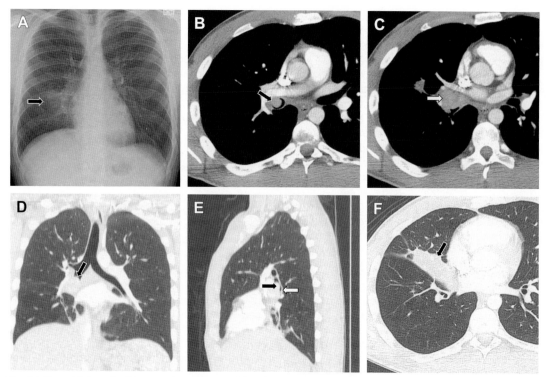

Fig. 13. Bronchial carcinoid tumor in a 17-year-old male who presented with a 2-year history of recurrent pneumonia. (*A*) Frontal radiograph after resolution of symptoms reveals a vague infrahilar and right middle lobe opacity (*arrow*). (*B*) Enhanced axial CT image shows a heterogeneously enhancing right hilar mass with an endobronchial component (*black arrow*). (*C*) Enhanced axial CT image inferior to (*B*) shows that the right hilar mass also has an extraluminal component (*arrow*). (*D*) Coronal reformatted CT image shows the endobronchial mass (*arrow*) located within the bronchus intermedius. (*E*) Sagittal reformatted CT image shows the endobronchial mass (*black arrow*) in the bronchus intermedius extending into the right middle lobe bronchus, with a narrowed but patent right lower lobe bronchus (*white arrow*). (*F*) Axial lung window CT image shows right middle lobe atelectasis (*black arrow*). Note that the lower lobe is aerated as a result of a patent right lower lobe bronchus seen in (*E*).

Complete surgical resection with primary reanastomosis or sleeve resection is regarded as the management of choice for the carcinoid tumors located within the large airway.[168]

Mucoepidermoid carcinoma

Mucoepidermoid carcinomas are composed of a mixture of mucus-secreting cells, squamous cells, and intermediate-type cells. Unlike in adults, the tumors tend to be low grade in children and remain localized for a long time with low metastatic potential.[169,170] As in adults, bronchial mucoepidermoid tumors in children typically arise in a mainstem bronchus or proximal portion of a lobar bronchus.[166] The most common presenting symptom in affected pediatric patients is recurrent pneumonia, but patients can also present with cough, wheezing, dyspnea, and hemoptysis, with duration of symptoms ranging from 1 week to 3.5 years.[169]

Chest radiographs typically show a central mass or endoluminal nodule with or without resultant obstructive pneumonia or atelectasis.[171] CT usually shows a smoothly oval or lobulated soft tissue mass, which adapts to the branching pattern of the airways (**Fig. 14**A, B). Punctate calcifications within the tumors may be seen in 50% of cases.[171,172] A recent report showed [18F]FDG accumulation in a mucoepidermoid carcinoma of the bronchus in a pediatric patient (**Fig. 14**C), a finding that may aid in distinguishing this type of malignancy from benign processes and a more common primary neoplasm in children such as carcinoid tumor, both of which typically show low FDG avidity.[173]

Surgical resection is the treatment of choice. The extent of surgery depends on location of the tumor, and ranges from segmental excision for tracheal lesions to lobectomy for lesions involving a lobar bronchus.[169,170]

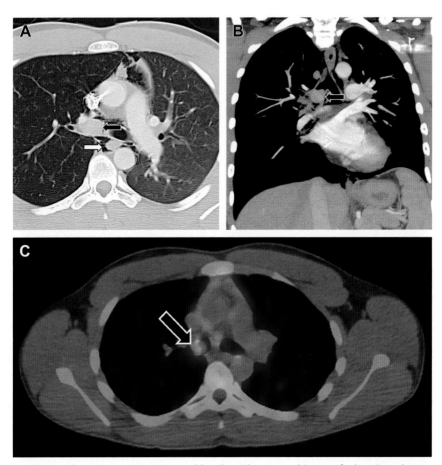

Fig. 14. Mucoepidermoid carcinoma in a 17-year-old male with a 1-year history of wheezing, shortness of breath, and occasional hemoptysis. The patient was initially diagnosed with asthma, and treated with an unspecified inhaler without resolution of symptoms. The patient subsequently developed chest pain and presented to the emergency department. (*A*) Axial lung window CT image shows pneumomediastinum (*white arrow*) and an obstructing endobronchial mass (*black arrow*) in the right mainstem bronchus. (*B*) Coronal reformatted enhanced CT image shows the obstructing endobronchial mass (*arrow*) in the right mainstem bronchus. The location and craniocaudal extension of this endobronchial mass is better visualized on this coronal reformatted CT image than axial CT image (*A*). (*C*) Fused image from [¹⁸F]FDG-PET-CT shows a mildly FDG-avid endobronchial lesion (*arrow*).

SUMMARY

The rarity of primary neoplasms of the lung and large airway may lead to a low index of suspicion for these lesions, with subsequent delay in achieving a correct diagnosis and initiation of effective treatment. In the case of malignant neoplasms, this delay can adversely affect prognosis by allowing progression of disease to an advanced stage. MDCT, with its improved efficiency and diagnostic capability compared with conventional CT, offers an important noninvasive imaging modality for confirmation and further characterization of these lesions in pediatric patients. Clear understanding of the proper MDCT techniques and the characteristic MDCT imaging appearance of primary lung and airway neoplasms aids in accurate

diagnosis and thus contributes to optimal pediatric patient care.

REFERENCES

1. Tischer W, Reddemann H, Herzog P, et al. Experience in surgical treatment of pulmonary and bronchial tumours in childhood. Prog Pediatr Surg 1987;21:118–35.
2. Lee EY, Greenberg SB, Boiselle PM. Multidetector computed tomography of pediatric large airway diseases: state-of-the-art. Radiol Clin North Am 2011;49(5):869–93.
3. Lee EY, Siegel MJ. MDCT of tracheobronchial narrowing in pediatric patients. J Thorac Imaging 2007;22(3):300–9.

4. Lee EY, Restrepo R, Dillman JR, et al. Imaging evaluation of pediatric trachea and bronchi: systematic review and updates. Semin Roentgenol 2012; 47(2):182–96.

5. Lee EY, Boiselle PM, Cleveland RH. Multidetector CT evaluation of congenital lung anomalies. Radiology 2008;247(3):632–48.

6. Coley BD. Chest sonography in children: current indications, techniques, and imaging findings. Radiol Clin North Am 2011;49(5):825–46.

7. Hellinger JC, Daubert M, Lee EY, et al. Congenital thoracic vascular anomalies: evaluation with state-of-the-art MR imaging and MDCT. Radiol Clin North Am 2011;49(5):969–96.

8. Lemos AA, Siegel MJ, Rossi G, et al. Single-versus multidetector-row CT: comparison of sedation rates, conventional angiograms and motion artefacts in young children following liver transplantation. Radiol Med 2006;111(7):911–20.

9. Lee EY, Dorkin H, Vargas SO. Congenital pulmonary malformations in pediatric patients: review and update on etiology, classification, and imaging findings. Radiol Clin North Am 2011;49(5):921–48.

10. Honda O, Johkoh T, Yamamoto S, et al. Comparison of quality of multiplanar reconstructions and direct coronal multidetector CT scans of the lung. AJR Am J Roentgenol 2002;179(4):875–9.

11. Dishop MK, Kuruvilla S. Primary and metastatic lung tumors in the pediatric population: a review and 25-year experience at a large children's hospital. Arch Pathol Lab Med 2008;132(7):1079–103.

12. Arrigoni MG, Woolner LB, Bernatz PE, et al. Benign tumors of the lung. A ten-year surgical experience. J Thorac Cardiovasc Surg 1970;60(4):589–99.

13. Hancock BJ, Di Lorenzo M, Youssef S, et al. Childhood primary pulmonary neoplasms. J Pediatr Surg 1993;28(9):1133–6.

14. Hartman GE, Shochat SJ. Primary pulmonary neoplasms of childhood: a review. Ann Thorac Surg 1983;36(1):108–19.

15. Meis-Kindblom JM, Kjellstrom C, Kindblom LG. Inflammatory fibrosarcoma: update, reappraisal, and perspective on its place in the spectrum of inflammatory myofibroblastic tumors. Semin Diagn Pathol 1998;15(2):133–43.

16. Gleason BC, Hornick JL. Inflammatory myofibroblastic tumours: where are we now? J Clin Pathol 2008;61(4):428–37.

17. Hedlund GL, Navoy JF, Galliani CA, et al. Aggressive manifestations of inflammatory pulmonary pseudotumor in children. Pediatr Radiol 1999; 29(2):112–6.

18. Akman C, Dincbas FO, Oz B, et al. Unusual cause of dysphagia: inflammatory pseudotumor of the lung. South Med J 2005;98(6):665–8.

19. Pettinato G, Manivel JC, De Rosa N, et al. Inflammatory myofibroblastic tumor (plasma cell granuloma). Clinicopathologic study of 20 cases with immunohistochemical and ultrastructural observations. Am J Clin Pathol 1990;94(5): 538–46.

20. Melloni G, Carretta A, Ciriaco P, et al. Inflammatory pseudotumor of the lung in adults. Ann Thorac Surg 2005;79(2):426–32.

21. Carillo C, Anile M, De Giacomo T, et al. Bilateral simultaneous inflammatory myofibroblastic tumor of the lung with distant metastatic spread. Interact Cardiovasc Thorac Surg 2011;13(2):246–7.

22. Corneli G, Alifano M, Forti Parri S, et al. Invasive inflammatory pseudo-tumor involving the lung and the mediastinum. Thorac Cardiovasc Surg 2001; 49(2):124–6.

23. Agrons GA, Rosado-de-Christenson ML, Kirejczyk WM, et al. Pulmonary inflammatory pseudotumor: radiologic features. Radiology 1998; 206(2):511–8.

24. Yao X, Alvarado Y, Brackeen J, et al. Plasma cell granuloma: a case report of multiple lesions in the lung and review of the literature. Am J Med Sci 2007;334(5):402–6.

25. Lee MH, Lee HB, Lee YC, et al. Bilateral multiple inflammatory myofibroblastic tumors of the lung successfully treated with corticosteroids. Lung 2011;189(5):433–5.

26. Matsubara O, Tan-Liu NS, Kenney RM, et al. Inflammatory pseudotumors of the lung: progression from organizing pneumonia to fibrous histiocytoma or to plasma cell granuloma in 32 cases. Hum Pathol 1988;19(7):807–14.

27. Berardi RS, Lee SS, Chen HP, et al. Inflammatory pseudotumors of the lung. Surg Gynecol Obstet 1983;156(1):89–96.

28. Bahadori M, Liebow AA. Plasma cell granulomas of the lung. Cancer 1973;31(1):191–208.

29. Spencer H. The pulmonary plasma cell/histiocytoma complex. Histopathology 1984;8(6):903–16.

30. Shapiro MP, Gale ME, Carter BL. Variable CT appearance of plasma cell granuloma of the lung. J Comput Assist Tomogr 1987;11(1):49–51.

31. Wells RG, Sty JR. Lung mass in a five-year-old girl. Chest 1986;89(5):747–8.

32. Verbeke JI, Verberne AA, Den Hollander JC, et al. Inflammatory myofibroblastic tumour of the lung manifesting as progressive atelectasis. Pediatr Radiol 1999;29(11):816–9.

33. Kim TS, Han J, Kim GY, et al. Pulmonary inflammatory pseudotumor (inflammatory myofibroblastic tumor): CT features with pathologic correlation. J Comput Assist Tomogr 2005;29(5):633–9.

34. Takayama Y, Yabuuchi H, Matsuo Y, et al. Computed tomographic and magnetic resonance features of inflammatory myofibroblastic tumor of the lung in children. Radiat Med 2008;26(10): 613–7.

35. Huellner MW, Schwizer B, Burger I, et al. Inflammatory pseudotumor of the lung with high FDG uptake. Clin Nucl Med 2010;35(9):722–3.

36. Higashi K, Ueda Y, Sakuma T, et al. Comparison of [(18)F]FDG PET and (201)Tl SPECT in evaluation of pulmonary nodules. J Nucl Med 2001;42(10): 1489–96.

37. Sulu E, Damadoglu E, Berk Takir H, et al. A case of endobronchial inflammatory pseudotumor invading the mediastinum. Tuberk Toraks 2011;59(1):77–80.

38. Slosman DO, Spiliopoulos A, Keller A, et al. Quantitative metabolic PET imaging of a plasma cell granuloma. J Thorac Imaging 1994;9(2):116–9.

39. Ishida T, Oka T, Nishino T, et al. Inflammatory pseudotumor of the lung in adults: radiographic and clinicopathological analysis. Ann Thorac Surg 1989;48(1):90–5.

40. Cerfolio RJ, Allen MS, Nascimento AG, et al. Inflammatory pseudotumors of the lung. Ann Thorac Surg 1999;67(4):933–6.

41. Copin MC, Gosselin BH, Ribet ME. Plasma cell granuloma of the lung: difficulties in diagnosis and prognosis. Ann Thorac Surg 1996;61(5): 1477–82.

42. Kim JH, Cho JH, Park MS, et al. Pulmonary inflammatory pseudotumor–a report of 28 cases. Korean J Intern Med 2002;17(4):252–8.

43. Matsubara T, Hirose K, Hatakeyama H, et al. Effect of the nonsteroidal anti-inflammatory drug 480156-S on hepatic drug-metabolizing activity and pharmacological action of diazepam and pentobarbital in rats. Nihon Yakurigaku Zasshi 1988;92(4):201–13.

44. Takeda S, Onishi Y, Kawamura T, et al. Clinical spectrum of pulmonary inflammatory myofibroblastic tumor. Interact Cardiovasc Thorac Surg 2008; 7(4):629–33.

45. Coffin CM, Watterson J, Priest JR, et al. Extrapulmonary inflammatory myofibroblastic tumor (inflammatory pseudotumor). A clinicopathologic and immunohistochemical study of 84 cases. Am J Surg Pathol 1995;19(8):859–72.

46. Sakurai H, Hasegawa T, Watanabe S, et al. Inflammatory myofibroblastic tumor of the lung. Eur J Cardiothorac Surg 2004;25(2):155–9.

47. Mondello B, Lentini S, Barone M, et al. Surgical management of pulmonary inflammatory pseudotumors: a single center experience. J Cardiothorac Surg 2011;6:18.

48. Fabre D, Fadel E, Singhal S, et al. Complete resection of pulmonary inflammatory pseudotumors has excellent long-term prognosis. J Thorac Cardiovasc Surg 2009;137(2):435–40.

49. Johansson M, Dietrich C, Mandahl N, et al. Recombinations of chromosomal bands 6p21 and 14q24 characterise pulmonary hamartomas. Br J Cancer 1993;67(6):1236–41.

50. Bateson EM. An analysis of 155 solitary lung lesions illustrating the differential diagnosis of mixed tumours of the lung. Clin Radiol 1965;16:51–65.

51. Bateson EM, Abbott EK. Mixed tumors of the lung, or hamarto-chondromas. A review of the radiological appearances of cases published in the literature and a report of fifteen new cases. Clin Radiol 1960;11:232–47.

52. Siegelman SS, Khouri NF, Scott WW Jr, et al. Pulmonary hamartoma: CT findings. Radiology 1986; 160(2):313–7.

53. Potente G, Macori F, Caimi M, et al. Noncalcified pulmonary hamartomas: computed tomography enhancement patterns with histologic correlation. J Thorac Imaging 1999;14(2):101–4.

54. Ledor K, Fish B, Chaise L, et al. CT diagnosis of pulmonary hamartomas. J Comput Tomogr 1981; 5(4):343–4.

55. Guo W, Zhao YP, Jiang YG, et al. Surgical treatment and outcome of pulmonary hamartoma: a retrospective study of 20-year experience. J Exp Clin Cancer Res 2008;27:8.

56. Sakai F, Sone S, Kiyono K, et al. MR of pulmonary hamartoma: pathologic correlation. J Thorac Imaging 1994;9(1):51–5.

57. Alexopoulou E, Economopoulos N, Priftis KN, et al. MR imaging findings of an atypical pulmonary hamartoma in a 12-year-old child. Pediatr Radiol 2008;38(10):1134–7.

58. Sminohara S, Hanagiri T, Kuwata T, et al. Clinical characteristics of pulmonary hamartoma resected surgically as undiagnosed pulmonary nodule. J UOEH 2012;34(1):41–6.

59. Hamper UM, Khouri NF, Stitik FP, et al. Pulmonary hamartoma: diagnosis by transthoracic needle-aspiration biopsy. Radiology 1985;155(1):15–8.

60. Dunbar F, Leiman G. The aspiration cytology of pulmonary hamartomas. Diagn Cytopathol 1989;5(2): 174–80.

61. Sinner WN. Fine-needle biopsy of hamartomas of the lung. AJR Am J Roentgenol 1982;138(1):65–9.

62. Dahlgren S. Needle biopsy of intrapulmonary hamartoma. Scand J Respir Dis 1966;47(3):187–94.

63. Hughes JH, Young NA, Wilbur DC, et al. Fine-needle aspiration of pulmonary hamartoma: a common source of false-positive diagnoses in the College of American Pathologists Interlaboratory Comparison Program in Nongynecologic Cytology. Arch Pathol Lab Med 2005;129(1):19–22.

64. van den Bosch JM, Wagenaar SS, Corrin B, et al. Mesenchymoma of the lung (so called hamartoma): a review of 154 parenchymal and endobronchial cases. Thorax 1987;42(10):790–3.

65. Devouassoux-Shisheboran M, Nicholson AG, Leslie K, et al. Sclerosing haemangioma. In: Travis WD, Brambilla E, Muller-Hemerlink HK, et al, editors. World Health Organization classification

of tumours. Pathology and genetics of tumours of the lung, pleura, thymus and heart. Lyon (France): IARC Press; 2004. p. 115–7.

66. Kuo KT, Hsu WH, Wu YC, et al. Sclerosing hemangioma of the lung: an analysis of 44 cases. J Chin Med Assoc 2003;66(1):33–8.

67. Sugio K, Yokoyama H, Kaneko S, et al. Sclerosing hemangioma of the lung: radiographic and pathological study. Ann Thorac Surg 1992;53(2): 295–300.

68. Liebow AA, Hubbell DS. Sclerosing hemangioma (histiocytoma, xanthoma) of the lung. Cancer 1956;9(1):53–75.

69. Devouassoux-Shisheboran M, Hayashi T, Linnoila RI, et al. A clinicopathologic study of 100 cases of pulmonary sclerosing hemangioma with immunohistochemical studies: TTF-1 is expressed in both round and surface cells, suggesting an origin from primitive respiratory epithelium. Am J Surg Pathol 2000;24(7):906–16.

70. Im JG, Kim WH, Han MC, et al. Sclerosing hemangiomas of the lung and interlobar fissures: CT findings. J Comput Assist Tomogr 1994;18(1):34–8.

71. Bahk YW, Shinn KS, Choi BS. The air meniscus sign in sclerosing hemangioma of the lung. Radiology 1978;128(1):27–9.

72. Nam JE, Ryu YH, Cho SH, et al. Air-trapping zone surrounding sclerosing hemangioma of the lung. J Comput Assist Tomogr 2002;26(3):358–61.

73. Sagara Y, Hayashi K, Shiraishi Y, et al. The pulmonary air meniscus sign in a case of sclerosing hemangioma. Nihon Kyobu Shikkan Gakkai Zasshi 1994;32(8):774–7.

74. Tanaka I, Inoue M, Matsui Y, et al. A case of pneumocytoma (so-called sclerosing hemangioma) with lymph node metastasis. Jpn J Clin Oncol 1986; 16(1):77–86.

75. Chen CS. Inflammatory pseudotumor and lung adenoma. Chin Med J (Engl) 1978;4(4):297–8.

76. Fujiyoshi F, Ichinari N, Fukukura Y, et al. Sclerosing hemangioma of the lung: MR findings and correlation with pathological features. J Comput Assist Tomogr 1998;22(6):1006–8.

77. Fujiyoshi F, Nakajo M, Ikeda K, et al. A case of sclerosing hemangioma of the lung: correlation of MR images with pathological findings. Radiat Med 1995;13(2):85–8.

78. Lee E, Park CM, Kang KW, et al. 18F-FDG PET/CT features of pulmonary sclerosing hemangioma. Acta Radiol 2012;54(1):24–9.

79. Keylock JB, Galvin JR, Franks TJ. Sclerosing hemangioma of the lung. Arch Pathol Lab Med 2009; 133(5):820–5.

80. Wang SE, Nieberg RK. Fine needle aspiration cytology of sclerosing hemangioma of the lung, a mimicker of bronchioloalveolar carcinoma. Acta Cytol 1986;30(1):51–4.

81. Chan AC, Chan JK. Can pulmonary sclerosing haemangioma be accurately diagnosed by intraoperative frozen section? Histopathology 2002; 41(5):392–403.

82. Gal AA, Nassar VH, Miller JI. Cytopathologic diagnosis of pulmonary sclerosing hemangioma. Diagn Cytopathol 2002;26(3):163–6.

83. Iyoda A, Baba M, Saitoh H, et al. Imprint cytologic features of pulmonary sclerosing hemangioma: comparison with well-differentiated papillary adenocarcinoma. Cancer 2002;96(3):146–9.

84. Wojcik EM, Sneige N, Lawrence DD, et al. Fine-needle aspiration cytology of sclerosing hemangioma of the lung: case report with immunohistochemical study. Diagn Cytopathol 1993;9(3):304–9.

85. Lei Y, Yong D, Jun-Zhong R, et al. Treatment of 28 patients with sclerosing hemangioma (SH) of the lung. J Cardiothorac Surg 2012;7(1):34.

86. Wei S, Tian J, Song X, et al. Recurrence of pulmonary sclerosing hemangioma. Thorac Cardiovasc Surg 2008;56(2):120–2.

87. Iyoda A, Hiroshima K, Shiba M, et al. Clinicopathological analysis of pulmonary sclerosing hemangioma. Ann Thorac Surg 2004;78(6): 1928–31.

88. Manivel JC, Priest JR, Watterson J, et al. Pleuropulmonary blastoma. The so-called pulmonary blastoma of childhood. Cancer 1988;62(8):1516–26.

89. Maris JM, Denny CT. Focus on embryonal malignancies. Cancer Cell 2002;2(6):447–50.

90. Priest JR, McDermott MB, Bhatia S, et al. Pleuropulmonary blastoma: a clinicopathologic study of 50 cases. Cancer 1997;80(1):147–61.

91. Wright JR Jr. Pleuropulmonary blastoma: a case report documenting transition from type I (cystic) to type III (solid). Cancer 2000;88(12):2853–8.

92. The pleuropulmonary blastoma registry. Signs and symptoms. [Web page]. 2009. Available at: http://ppbregistry.org/doctors/signs.htm. Accessed November 7, 2012.

93. Naffaa LN, Donnelly LF. Imaging findings in pleuropulmonary blastoma. Pediatr Radiol 2005;35(4): 387–91.

94. Griffin N, Devaraj A, Goldstraw P, et al. CT and histopathological correlation of congenital cystic pulmonary lesions: a common pathogenesis? Clin Radiol 2008;63(9):995–1005.

95. Orazi C, Inserra A, Schingo PM, et al. Pleuropulmonary blastoma, a distinctive neoplasm of childhood: report of three cases. Pediatr Radiol 2007; 37(4):337–44.

96. Geiger J, Walter K, Uhl M, et al. Imaging findings in a 3-year-old girl with type III pleuropulmonary blastoma. In Vivo 2007;21(6):1119–22.

97. Indolfi P, Bisogno G, Casale F, et al. Prognostic factors in pleuro-pulmonary blastoma. Pediatr Blood Cancer 2007;48(3):318–23.

98. Venkatramani R, Malogolowkin MH, Wang L, et al. Pleuropulmonary blastoma: a single-institution experience. J Pediatr Hematol Oncol 2012;34(5): e182–5.

99. The pleuropulmonary blastoma registry. Prognosis. [Web page]. 2009. Available at: http://ppbregistry.org/doctors/prognosis.htm. Accessed November 7, 2012.

100. Travis WD. The concept of pulmonary neuroendocrine tumours. In: Travis WD, Brambilla E, Muller-Hemerlink HK, et al, editors. World Health Organization classification of tumours. Pathology and genetics of tumours of the lung, pleura, thymus and heart. Lyon (France): IARC Press; 2004. p. 19–20.

101. Okike N, Bernatz PE, Woolner LB. Carcinoid tumors of the lung. Ann Thorac Surg 1976;22(3):270–7.

102. Travis WD, Rush W, Flieder DB, et al. Survival analysis of 200 pulmonary neuroendocrine tumors with clarification of criteria for atypical carcinoid and its separation from typical carcinoid. Am J Surg Pathol 1998;22(8):934–44.

103. Yu DC, Grabowski MJ, Kozakewich HP, et al. Primary lung tumors in children and adolescents: a 90-year experience. J Pediatr Surg 2010;45(6): 1090–5.

104. Zwiebel BR, Austin JH, Grimes MM. Bronchial carcinoid tumors: assessment with CT of location and intratumoral calcification in 31 patients. Radiology 1991;179(2):483–6.

105. Chong S, Lee KS, Chung MJ, et al. Neuroendocrine tumors of the lung: clinical, pathologic, and imaging findings. Radiographics 2006;26(1): 41–57 [discussion: 57–8].

106. Rosado de Christenson ML, Abbott GF, Kirejczyk WM, et al. Thoracic carcinoids: radiologic-pathologic correlation. Radiographics 1999;19(3):707–36.

107. Collins BT, Cramer HM. Fine needle aspiration cytology of carcinoid tumors. Acta Cytol 1996; 40(4):695–707.

108. McCaughan BC, Martini N, Bains MS. Bronchial carcinoids. Review of 124 cases. J Thorac Cardiovasc Surg 1985;89(1):8–17.

109. Rea F, Rizzardi G, Zuin A, et al. Outcome and surgical strategy in bronchial carcinoid tumors: single institution experience with 252 patients. Eur J Cardiothorac Surg 2007;31(2):186–91.

110. Rizzardi G, Marulli G, Calabrese F, et al. Bronchial carcinoid tumours in children: surgical treatment and outcome in a single institution. Eur J Pediatr Surg 2009;19(4):228–31.

111. Jackman DM, Johnson BE. Small-cell lung cancer. Lancet 2005;366(9494):1385–96.

112. Tronnes H, Haugland HK, Bekassy AN, et al. Small cell lung cancer in a 14-year-old girl. J Pediatr Hematol Oncol 2012;34(2):e86–8.

113. Kim CK, Chung CY, Koh YY. Primary small cell bronchogenic carcinoma in a 14-year-old boy. Pediatr Pulmonol 2000;29(4):317–20.

114. Walker WP, Wittchow RJ, Bottles K, et al. Paranuclear blue inclusions in small cell undifferentiated carcinoma: a diagnostically useful finding demonstrated in fine-needle aspiration biopsy smears. Diagn Cytopathol 1994;10(3):212–5.

115. Siddiqui MT. Pulmonary neuroendocrine neoplasms: a review of clinicopathologic and cytologic features. Diagn Cytopathol 2010;38(8):607–17.

116. Renshaw AA, Haja J, Lozano RL, et al. Distinguishing carcinoid tumor from small cell carcinoma of the lung: correlating cytologic features and performance in the College of American Pathologists Non-Gynecologic Cytology Program. Arch Pathol Lab Med 2005;129(5):614–8.

117. Schild SE, Bonner JA, Shanahan TG, et al. Long-term results of a phase III trial comparing once-daily radiotherapy with twice-daily radiotherapy in limited-stage small-cell lung cancer. Int J Radiat Oncol Biol Phys 2004;59(4):943–51.

118. Turrisi AT 3rd, Kim K, Blum R, et al. Twice-daily compared with once-daily thoracic radiotherapy in limited small-cell lung cancer treated concurrently with cisplatin and etoposide. N Engl J Med 1999;340(4):265–71.

119. Ramos SG, Barbosa GH, Tavora FR, et al. Bronchioloalveolar carcinoma arising in a congenital pulmonary airway malformation in a child: case report with an update of this association. J Pediatr Surg 2007;42(5):E1–4.

120. Guddati AK, Marak CP. Pediatric primary lung adenocarcinoma in the absence of congenital pulmonary airway malformation. Med Oncol 2012; 29(4):2661–3.

121. Lal DR, Clark I, Shalkow J, et al. Primary epithelial lung malignancies in the pediatric population. Pediatr Blood Cancer 2005;45(5):683–6.

122. Kodama T, Shimosato Y, Watanabe S, et al. Six cases of well-differentiated adenocarcinoma simulating fetal lung tubules in pseudoglandular stage. Comparison with pulmonary blastoma. Am J Surg Pathol 1984;8(10):735–44.

123. Niitu Y, Kubota H, Hasegawa S, et al. Lung cancer (squamous cell carcinoma) in adolescence. Am J Dis Child 1974;127(1):108–11.

124. Asamura H, Nakayama H, Kondo H, et al. AFP-producing squamous cell carcinoma of the lung in an adolescent. Jpn J Clin Oncol 1996;26(2):103–6.

125. Kim HS, Lee JJ, Cho AR, et al. Squamous cell carcinoma of the lung in an autistic child who has never smoked. J Pediatr Hematol Oncol 2011; 33(5):e216–9.

126. La Salle AJ, Andrassy RJ, Stanford W. Bronchogenic squamous cell carcinoma in childhood; a case report. J Pediatr Surg 1977;12(4):519–21.

127. Sharma R, Stein D, Khan W. Primary squamous cell carcinoma of lung in a 7-year-old boy: a case report. J Pediatr Hematol Oncol 2011;33(7): e307–9.

128. Shelley BE, Lorenzo RL. Primary squamous cell carcinoma of the lung in childhood. Pediatr Radiol 1983;13(2):92–4.

129. Abuzetun JY, Hazin R, Suker M, et al. Primary squamous cell carcinoma of the lung with bony metastasis in a 13-year-old boy: case report and review of literature. J Pediatr Hematol Oncol 2008;30(8):635–7.

130. Keita O, Lagrange JL, Michiels JF, et al. Primary bronchogenic squamous cell carcinoma in children: report of a case and review of the literature. Med Pediatr Oncol 1995;24(1):50–2.

131. Park JA, Park HJ, Lee JS, et al. Adenocarcinoma of lung in never smoked children. Lung Cancer 2008; 61(2):266–9.

132. Kayton ML, He M, Zakowski MF, et al. Primary lung adenocarcinomas in children and adolescents treated for pediatric malignancies. J Thorac Oncol 2010;5(11):1764–71.

133. Tanaka R, Horikoshi H, Nakazato Y, et al. Magnetic resonance imaging in peripheral lung adenocarcinoma: correlation with histopathologic features. J Thorac Imaging 2009;24(1):4–9.

134. Lack EE, Harris GB, Eraklis AJ, et al. Primary bronchial tumors in childhood. A clinicopathologic study of six cases. Cancer 1983;51(3):492–7.

135. Roby BB, Drehner D, Sidman JD. Pediatric tracheal and endobronchial tumors: an institutional experience. Arch Otolaryngol Head Neck Surg 2011; 137(9):925–9.

136. Armstrong LR, Preston EJ, Reichert M, et al. Incidence and prevalence of recurrent respiratory papillomatosis among children in Atlanta and Seattle. Clin Infect Dis 2000;31(1):107–9.

137. Gabbott M, Cossart YE, Kan A, et al. Human papillomavirus and host variables as predictors of clinical course in patients with juvenile-onset recurrent respiratory papillomatosis. J Clin Microbiol 1997; 35(12):3098–103.

138. Wilson RW, Kirejczyk W. Pathological and radiological correlation of endobronchial neoplasms: part I, Benign tumors. Ann Diagn Pathol 1997; 1(1):31–46.

139. Derkay CS. Task force on recurrent respiratory papillomas. A preliminary report. Arch Otolaryngol Head Neck Surg 1995;121(12):1386–91.

140. Jones SR, Myers EN, Barnes L. Benign neoplasms of the larynx. Otolaryngol Clin North Am 1984; 17(1):151–78.

141. Zacharisen MC, Conley SF. Recurrent respiratory papillomatosis in children: masquerader of common respiratory diseases. Pediatrics 2006;118(5): 1925–31.

142. John SD, Swischuk LE. Stridor and upper airway obstruction in infants and children. Radiographics 1992;12(4):625–43 [discussion: 644].

143. Kawanami T, Bowen A. Juvenile laryngeal papillomatosis with pulmonary parenchymal spread. Case report and review of the literature. Pediatr Radiol 1985;15(2):102–4.

144. Kramer SS, Wehunt WD, Stocker JT, et al. Pulmonary manifestations of juvenile laryngotracheal papillomatosis. AJR Am J Roentgenol 1985; 144(4):687–94.

145. Majoros M, Parkhill EM, Devine KD. Papilloma of the larynx in children. A clinicopathologic study. Am J Surg 1964;108:470–5.

146. Lindeberg H, Elbrond O. Malignant tumours in patients with a history of multiple laryngeal papillomas: the significance of irradiation. Clin Otolaryngol Allied Sci 1991;16(2):149–51.

147. Ruan SY, Chen KY, Yang PC. Recurrent respiratory papillomatosis with pulmonary involvement: a case report and review of the literature. Respirology 2009;14(1):137–40.

148. Chang CH, Wang HC, Wu MT, et al. Virtual bronchoscopy for diagnosis of recurrent respiratory papillomatosis. J Formos Med Assoc 2006;105(6): 508–11.

149. Xue Q, Wang H, Wang J. Recurrent respiratory papillomatosis: an overview. Eur J Clin Microbiol Infect Dis 2010;29(9):1051–4.

150. Ongkasuwan J, Friedman EM. Juvenile recurrent respiratory papilloma: variable intersurgical intervals. Laryngoscope 2012;122(12):2844–9.

151. Wiatrak BJ, Wiatrak DW, Broker TR, et al. Recurrent respiratory papillomatosis: a longitudinal study comparing severity associated with human papilloma viral types 6 and 11 and other risk factors in a large pediatric population. Laryngoscope 2004; 114(11 Pt 2 Suppl 104):1–23.

152. Koplewitz BZ, Springer C, Slasky BS, et al. CT of hemangiomas of the upper airways in children. AJR Am J Roentgenol 2005;184(2):663–70.

153. Holinger PH, Brown WT. Congenital webs, cysts, laryngoceles and other anomalies of the larynx. Ann Otol Rhinol Laryngol 1967;76(4):744–52.

154. Shikhani AH, Jones MM, Marsh BR, et al. Infantile subglottic hemangiomas. An update. Ann Otol Rhinol Laryngol 1986;95(4 Pt 1):336–47.

155. Blei F. Vascular anomalies: from bedside to bench and back again. Curr Probl Pediatr Adolesc Health Care 2002;32(3):72–93.

156. Orlow SJ, Isakoff MS, Blei F. Increased risk of symptomatic hemangiomas of the airway in association with cutaneous hemangiomas in a "beard" distribution. J Pediatr 1997;131(4):643–6.

157. Sutton TJ, Nogrady MB. Radiologic diagnosis of subglottic hemangioma in infants. Pediatr Radiol 1973;1(4):211–6.

158. Cooper M, Slovis TL, Madgy DN, et al. Congenital subglottic hemangioma: frequency of symmetric subglottic narrowing on frontal radiographs of the neck. AJR Am J Roentgenol 1992;159(6): 1269–71.

159. Rutter MJ. Evaluation and management of upper airway disorders in children. Semin Pediatr Surg 2006;15(2):116–23.

160. Bajaj Y, Hartley BE, Wyatt ME, et al. Subglottic haemangioma in children: experience with open surgical excision. J Laryngol Otol 2006;120(12): 1033–7.

161. Chen D, Ryan G, Edwards M. Bronchial sleeve resection for a patient with an inflammatory pseudotumour. ANZ J Surg 2001;71(3):187–9.

162. Hoseok I, Joungho H, Ahn KM, et al. Complete surgical resection of inflammatory myofibroblastic tumor with carinal reconstruction in a 4-year-old boy. J Pediatr Surg 2005;40(12):e23–5.

163. Maeda M, Matsuzaki Y, Edagawa M, et al. Successful treatment of a bronchial inflammatory pseudotumor by bronchoplasty in an 8-year-old boy: report of a case. Surg Today 2000;30(5):465–8.

164. Uchida DA, Hawkins JA, Coffin CM, et al. Inflammatory myofibroblastic tumor in the airway of a child. Ann Thorac Surg 2009;87(2):610–3.

165. Boloursaz MR, Khalilzadeh S, Dezfoli AA, et al. Inflammatory myofibroblastic tumor of the trachea. Pediatr Surg Int 2011;27(8):895–7.

166. Bellah RD, Mahboubi S, Berdon WE. Malignant endobronchial lesions of adolescence. Pediatr Radiol 1992;22(8):563–7.

167. Hurt R, Bates M. Carcinoid tumours of the bronchus: a 33 year experience. Thorax 1984;39(8): 617–23.

168. Bagheri R, Mashhadi M, Haghi SZ, et al. Tracheobronchopulmonary carcinoid tumors: analysis of 40 patients. Ann Thorac Cardiovasc Surg 2011; 17(1):7–12.

169. Torres AM, Ryckman FC. Childhood tracheobronchial mucoepidermoid carcinoma: a case report and review of the literature. J Pediatr Surg 1988; 23(4):367–70.

170. Leiberman A, Bar-Ziv J, Zirkin HJ. Low grade mucoepidermoid tumour of the bronchus in childhood: a therapeutic dilemma. Eur J Pediatr 1986; 145(1–2):130–2.

171. Kim TS, Lee KS, Han J, et al. Mucoepidermoid carcinoma of the tracheobronchial tree: radiographic and CT findings in 12 patients. Radiology 1999; 212(3):643–8.

172. Desai DP, Holinger LD, Gonzalez-Crussi F. Tracheal neoplasms in children. Ann Otol Rhinol Laryngol 1998;107(9 Pt 1):790–6.

173. Lee EY, Vargas SO, Sawicki GS, et al. Mucoepidermoid carcinoma of bronchus in a pediatric patient: (18)F-FDG PET findings. Pediatr Radiol 2007; 37(12):1278–82.

Vascular Anomalies in Pediatric Patients
Updated Classification, Imaging, and Therapy

Ramya Kollipara, BA[a], Ashika Odhav, BA[a],
Kenny E. Rentas, MD[b], Douglas C. Rivard, DO[c],
Lisa H. Lowe, MD[c],*, Laura Dinneen, MD[c]

KEYWORDS

- Vascular anomalies • Pediatric patients • Classification • Imaging • Therapy

KEY POINTS

- The International Society for the Study of Vascular Anomalies classifies vascular anomalies into 2 categories: vascular neoplasms and vascular malformations.
- It has been widely adopted by various pediatric subspecialists, because it reliably correlates patient presentation and disease progression, with more accurate histology, diagnosis, imaging, and treatment.

INTRODUCTION

Recent advances in knowledge regarding histopathology, cause, and treatment of pediatric vascular anomalies have led to substantial changes in classification and terminology. Over the past 2 decades, various subspecialists have adopted a new classification system proposed by the International Society for the Study of Vascular Anomalies (ISSVA), which divides vascular anomalies into 2 main categories: neoplasms and malformations.[1] This system provides a systematic approach to vascular malformations that correlates histopathology with clinical course and therapy. However, the inconsistent use of the new system, as well as use of older terms, continues to cause confusion in the medical community.[2]

The need for uniformity has become important to prevent misdiagnosis and inaccurate management. This review article has 2 aims: first, to review the ISSVA classification of vascular anomalies by discussing representative lesions in each category, including their histopathogenesis, essential imaging features, and current treatment approach; second, to clarify the nomenclature used in the ISSVA system compared with previous classification systems.

CURRENT CLASSIFICATION AND NOMENCLATURE OF VASCULAR ANOMALIES

The binary classification system for vascular anomalies was originally introduced in 1982 by Mulliken and Glowacki and later, adopted and

[a] University of Missouri-Kansas City SOM, Kansas City, MO 64108, USA; [b] Department of Radiology, Saint Luke's Hospital and The University of Missouri-Kansas City, 4401 Wornall Road, Kansas City, MO 64112, USA; [c] Department of Radiology, Children's Mercy Hospital and Clinics and The University of Missouri-Kansas City, 2401 Gillham Road, Kansas City, MO 64108, USA
* Corresponding author.
E-mail address: lhlowe@cmh.edu

Radiol Clin N Am 51 (2013) 659–672
http://dx.doi.org/10.1016/j.rcl.2013.04.002

revised by the ISSVA in 1996.[1-3] This system, which is now widely accepted by pediatric subspecialists who care for children with these anomalies, divides anomalies into 2 major histopathologic categories: vasoproliferative (or vascular) neoplasms and vascular malformations (Table 1).[1,3] The key distinction between the 2 groups is the presence or absence of increased endothelial cell turnover (mitosis). Vascular neoplasms have mitosis, and vascular malformations do not. Vascular malformations are congenitally malformed capillary, lymphatic, venous, and arterial vessels.[1] Growth of vasoproliferative neoplasms is caused by mitotic activity leading to an increased number of cells within the lesion. Conversely, vascular malformations grow with the child and may enlarge as a result of vessel distention caused by hemorrhage, infection, or inflammation.[4] The ISSVA system classifies hemangiomas, the most common vascular neoplasm, as infantile or congenital based on histopathologic markers and age of presentation. Specifically, infantile hemangiomas are positive for the glucose 1 transporter protein (GLUT1+) and congenital hemangiomas are glucose 1 transporter protein negative (GLUT1−).[5] Because most hemangiomas are not biopsied, the age of presentation is critical. Although infantile hemangiomas typically present from 2 weeks to 2 months of age, all congenital hemangiomas are present on day 1 of life.[4]

The new classification system includes changes in terminology that have focused on replacing misleading terms with descriptors that more accurately reflect the pathologic findings and lesion clinical course. In the past, the term hemangioma has been used to describe a variety of vascular malformations that present in adults, do not proliferate or involute, and have no mitosis (are not neoplasms). On histopathology, these GLUT1− lesions are proved to be primarily venous malformations rather than neoplasms. Specifically, the lesions formerly described as vertebral, hepatic, and intraosseous hemangiomas are all now GLUT1− pathologically proved venous malformations, composed of malformed venous channels.[6] Similarly, the term cavernous hemangioma has been removed from the new classification system, because it is not a GLUT1+ neoplasm, but is composed of malformed vessels, thus is a vascular malformation.[5,7] Nonneoplastic lesions composed of malformed lymphatic channels that contain the suffix -oma (cystic hygroma and lymphangioma), which erroneously implies neoplasm, have been replaced with the more accurate term lymphatic malformation.[8] Similarly, the nonneoplastic lesion termed cavernoma is also a venous malformation.[9]

Table 1
ISSVA classification system and treatment of vascular anomalies

Vascular Anomaly	Treatment
Vascular Neoplasms	
Infantile hemangioma	Ranges from conservative observation, propanolol or steroids to vincristine, embolization, and liver transplant (rare)
Congenital hemangioma	
RICH	Same treatment as infantile hemangiomas
NICH	Surgical resection
Hemangioendothelioma: all variants such as kaposiform, spindle cell, epithelioid	Surgical resection and/or chemotherapy depending on the specific pathology
Angiosarcoma	Surgical resection or chemotherapy depending on the specific pathology
Vascular Malformations	
Slow flow	
Lymphatic	Sclerotherapy
Venous	Surgery
Venolymphatic	Sclerotherapy and/or surgery
Fast-flow arterial abnormalities	
AVM, AVF, and combined vascular malformations	Embolization and/or surgery

Abbreviations: AVF, arteriovenous fistula; AVM, arteriovenous malformation; NICH, noninvoluting congenital hemangioma; RICH, rapidly involuting congenital hemangioma.

IMAGING TECHNIQUES

Typically, the diagnosis of vascular anomalies is made clinically. However, imaging is used to clarify difficult cases and aid in the planning of potential endovascular or surgical intervention. The choice of imaging modality varies based on the clinical scenario and specific lesion; the 3 main noninvasive imaging modalities used are ultrasonography (US), magnetic resonance (MR) imaging, and computed tomography (CT).[10,11]

US is often used as the initial screening study, because of its wide availability and ease of performance, without requirement for sedation or ionizing radiation. Use of color and spectral Doppler in addition to longitudinal and transverse grayscale imaging allows interrogation of lesion vascularity and type of vessels present. Probe selection depends on anatomic location of the lesion. Vascular anomalies that are most amenable to sonography include small superficial and solid visceral lesions. In general, sonography can be used to determine the type of lesion present, which is useful to guide initial therapy, and plan further imaging evaluation.[11–13] Also, sonography may be used during image-guided biopsy and intervention in some cases.[14]

CT and MR imaging are useful to evaluate the extent of larger lesions and their relationships to adjacent structures before treatment.[11] CT, particularly multidetector CT, is advantageous, because of its fast speed, wide availability, and decreased requirement for sedation. It is especially useful in situations requiring urgent imaging and lesions with osseous involvement.[13] Care must be taken in children to use as little ionizing radiation as possible closely, following the ALARA (As Low As Reasonably Achievable) principle. To achieve a low radiation dose, the coverage of the CT study should be limited only to the region of interest and multiphase imaging must be avoided. Contrast is typically used for assessing the vascular component of lesions. MR imaging and time-resolved MR angiography techniques also help characterize pertinent vascular anatomy.[15] Specific MR imaging protocols depend on the type of vascular anomaly suspected and its location. However, in general, lesions are imaged to determine lesion extent using multiplanar T1, T2, inversion recovery, and gradient echo techniques with contrast administration. Fat suppression is used liberally as well. Diffusion and susceptibility imaging may help narrow the differential diagnosis.

Radiography may show organomegaly, calcifications, soft tissue masses, and osseous changes. Angiography, although rarely performed, can reflect the histopathology of the vascular lesions, including providing the necessary information to differentiate hemangiomas (organized, glandlike neoplasms with parenchymal involvement) from malformations, which are abnormal vessels without parenchymal staining.[8]

SPECTRUM OF IMAGING FINDINGS
Vascular Neoplasms

Several representative vascular neoplasms are discussed herein, including infantile hemangiomas, congenital hemangiomas (rapidly involuting congenital hemangiomas [RICH], and noninvoluting congenital hemangiomas [NICH]), kaposiform hemangioendotheliomas (KHs), and angiosarcoma.[16,17] Vascular anomalies, including tufted angioma, hemangiopericytoma, and various types of hemangioendotheliomas are usually diagnosed with biopsy rather than imaging and are not discussed further.

Theories and observations related to vascular tumor origin

Vascular neoplasms result from vasculogenesis (primitive blood vessels arising from angioblasts) rather than angiogenesis (proliferation of vessels from previously existing vessels), as previously believed.[9,10,18] A cellular marker that supports this process is the presence of vascular endothelial growth factor, which is increased in proliferating rather than involuting hemangiomas.[19–21] Involuting vascular tumors histologically show amplified apoptosis of vascular lumens, stem cell differentiation into adipose cells, and mast cells.[4,22,23]

One hypothesis on the origin of hemangiomas indicates that they arise from embolized placental tissue. This hypothesis is supported by the observation that a higher rate of hemangiomas arise in infants who have undergone in utero procedures, as well as the fact that the life cycle of placental tissue and hemangiomas is similar.[17,19,22,24] Furthermore, the placenta is the only tissue in the human body that expresses the GLUT1 protein, which is also found in infantile hemangiomas.[4,25] Congenital hemangiomas are GLUT1−, a difference that may be caused by somatic mutations and differences in the fetal environment.[18,26–29] Transformation of RICH into NICH and combined congenital and infantile hemangiomas has been described.[4,27] Other recent theories suggest that hemangiomas arise in segmental or regional distributions along embryonic prominences and fusion lines, where a great amount of neuromesenchyme is present, such as the head and neck.[22,29,30] Neuromesenchyme promotes spread of hemangioblasts to these sites.[22]

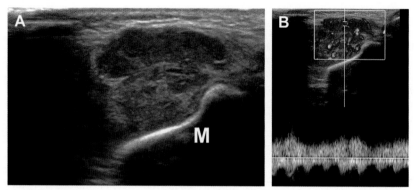

Fig. 1. Infantile hemangioma in a 2-month-old girl with swelling at the angle of the mandible (M). Longitudinal (*A*) grayscale and (*B*) Doppler sonographic images reveal a well-defined, solid, hypervascular mass with internal arterial and venous wave forms.

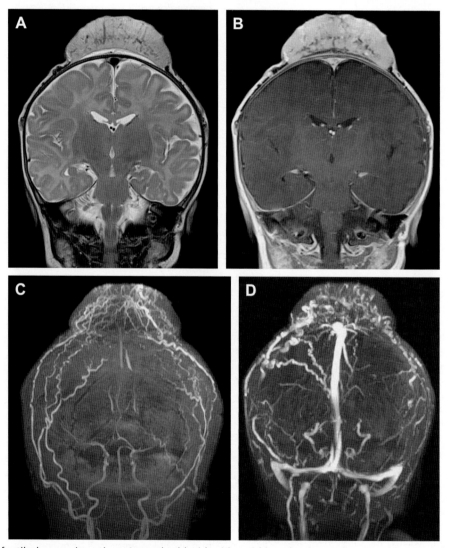

Fig. 2. Infantile hemangioma in a 4-month-old girl with quickly enlarging scalp mass since 2 weeks of age. Coronal (*A*) T2-weighted and (*B*) fat-suppressed T1-postcontrast enhanced MR images reveal a well-defined, hyperintense, vigorously enhancing scalp mass with multiple internal flow voids. (*C*) MR arteriogram shows a markedly hypervascular mass, which is supplied by innumerable external carotid artery branches. (*D*) Similarly, MR venogram reveals numerous prominent draining veins.

Infantile hemangioma

Although the presentation of infantile hemangiomas can be variable, they present most often in premature White females between 2 weeks and 2 months of life.[31–33] They can be single (31%), multiple (10%–25%), regional, segmental, or diffuse and occur most frequently on the skin or in the liver.[33–35] Associated liver lesions are found in 31% of infants with cutaneous hemangiomas,[35] and the most common cutaneous sites are the head, neck, trunk, and extremities.[22,33] Previously, hemangiomas had been reported as intraosseous in location.[27] However, these GLUT1− lesions have been pathologically reclassified as venous malformations (discussed later).[6,36]

Hemangiomas have 2 predictable phases of growth: (1) rapid growth (proliferative phase) up to 1 year of age, and (2) regression (involution phase), occurring from age 1 to 8 years, with gradual resolution of any remaining disease in some children after 8 years of age.[14,20,37]

Most infantile hemangiomas are diagnosed clinically.[1,2] If imaging is required, color Doppler US with spectral interrogation is useful to obtain an initial diagnosis without sedation or radiation exposure. In small, superficial lesions, US may be sufficient (**Fig. 1**). More frequently, MR is

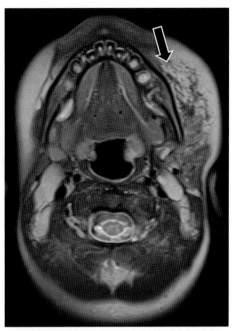

Fig. 3. Involuting infantile hemangioma in a 6-year-old boy. Axial T2-weighted MR image shows poorly defined T2 hypointense stranding through the left cheek subcutaneous fat anterior to the parotid gland (*arrow*).

Table 2
Summary of US and MR imaging features of vascular anomalies

	Vascular Neoplasms	Slow-Flow Malformations	Fast-Flow Malformations
Grayscale US	Well-defined Solid Mixed echogenicity	Venous: multispatial, compressible, solid, echogenic, phleboliths Lymphatic: multispatial, multicystic ± fluid ± debris Venolymphatic: combined features	Cluster of vessels Little if any solid mass
Doppler US	Arterial and venous spectra Hypervascular	Venous: venous waveforms Lymphatic: venous flow in septae Venolymphatic: combined features	Arterial and venous waveforms Arterialization of venous waveforms
MR imaging	T1 intermediate intensity T2 hyperintense Vigorously enhancing Intralesional flow voids	Venous: heterogeneous, intermediate intensity on T1, no flow voids, high intensity on T2, enhance Lymphatic: low to intermediate intensity on T1W, high intensity on T2W, Enhancement only in septae Venolymphatic: combined features	Serpiginous flow voids on T1W and T2W Little if any solid mass

Abbreviations: T1W, T1-weighted; T2W, T2-weighted.

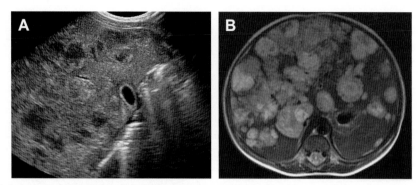

Fig. 4. Multiple hepatic infantile hemangiomas in a 4-month-old girl with several cutaneous hemangiomas. (*A*) Transverse grayscale sonogram of the liver shows multiple well-circumscribed, variable sized, hypoechoic hepatic masses. Lesions were hypervascular on color Doppler (*not shown*). (*B*) Axial T2-weighted MR image confirms multiple well-defined, T2 hyperintense masses containing flow voids scattered throughout the liver. Splenic lesions are noted as well.

required to better portray lesion extent. CT can be used to evaluate lesions that may require emergent intervention.[4,33,38]

Cross-sectional imaging typically shows single or multiple, lobulated, highly vascular, enhancing masses with internal flow voids containing arterial and venous spectra on Doppler sonography (**Fig. 2**). During involution, infantile hemangiomas become gradually more heterogeneous as a result of apoptosis and fatty replacement (**Fig. 3**).[4] **Table 2** summarizes imaging findings in vascular lesions.

The main differential diagnosis for multiple infantile hemangiomas, especially with extensive hepatic involvement, is metastatic neuroblastoma (**Fig. 4**).[38] In the past, multiphase CT or MR imaging was recommended for diagnosis based on pattern of enhancement. However, enhancement patterns in infantile hemangiomas are nonspecific and unreliable.[38] Performance of multiphasic CT should be avoided in children because of high ionizing radiation doses.[1,2] Instead, urine catecholamines should be collected and abdominal sonography performed to search for an adrenal mass.

Management of infantile hemangiomas varies widely depending on the patient's symptoms, which are influenced by the location and number of lesions. Conservative management with observation is the mainstay for uncomplicated hemangiomas.[39–42] Skin ulceration is the most common complication identified, and is usually managed

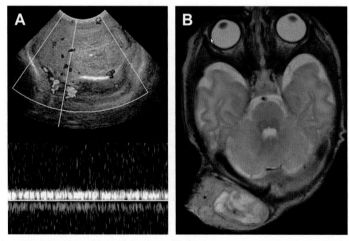

Fig. 5. RICH in a 1-day-old girl with scalp mass seen on third-trimester prenatal sonogram. (*A*) Axial color Doppler sonogram with spectral tracing shows a vascular mass with venous waveforms. Arterial wave forms are also present within the lesion (*not shown*). (*B*) Axial T2-weighted MR image reveals a well-defined T2 hyperintense right-sided posterior occipital scalp mass.

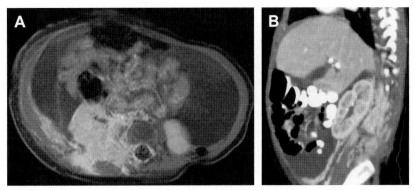

Fig. 6. Kaposiform hemangioendothelioma in a 1-day-old girl with a blanching nonpulsatile abdominal wall mass. Axial (A) and (B) sagittal contrast-enhanced CT images show an ill-defined, vigorously enhancing infiltrative mass involving the right paraspinous soft tissues. The lesion involves the iliopsoas muscle, erector spinae muscle, and paraspinous and subcutaneous fat and extends into the adjacent spinal canal.

with laser therapy.[13] Other complications include thrombocytopenia, heart failure, respiratory compromise, hypothyroidism, and hemorrhage. Depending on severity, treatment of complications range from antiangiogenic drugs (propranolol and steroids more so than vincristine), to embolization, surgery, and rarely, liver transplant.[13,43–45]

Congenital hemangioma

In contrast to infantile hemangiomas, congenital hemangiomas are GLUT1− and are present at birth.[33,46] Congenital hemangiomas begin their proliferative growth phase in utero and thus can be detected on prenatal imaging.[46–48] They are divided into 2 subtypes based on their clinical

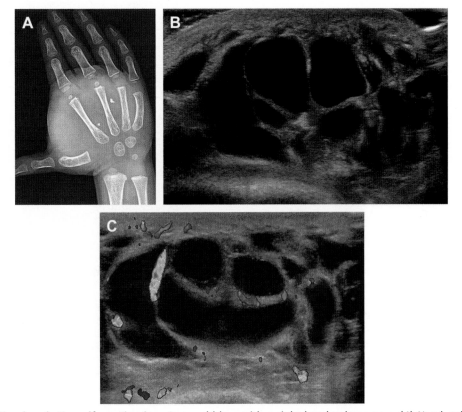

Fig. 7. Venolymphatic malformation in a 4-year-old boy with a right hand palmar mass. (A) Hand radiograph shows 2 calcified phleboliths on either side of the second metacarpal bone. Longitudinal (B) grayscale and (C) color Doppler sonographic images of the mass show a multicystic mass with flow in the septations of the lesion.

course: (1) RICH and NICH.[16,17,27] Although RICH regress quickly by 1 to 2 years of age, NICH remain stable or gradually increase in size. Because biopsy of congenital hemangiomas is typically deferred, the lesions are classified based on their presentation and clinical course.[27]

On imaging, congenital hemangiomas are similar to infantile hemangiomas (**Fig. 5**).[4] Imaging features of RICH and NICH have been described, including heterogeneity (62.5% vs 72%), visible vessels (62.5% vs 72%), and calcifications (37.5% vs 17%), respectively.[49] Angiography of RICH shows well-defined, deeply stained lobules encompassed by large systemic arteries, but is rarely a component of the currently recommended diagnostic workup.[45]

Because RICH tend to regress over time, management is similar to that of infantile hemangioma.[50,51] Conversely, surgery is often needed for NICH, because they do not regress.[51]

Kaposiform hemangioendothelioma

KH is a vascular neoplasm that histologically consists of GLUT1− nodules of vascular and lymphatic vessels. KH commonly presents shortly after birth, usually on the trunk, extremities, head, neck, and retroperitoneum, with spread to neighboring lymph nodes and soft tissue structures. Metastases to distant sites are extremely rare.[52] KH, if arising as part of Kasabach-Merritt syndrome, can present in conjunction with consumptive coagulopathy secondary to platelet sequestration, leading to thrombocytopenia.[53] Key imaging features of KH reveal large, infiltrative, poorly defined, multinodular, vascular lesions (**Fig. 6**). KHs tend to be large and contain multiple draining vessels with striking internal flow voids.[33] They have a poor prognosis and are difficult to treat.[42] When KH presents without Kasabach-Merritt syndrome, management ranges from wide local excision to embolization to supportive care.[54,55]

Angiosarcoma

Angiosarcomas are rare vascular neoplasms of the liver that confer a poor prognosis despite treatment. These tumors commonly arise in females, with an average age of presentation of 3.7 years. Eight of 38 cases reported before 2008 occurred in combination with hemangiomas.[35] Angiosarcomas are heterogeneous on imaging and usually present with significant enhancement, with lakes of contrast pooling.[4] Multiple synchronous primary hepatic tumors or metastases may occur.[35]

Vascular Malformations

Vascular malformations, the second major category in the ISSVA classification, are congenital

lesions that often present at birth, but can present at any age. Even although they may not be clinically recognized until later in life, they tend to grow in proportion to the child, and do not regress.[8] Spontaneous enlargement can occur secondary to arteriovenous communications, thrombosis, trauma, hormonal changes, internal hemorrhage, and infection.[8] Vascular malformations are subdivided into slow-flow versus fast-flow (or low-flow vs high-flow) malformations. Slow-flow (or low-flow) malformations encompass vessels of capillary, lymphatic, or venous origin. In contrast, fast (or high) flow denotes an arterial origin mixed with other vascular components.[1] Capillary components of vascular malformations involve the superficial layers of the skin and are better visualized on physical examination than imaging. Because of the lack of imaging findings, capillary malformations are not discussed further.[1]

Slow-flow malformations

Slow-flow malformations consist of congenitally malformed venous or lymphatic vessels.[16] These lesions are differentiated from neoplasms because they are GLUT1− and do not have mitoses (are not

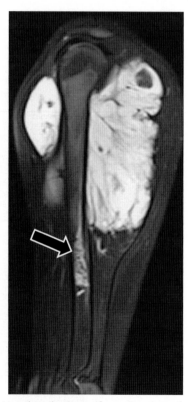

Fig. 8. Venolymphatic malformation in a 4-year-old girl with right arm pain and swelling. Sagittal T2-weighted fat-suppressed MR image reveals a multispatial, mixed solid and multicystic lesion with phleboliths and intraosseous extension (*arrow*).

neoplasms).[6,36] Often, these malformations affect the face, limbs and trunk, followed by internal viscera, bones, and skeletal muscle.[36,56] The clinical presentation varies depending on size, location, and age of onset.[14] Typical clinical features include sudden, sometimes painful, masses, which are easily compressible and increase in size with Valsalva and change in position.[13]

Imaging of slow-flow anomalies begins with color Doppler sonography, with interrogation to characterize the lesion. Lesions can be described as mostly solid (venous), multicystic (lymphatic), and multispatial with venous wave forms (**Fig. 7**).[16] Additional MR imaging is often needed to determine severity and extent of involvement to help guide therapy and determine need for intervention (**Figs. 8** and **9**). Calcifications within slow-flow vascular lesions (phleboliths) can be seen on radiography and, more often, on MR imaging. See **Table 2** for summarized imaging findings.[10,16]

Treatment plans vary based on lesion location and effects on the surrounding structures. Many slow-flow malformations are managed conservatively with observation when small. Compression garments may be used in some cases to relieve pain and swelling. When the lesion is harmful because of its location, is rapidly enlarging, is causing a significant cosmetic deformity, or is causing possible increased morbidity by affecting surrounding structures (eg, airway compression), invasive treatments may be considered. Sclerotherapy is the most common form of treatment, for both venous and lymphatic malformations, sometimes requiring multiple sessions based on response to therapy and recurrence of symptoms.[57,58]

High-flow vascular malformations

High-flow malformations contain arterial and venous structures clustered together without an intervening solid mass. They are subdivided into 2 groups based on their origin and anatomy as arteriovenous malformations (AVM) and arteriovenous fistulas (AVF). On clinical examination, they present as warm pink patches associated with a thrill on palpation or vascular murmur on auscultation.[13] These lesions can present with complications of pain, hemorrhage, ulceration, or ischemic changes and, in some cases, increase risk for congestive heart failure, seizure, and neurologic complaints, depending on location.[59]

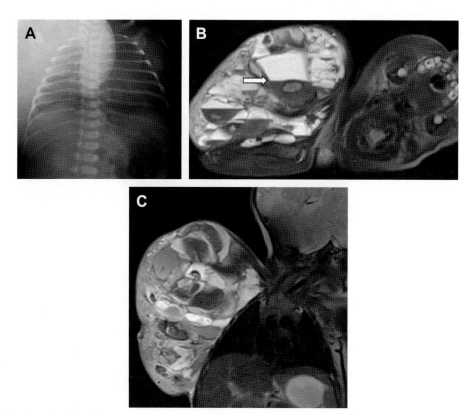

Fig. 9. Venolymphatic malformation in a 1-day-old boy with in utero identification of neck mass. (*A*) Chest radiograph shows a large soft tissue mass over the right neck and chest. (*B*) Axial and (*C*) coronal T2-weighted fat-suppressed MR images reveal a large multispatial, mixed solid and multicystic mass containing scattered fluid-fluid levels (*arrow*).

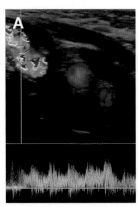
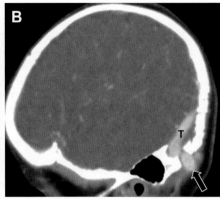
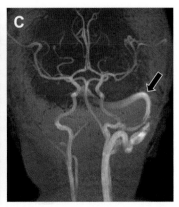

Fig. 10. AVF in a 6-month-old boy with a left retroauricular pulsatile thrill. (*A*) Color Doppler sonogram with spectral tracing shows a tortuous tubular vessel in the left retroauricular scalp with high-velocity pulsatile flow. (*B*) Sagittal reconstructed CT angiogram confirms the large artery (*straight arrow*) seen on sonography and shows communication with the transverse sinus (T) via the occipital bone. (*C*) Frontal image from a three-dimensional time-of-flight MR angiogram confirms a large artery over the left ear with early venous filling of the left transverse sinus (*arrow*) and jugular vein.

On histologic examination, both subtypes are made of dysplastic arteries that drain into arterialized veins in absence of capillary beds.[23]

AVMs are congenital lesions that contain a nidus between the arterial and venous components. These lesions are commonly seen in the muscle, subcutaneous fat, bone, and cranium. AVMs can present as single or multiple lesions, and can be associated with a genetic disorder. In contrast, AVFs do not contain a nidus, are often acquired, and are more commonly found in the brain.[13]

With high-flow lesions, Doppler US, MR imaging, and contrast-enhanced CT are often used. Similar to other vascular anomalies, US is the best initial test and can provide information to make a diagnosis and plan for further treatment, followed by CT or MR imaging with angiography, to determine the severity and extent of the lesion (**Figs. 10** and **11**). AVMs and AVFs are hypervascular and often multispatial. CT has the advantage of rapid evaluation and identification of bone involvement, whereas MR imaging does not require ionizing radiation exposure. All cross-sectional imaging studies show a cluster of vessels with no intervening solid mass.[10]

Before therapy for high-flow malformations, angiography is helpful to assess the lesion vascularity. Embolization, followed by surgery, is most commonly used.[13] Combination therapies are often used, especially in children.[17,25]

Regional Associations and Diffuse Syndromes

Typically, vascular anomalies appear as a solitary lesion, but physicians should be aware of their tendency toward regional and diffuse involvement. Treatment of regional and diffuse syndromes

varies based on symptoms, type of vascular lesion and involved anatomy.[10,19,24] Regional syndromes include several associated vascular malformations that occur in a segmental or regional distribution. Common examples include Sturge-Weber, Klippel-Trénaunay, and Parkes Weber syndromes, in which imaging findings are regional, often affecting a dermatomal distribution (**Fig. 12**). Some regional and diffuse syndromes, for example, PHACES (posterior fossa malformations, hemangiomas, arterial anomalies, cardiac defects,

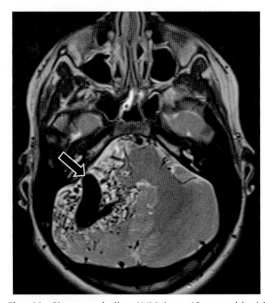

Fig. 11. Giant cerebellar AVM in a 12-year-old girl found incidentally during a trauma workup. Axial T2-weighted MR image shows multiple intra-axial and extra-axial vascular channels with a central large caliber draining venous flow void (*arrow*).

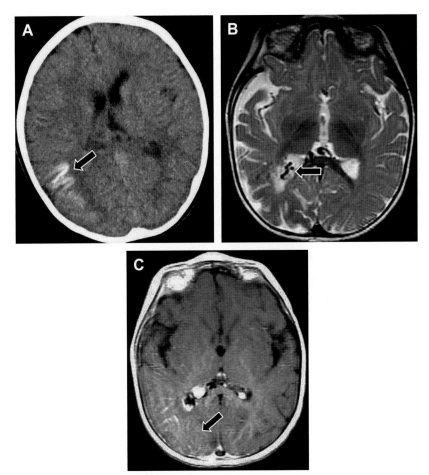

Fig. 12. Sturge-Weber syndrome in a 5-year-old boy with worsening seizures. (*A*) Axial CT image reveals right parietal gyriform calcification (*arrow*). Axial (*B*) T2-weighted and (*C*) postcontrast enhanced T1-weighted images show right cerebral atrophy and an enlarged choroid plexus containing a large draining vein (*arrow*). Choroid plexus and leptomeningeal enhancement (*arrow*) of the right parieto-occipital lobe are also shown.

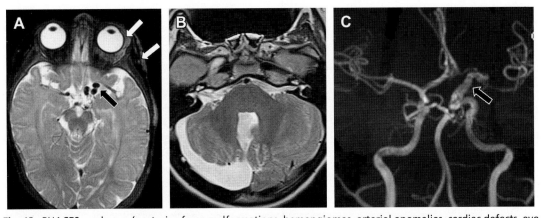

Fig. 13. PHACES syndrome (posterior fossa malformations, hemangiomas, arterial anomalies, cardiac defects, eye abnormalities, sternal cleft, and supraumbilical raphe syndrome) in a 10-year-old girl with a slowly resolving left facial hemangioma. (*A*) Axial fat-suppressed T2-weighted MR image through the orbital roof shows a hyperintense mass in the left lateral orbit that extends into the left subcutaneous fat (*white arrows*). An ectatic tortuous supraclinoid internal carotid artery (*black arrow*) is also seen. (*B*) Axial T2-weighted image through the posterior fossa reveals right cerebellar and vermian hypoplasia. (*C*) Three-dimensional time-of-flight MR arteriogram confirms ectasia of the left internal carotid artery (*arrow*).

eye abnormalities, sternal cleft, and supraumbilical raphe syndrome) and LUMBAR (lower body hemangiomas, urogenital anomalies, myelopathy, bony deformities, anorectal and arterial anomalies, renal anomalies) syndromes, include several anomalies as well as associated vascular neoplasms (**Fig. 13**).[10,24]

Diffuse syndromes are combinations of vascular malformations that occur with fast-flow and slow-flow anomalies. These vascular lesions can be found throughout the body. Although a complete discussion is beyond the scope of this manuscript, some common examples of diffuse syndromes include hereditary hemorrhagic telangiectasia and epidermal nevus syndrome, which are listed along with the category of associated vascular malformation in **Box 1**.[10,24]

SUMMARY

The ISSVA classification of vascular anomalies divides vascular anomalies into 2 categories: vascular neoplasms and vascular malformations. It has been widely adopted by various pediatric subspecialists, because it reliably correlates patient presentation and disease progression, with more accurate histology, diagnosis, imaging, and treatment.

Box 1
Summary of regional and diffuse syndromes

Regional syndromes with associated vascular neoplasms

PHACES

- Posterior fossa abnormalities
- Hemangioma in cranial nerve 5 distribution
- Intracranial arterial anomalies
- Cardiac anomalies or coarctation of aorta
- Eye anomalies
- Sternal defects

LUMBAR

- Lower body hemangiomas
- Urogenital anomalies
- Myelopathy
- Bony deformities
- Anorectal and arterial anomalies
- Renal anomalies

Regional syndromes without associated vascular neoplasms

Sturge-Weber

Klippel-Trénaunay

Parkes Weber

Diffuse syndromes

Associated with fast-flow malformations

- Hereditary hemorrhagic telangiectasia (Osler-Weber-Rendu)

Associated with slow-flow malformations

- Proteus syndrome
- Blue rubber bleb nevus syndrome
- Bannayan-Riley-Ruvalcaba syndrome

REFERENCES

1. Mulliken JB, Glowacki J. Hemangiomas and vascular malformations in infants and children: a classification based on endothelial characteristics. Plast Reconstr Surg 1982;69(3):412–22.
2. Hassanein AH, Mulliken JB, Fishman SJ, et al. Evaluation of terminology for vascular anomalies in current literature. Plast Reconstr Surg 2011;127(1): 347–51.
3. Mulliken JB, Glowacki J. Classification of pediatric vascular lesions. Plast Reconstr Surg 1982;70(1): 120–1.
4. Lowe LH, Marchant TC, Rivard DC, et al. Vascular malformations: classification and terminology the radiologist needs to know. Semin Roentgenol 2012;47(2):106–17.
5. Hand JL, Frieden IJ. Vascular birthmarks of infancy: resolving nosologic confusion. Am J Med Genet 2002;108(4):257–64.
6. Greene AK, Rogers GF, Mulliken JB. Intraosseous "hemangiomas" are malformations and not tumors. Plast Reconstr Surg 2007;119(6):1949–50 [author reply: 1950].
7. Frieden IJ, Haggstrom AN, Drolet BA, et al. Infantile hemangiomas: current knowledge, future directions. Proceedings of a research workshop on infantile hemangiomas, April 7-9, 2005, Bethesda, Maryland, USA. Pediatr Dermatol 2005;22(5):383–406.
8. Burrows PE, Mulliken JB, Fellows KE, et al. Childhood hemangiomas and vascular malformations: angiographic differentiation. AJR Am J Roentgenol 1983;141(3):483–8.
9. Nguyen VA, Furhapter C, Romani N, et al. Infantile hemangioma is a proliferation of beta 4-negative endothelial cells adjacent to HLA-DR-positive cells with dendritic cell morphology. Hum Pathol 2004; 35(6):739–44.
10. Cohen MM Jr. Vasculogenesis, angiogenesis, hemangiomas, and vascular malformations. Am J Med Genet 2002;108(4):265–74.
11. Dubois J, Garel L. Imaging and therapeutic approach of hemangiomas and vascular

malformations in the pediatric age group. Pediatr Radiol 1999;29(12):879–93.

12. Dubois J, Patriquin HB, Garel L, et al. Soft-tissue hemangiomas in infants and children: diagnosis using Doppler sonography. AJR Am J Roentgenol 1998;171(1):247–52.

13. Legiehn GM, Heran MK. Classification, diagnosis, and interventional radiologic management of vascular malformations. Orthop Clin North Am 2006;37(3):435–74, vii–viii.

14. Legiehn GM, Heran MK. Venous malformations: classification, development, diagnosis, and interventional radiologic management. Radiol Clin North Am 2008;46(3):545–97, vi.

15. Kim JS, Chandler A, Borzykowski R, et al. Maximizing time-resolved MRA for differentiation of hemangiomas, vascular malformations and vascularized tumors. Pediatr Radiol 2012;42(7): 775–84.

16. Eifert S, Villavicencio JL, Kao TC, et al. Prevalence of deep venous anomalies in congenital vascular malformations of venous predominance. J Vasc Surg 2000;31(3):462–71.

17. North PE, Waner M, Mizeracki A, et al. A unique microvascular phenotype shared by juvenile hemangiomas and human placenta. Arch Dermatol 2001;137(5):559–70.

18. Boye E, Yu Y, Paranya G, et al. Clonality and altered behavior of endothelial cells from hemangiomas. J Clin Invest 2001;107(6):745–52.

19. Ritter MR, Dorrell MI, Edmonds J, et al. Insulin-like growth factor 2 and potential regulators of hemangioma growth and involution identified by large-scale expression analysis. Proc Natl Acad Sci U S A 2002;99(11):7455–60.

20. Takahashi K, Mulliken JB, Kozakewich HP, et al. Cellular markers that distinguish the phases of hemangioma during infancy and childhood. J Clin Invest 1994;93(6):2357–64.

21. Zhang L, Lin X, Wang W, et al. Circulating level of vascular endothelial growth factor in differentiating hemangioma from vascular malformation patients. Plast Reconstr Surg 2005;116(1):200–4.

22. Lo K, Mihm M, Fay A. Current theories on the pathogenesis of infantile hemangioma. Semin Ophthalmol 2009;24(3):172–7.

23. Yu Y, Fuhr J, Boye E, et al. Mesenchymal stem cells and adipogenesis in hemangioma involution. Stem Cells 2006;24(6):1605–12.

24. Friedlander SF, Ritter MR, Friedlander M. Recent progress in our understanding of the pathogenesis of infantile hemangiomas. Lymphat Res Biol 2005; 3(4):219–25.

25. North PE, Waner M, Mizeracki A, et al. GLUT1: a newly discovered immunohistochemical marker for juvenile hemangiomas. Hum Pathol 2000; 31(1):11–22.

26. Chang EI, Thangarajah H, Hamou C, et al. Hypoxia, hormones, and endothelial progenitor cells in hemangioma. Lymphat Res Biol 2007;5(4):237–43.

27. Mulliken JB, Enjolras O. Congenital hemangiomas and infantile hemangioma: missing links. J Am Acad Dermatol 2004;50(6):875–82.

28. Walter JW, North PE, Waner M, et al. Somatic mutation of vascular endothelial growth factor receptors in juvenile hemangioma. Genes Chromosomes Cancer 2002;33(3):295–303.

29. Waner M, North PE, Scherer KA, et al. The nonrandom distribution of facial hemangiomas. Arch Dermatol 2003;139(7):869–75.

30. Haggstrom AN, Drolet BA, Baselga E, et al. Prospective study of infantile hemangiomas: clinical characteristics predicting complications and treatment. Pediatrics 2006;118(3):882–7.

31. Bruckner AL, Frieden IJ. Hemangiomas of infancy. J Am Acad Dermatol 2003;48(4):477–93 [quiz: 494–6].

32. Holmdahl K. Cutaneous hemangiomas in premature and mature infants. Acta Paediatr 1955;44(4): 370–9.

33. Slovis T. Caffey's pediatric diagnostic imaging. 11th edition. Philadelphia: Mosby Elsevier; 2008.

34. Chiller KG, Passaro D, Frieden IJ. Hemangiomas of infancy: clinical characteristics, morphologic subtypes, and their relationship to race, ethnicity, and sex. Arch Dermatol 2002;138(12):1567–76.

35. Nord KM, Kandel J, Lefkowitch JH, et al. Multiple cutaneous infantile hemangiomas associated with hepatic angiosarcoma: case report and review of the literature. Pediatrics 2006;118(3):e907–13.

36. Bruder E, Perez-Atayde AR, Jundt G, et al. Vascular lesions of bone in children, adolescents, and young adults. A clinicopathologic reappraisal and application of the ISSVA classification. Virchows Arch 2009;454(2):161–79.

37. Donnelly LF, Adams DM, Bisset GS 3rd. Vascular malformations and hemangiomas: a practical approach in a multidisciplinary clinic. AJR Am J Roentgenol 2000;174(3):597–608.

38. Rivard DC, Lowe LH. Radiological reasoning: multiple hepatic masses in an infant. AJR Am J Roentgenol 2008;190(Suppl 6):S46–52.

39. Kalpatthi R, Germak J, Mizelle K, et al. Thyroid abnormalities in infantile hepatic hemangioendothelioma. Pediatr Blood Cancer 2007;49(7): 1021–4.

40. Kassarjian A, Zurakowski D, Dubois J, et al. Infantile hepatic hemangiomas: clinical and imaging findings and their correlation with therapy. AJR Am J Roentgenol 2004;182(3):785–95.

41. Ruppe MD, Huang SA, Jan de Beur SM. Consumptive hypothyroidism caused by paraneoplastic production of type 3 iodothyronine deiodinase. Thyroid 2005;15(12):1369–72.

42. Sarkar M, Mulliken JB, Kozakewich HP, et al. Thrombocytopenic coagulopathy (Kasabach-Merritt phenomenon) is associated with kaposiform hemangioendothelioma and not with common infantile hemangioma. Plast Reconstr Surg 1997; 100(6):1377–86.

43. Denoyelle F, Leboulanger N, Enjolras O, et al. Role of propranolol in the therapeutic strategy of infantile laryngotracheal hemangioma. Int J Pediatr Otorhinolaryngol 2009;73(8):1168–72.

44. Konez O, Burrows PE, Mulliken JB, et al. Angiographic features of rapidly involuting congenital hemangioma (RICH). Pediatr Radiol 2003;33(1): 15–9.

45. Leaute-Labreze C, Dumas de la Roque E, Hubiche T, et al. Propranolol for severe hemangiomas of infancy. N Engl J Med 2008;358(24): 2649–51.

46. Krol A, MacArthur CJ. Congenital hemangiomas: rapidly involuting and noninvoluting congenital hemangiomas. Arch Facial Plast Surg 2005;7(5):307–11.

47. Gorincour G, Kokta V, Rypens F, et al. Imaging characteristics of two subtypes of congenital hemangiomas: rapidly involuting congenital hemangiomas and non-involuting congenital hemangiomas. Pediatr Radiol 2005;35(12):1178–85.

48. Marler JJ, Fishman SJ, Upton J, et al. Prenatal diagnosis of vascular anomalies. J Pediatr Surg 2002;37(3):318–26.

49. Rogers M, Lam A, Fischer G. Sonographic findings in a series of rapidly involuting congenital hemangiomas (RICH). Pediatr Dermatol 2002;19(1):5–11.

50. Boon LM, Enjolras O, Mulliken JB. Congenital hemangioma: evidence of accelerated involution. J Pediatr 1996;128(3):329–35.

51. Lopez-Gutierrez JC, Diaz M, Ros Z. Giant rapidly involuting congenital hemangioma of the face: 15-year follow-up. Arch Facial Plast Surg 2005; 7(5):316–8.

52. Lyons LL, North PE, Mac-Moune Lai F, et al. Kaposiform hemangioendothelioma: a study of 33 cases emphasizing its pathologic, immunophenotypic, and biologic uniqueness from juvenile hemangioma. Am J Surg Pathol 2004;28(5):559–68.

53. Enjolras O. Color atlas of vascular tumors and vascular malformations. West Nyack (NY): Cambridge University Press; 2007.

54. Vin-Christian K, McCalmont TH, Frieden IJ. Kaposiform hemangioendothelioma. An aggressive, locally invasive vascular tumor that can mimic hemangioma of infancy. Arch Dermatol 1997;133(12): 1573–8.

55. Zukerberg LR, Nickoloff BJ, Weiss SW. Kaposiform hemangioendothelioma of infancy and childhood. An aggressive neoplasm associated with Kasabach-Merritt syndrome and lymphangiomatosis. Am J Surg Pathol 1993;17(4):321–8.

56. Hein KD, Mulliken JB, Kozakewich HP, et al. Venous malformations of skeletal muscle. Plast Reconstr Surg 2002;110(7):1625–35.

57. Pappas DC Jr, Persky MS, Berenstein A. Evaluation and treatment of head and neck venous vascular malformations. Ear Nose Throat J 1998;77(11): 914–6, 918–22.

58. Pascarella L, Bergan JJ, Yamada C, et al. Venous angiomata: treatment with sclerosant foam. Ann Vasc Surg 2005;19(4):457–64.

59. Stapf C, Mohr JP, Pile-Spellman J, et al. Epidemiology and natural history of arteriovenous malformations. Neurosurg Focus 2001;11(5):e1.

Practical Magnetic Resonance Imaging Evaluation of Peripheral Nerves in Children

Magnetic Resonance Neurography

Cesar Cortes, MD[a], Yanerys Ramos, MD[b],
Ricardo Restrepo, MD[c], Jose Andres Restrepo, MD[d],
John A.I. Grossman, MD[c], Edward Y. Lee, MD, MPH[e],*

KEYWORDS

- Magnetic resonance imaging (MRI) • MR neurography • Peripheral nerves • Pediatric patients

KEY POINTS

- Various underlying pathologies can affect the peripheral nerves of children, and the difficulties of evaluating peripheral nerves are heightened in children due to their smaller size and rarity of the potential pathologies relative to adults.
- Careful imaging planning between the radiologist and the referring physician is important before a magnetic resonance (MR) neurography to maximize the yield of the examination and keep the imaging time to a minimum.
- The findings of peripheral nerve pathology include direct findings in the nerve and indirect findings in the denervated muscles.
- MR imaging, which is a noninvasive imaging modality and not associated with ionizing radiation, is an excellent imaging tool for detecting both direct and indirect findings associated with peripheral nerve pathology particularly in the pediatric population.
- Clear understanding of clinical indications, MR imaging technique, and MR imaging findings of both normal and abnormal peripheral nerves in the pediatric population can lead to early diagnosis and optimal patient care.

INTRODUCTION

The underlying causes of nerve pathology in the pediatric age group encompass a spectrum of intrinsic and extrinsic conditions, including hereditary disorders, benign and malignant neoplasms, infection, inflammation, and trauma. Imaging evaluation of peripheral nerves is often challenging due to the small size and the often meandering course of these structures. In children, this is further complicated by the smaller size of the patients and the relative infrequency of these pathologic conditions with little information available in the radiology literature.

Magnetic resonance (MR) neurography, which is a noninvasive imaging modality, is an excellent imaging tool to assess the detail of peripheral nerves. It should be considered when evaluating

[a] Department of Diagnostic Radiology, University of Puerto Rico School of Medicine, PO Box 365067, San Juan, PR 00936-5067, USA; [b] Department of Radiology, Cincinnati Children's Hospital Medical Center, 3333 Burnet Avenue, Cincinnati, OH 45229, USA; [c] Department of Radiology, Miami Children's Hospital, 3100 Southwest 62nd Avenue, Miami, FL 33155, USA; [d] Department of Rehabilitation Medicine, Humana, CAC Florida Medical Center, 525 East 25th Street, Miami, FL 33013, USA; [e] Division of Magnetic Resonance and Thoracic Imaging, Department of Radiology, Boston Children's Hospital, Harvard Medical School, 300 Longwood Avenue, Boston, MA 02115, USA
* Corresponding author.
E-mail address: Edward.Lee@childrens.harvard.edu

Radiol Clin N Am 51 (2013) 673–688
http://dx.doi.org/10.1016/j.rcl.2013.04.006
0033-8389/13/$ – see front matter © 2013 Elsevier Inc. All rights reserved.

pediatric patients with clinically suspected underlying peripheral neurologic disorders. Particularly when the cause of neuropathy is not clear from the clinical findings and electromyography, MR neurography may demonstrate changes that are more suggestive of specific neuropathies, identify the specific location of an injury or tumor, or show normal-appearing nerves, narrowing the differential diagnosis.

For evaluating peripheral nerve pathology with MR imaging, radiologists must be not only familiar with the different underlying disorders affecting peripheral nerves in children but also prepared to use an optimal MR imaging protocol.[1] Such optimized MR imaging protocol can decrease the scanning time and eliminate the need for additional imaging.[1] The overarching goal of this article is to review the current MR imaging technique, clinical indication, normal anatomy, and common disorders that affect peripheral nerves in the pediatric population. Such knowledge has a great potential for early diagnosis, which, in turn, can lead to optimal pediatric patient care.

MR Imaging Technique

The MR technique used for the evaluation of peripheral nerves of the extremities (ie, MR neurography) in children is similar to that used in adults. However, the smaller size of the structures and inability to stay still in infants and young children make it more challenging. A 3-T instead of 1.5-T MR imaging scanner is preferred because of the higher signal-to-noise ratio of the 3-T MR imaging scanner.[2] To decrease motion, infants and young children (<7 years) who cannot follow instructions need either sedation or general anesthesia.

Before the MR neurography, clear communication between the radiologist and the ordering physician is essential so that the examination can be focused on a specific area of interest, which can help determine the type of MR imaging coil to be used. Evaluation of peripheral nerves with MR imaging can be performed with the smallest body coil, such as a phased-array coil, that fits tightly around the area of interest.

In the authors' institution, the standard MR neurography protocol includes the use of high-resolution T1-weigheted sequences for the evaluation of the regional anatomy and landmarks in combination with fluid-sensitive sequences with fat saturation whereby pathologic changes are more conspicuous (Box 1, Fig. 1A). Of the fluid-sensitive sequences, short tau inversion recovery (STIR) images have more uniform fat suppression and excellent T2 contrast. However, they have an intrinsic low signal-to-noise ratio and are more sensitive to blood

---

Box 1
MR neurography technique

High-resolution T1-weighted images

- Isotropic images (submillimeter voxel size) to allow 3D reconstruction
- Best for anatomic evaluation: size, shape, course
- At least 2 planes: perpendicular and along the long axis of nerve
- Usually no intravenous contrast, except in cases of tumor, infection or after surgery

Fluid-sensitive sequence

- Makes pathologic conditions more conspicuous
- T2FS: Higher signal-to-noise ratio, less affected by blood flow artifacts
- STIR: More homogeneous fat suppression

Abbreviations: STIR, short tau inversion recovery; T2FS, frequency selected T2 fat-saturated.

---

flow artifacts that could be detrimental as peripheral nerves travel in the neurovascular bundle (see Fig. 1B). Frequency-selected T2 fat-saturated images have higher signal-to-noise ratio and are less affected by blood flow artifacts, but the fat saturation is more inhomogeneous (see Fig. 1C).[1] Intravenous gadolinium is not routinely used but may be helpful in differentiating nerves from adjacent vessels, and in the assessment of tumors, infection, and postsurgical patients.

Images should be evaluated in at least 2 planes to follow the entire nerve trajectory with confidence. One plane must be perpendicular to the nerve to show its cross-sectional appearance for the evaluation of fascicular pattern, nerve size, and shape. This plane is less susceptible to volume averaging. The other plane should be along the long axis of the nerve for evaluation of the trajectory, mass effect, displacement, and focal enlargement. The long-axis images can be reformatted oblique maximum-intensity projection images generated during postprocessing.[3]

Clinical Indications for MR Neurography

It is important to understand that the causes of peripheral neuropathy differ between children and adults, with most causes being inherited in children and acquired in adults. Even the causes of acquired neuropathies differ between children and adults, the latter being mostly due to entrapment, chronic and toxic injury, or systemic disease, whereas in children they are mostly due to infection, inflammation, and trauma. Understanding these

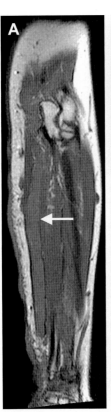
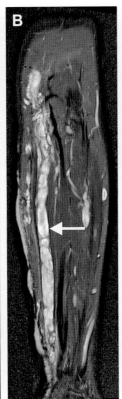
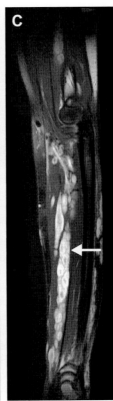

Fig. 1. Plexiform neurofibroma in a 5-year-old girl. (*A*) Coronal T1-weighted MR image of the forearm shows abnormalities of the caliber and the shape of the ulnar nerve (*arrow*) with minimal signal alteration. (*B*) Coronal STIR and (*C*) sagittal T2-weighted MR images with fat saturation clearly show the abnormal signal intensity of the nerve (*arrow*). Note the less homogeneous fat saturation of the T2-weighted MR image (*C*) at the edges of the image.

differences between children and adults are essential for the proper evaluation of peripheral nerve pathologies in the pediatric population.

The main clinical indications for initial MR neurography in the pediatric age group include the following: (1) children with underlying hereditary conditions that predispose to or are associated with the development of neuropathy; (2) explained neuropathy in pediatric patients without underlying predisposing conditions; and (3) neuropathy in pediatric patients with a history of infection, inflammation, or trauma. In addition, MR neurography can provide important information regarding the response to treatment or surgery, sometimes before there is clinical recovery or physical examination findings.[4]

Histology of Peripheral Nerves

The peripheral nerve consists of functional units of axons. Each axon is either myelinated or unmyelinated and can receive afferent signals or send efferent signals. A peripheral nerve is composed of fascicles, which consist of motor, sensory, and sympathetic fibers. Large peripheral nerves consist of 3 layers of connective tissue, the innermost endoneurium, the perineurium surrounding each fascicle, and the epineurium surrounding the nerve. The endoneurium consists of loose vascular connective tissue and extracellular fluid. The perineurium consists of tightly adherent epithelial-like cells and endothelial cells that provide a protective barrier against infectious or toxic agents. The epineurium is the outer connective tissue providing support for the nerve (**Fig. 2**).[1]

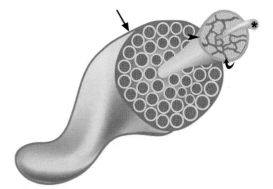

Fig. 2. Drawing illustrating the layers of a peripheral nerve: The epineurium (*straight black arrow*) is the outer connective tissue that provides mechanical support to the nerve; the perineurium (*arrowhead*) surrounds each fascicle and is a barrier against infectious or toxic agents; the endoneurium (*curved arrow*) consists of loose vascular connective tissue and extracellular fluid, which invests the axon (*asterisk*), the basic unit of the peripheral nerve.

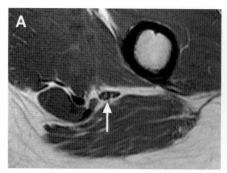
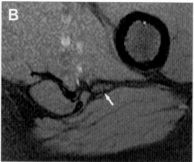

Fig. 3. Normal MR appearance of the sciatic nerve in an adolescent boy. (A) Axial T1-weighted MR image of the proximal thigh demonstrates the normal ovoid-shaped sciatic nerve (*arrow*) surrounded by fat. (B) Axial T2-weighted MR image with fat saturation at the same level demonstrates the normal slightly hyperintense sciatic nerve (*arrow*). In both MR sequences, the homogeneous fascicular size of the nerve is evident.

MR imaging Appearance of Peripheral Nerves

The evaluation of nerve pathology with MR neurography requires the identification of both direct and indirect imaging findings of nerve injury. Direct findings are seen in the nerve itself, and indirect findings are found in denervated muscles.

On axial T1-weighted MR images, a normal nerve appears as a round to ovoid structure iso-intense to muscle surrounded by fat (**Fig. 3**). On long-axis MR images, the shape and size of the nerve tend to be uniform except in places of normal turns or expected change of trajectory (**Fig. 4**). In larger nerves, a homogeneous fascicular pattern can be appreciated (see **Fig. 3**). The T1 signal intensity of

the nerve does not change substantially when affected; instead, focal changes in thickness and shape can be appreciated (see **Fig. 4**). If contrast is administered, a normal nerve should not enhance, as it is isolated by the blood-nerve barrier.[5] On T2-weighted MR images, normal nerves are iso-intense to slightly hyperintense to muscle (see **Fig. 3**B).

Intrinsic MR findings of nerve pathology include abnormal shape, such as focal or diffuse enlargement, stretching or interruption, diffuse or focal accentuated increased T2 signal, contrast enhancement, and an altered fascicular pattern, such as enlarged fascicles and cystic changes (see **Figs. 1** and **4–7**). Other imaging findings

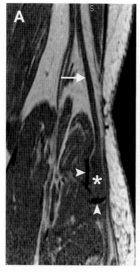
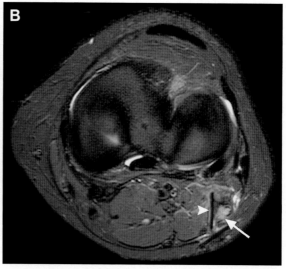

Fig. 4. A 14-year-old girl after a glass laceration of the knee. (A) T1-weighted coronal oblique MR image of the leg shows the normal T1 appearance of the unaffected common peroneal nerve proximally (*arrow*), with nerve transection by the glass fragments distally (*arrowheads*) and focal nerve thickening representing a neuroma (*asterisk*). (B) Axial STIR image demonstrates an abnormally thickened and hyperintense common peroneal nerve (*arrow*) at the neuroma site surrounded by glass fragments (*arrowhead*).

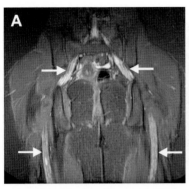
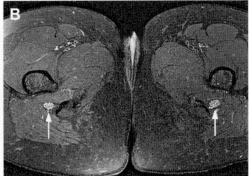

Fig. 5. A 16-year-old girl with Charcot-Marie-Tooth neuropathy. (*A*) Coronal STIR and (*B*) axial T2-weighted MR images with fat saturation of the pelvis demonstrate diffuse enlargement, accentuated heterogeneous fascicular pattern, and increased signal intensity of the sciatic nerves (*arrows*).

suggestive of nerve pathology include loss of surrounding fat planes and mass effect with altered trajectory. In general, nerve pathology leads to a further increase in T2 signal intensity; however, abnormal T2 signal intensity seen within the nerves may be due to the magic angle effect, which is a potential source of false-positive pathologic condition.[6]

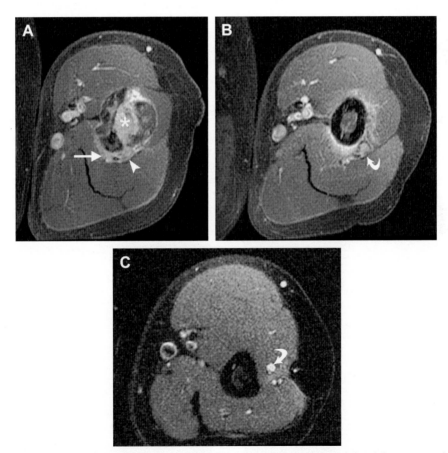

Fig. 6. Radial nerve injury after a humeral shaft fracture in an adolescent boy. (*A*) Axial contrast-enhanced T1-weighted MR image with fat saturation of the proximal arm shows a healing fracture (*asterisk*) with callus (*arrow*) encasing the amorphous, abnormally enhancing radial nerve (*arrowhead*) at the radial sulcus. (*B*) Axial contrast-enhanced T1-weighted MR image with fat saturation at a slightly more distal location shows thickening and abnormal enhancement of the nerve (*curved arrow*). (*C*) Axial STIR image just proximal to the elbow shows an abnormally increased signal intensity of the nerve (*curved arrow*).

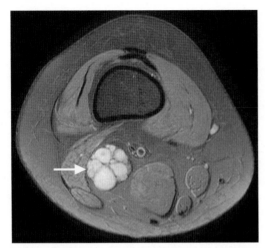

Fig. 7. Adolescent boy with neurofibromatosis type I. Axial T2-weighted MR image with fat saturation of the thigh shows an abnormal exaggerated fascicular pattern of the distal sciatic nerve (*arrow*) with heterogeneous enlargement and increased signal of the fascicles.

The imaging findings of muscle denervation depend on the time elapsed since the injury. In acute injury (<1 month), MR may show no changes. During the subacute phase (~1–12 months), muscle is T2 hyperintense (**Fig. 8**). This T2 hyperintense muscle is not pathognomonic and can be seen with multiple pathologic conditions besides denervation, such as infectious or inflammatory myositis or after direct trauma. Such MR signal change is

thought to be due to an increase in the fraction of extracellular water within the muscle with concomitant decreased fraction of intracellular water and muscle fiber size. In chronic muscle denervation (>12 months), there is muscle atrophy and fatty infiltration, which is best seen on T1-weighted MR images (**Fig. 9**).[7] The timing of these MR signal changes can vary. MR imaging is also useful in identifying muscles not typically expected in the territory of an injured nerve due to the variability of motor nerve unit anatomy that can be undiagnosed with electromyography.

SPECTRUM OF PERIPHERAL NERVE DISORDERS

Neuropathies are characterized by nerve dysfunction resulting in numbness, weakness, pain, and loss of reflexes. The underlying causes of peripheral neuropathies differ between adults and children. In adults, most cases of neuropathies are acquired (60%) and related to entrapment or acute/chronic injury from playing sports or participating in occupational activities. In children, more than 70% of neuropathies are related to inherited causes (**Box 2**).[8] Among the acquired causes, children are less likely to have toxic or systemic disease-related neuropathies.[8]

There are several ways to categorize neuropathies, including the number of affected nerves, type of nerve affected, acuity of symptoms, inheritance pattern, location of the injury within the nerve, or cause (see **Box 2**). For practical purposes, this article categorizes the peripheral neuropathies into 2 groups: intrinsic and extrinsic to the affected nerves.

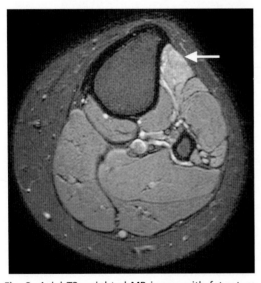

Fig. 8. Axial T2-weighted MR image with fat saturation of the leg of the pediatric patient from **Fig. 4** shows localized increased signal intensity of the anterior tibialis muscle consistent with subacute denervation (*arrow*).

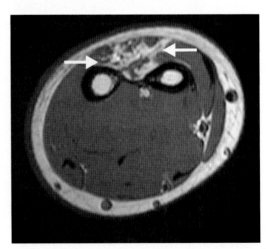

Fig. 9. Axial T1-weighted MR image of the forearm of an adolescent girl with a proximal radial nerve injury shows extreme atrophy with fatty replacement of the muscles (*arrows*) of the extensor compartment.

Box 2
Peripheral neuropathies in children

Hereditary (71.2%)

  Hereditary motor and sensory neuropathy (HMSN ≈ CMT)[a]

    Includes Charcot Marie Tooth, Dejerine Sotas

  Inherited (others)

    Ataxic and sensory neuropathies (familial dysautonomia-reflex sympathetic dystrophy included)

  Inherited central nervous system disease and neuropathy

  Inherited metabolic (leukodystrophies, lipid storage disease, peroxisomal disorder, mitochondrial disorders)

Acquired (10.4%)

  Traumatic

  Toxic

  Inflammatory/infectious

  Systemic disease (autoimmune-AIDP and CIDP)

  Idiopathic

Uncertain (18.4%)

Abbreviations: AIDP, acute inflammatory demyelinating disease (Guillan-Barre); CIDP, chronic inflammatory demyelinating disease.

[a] HSMN and Charcot-Marie-Tooth (CMT) classifications are used interchangeably, except for HMSN IV, which should not be used anymore (Refsum disease) and CMT IV, which is a group of recessively inherited polyneuropathies.

Adapted from Ouvrier RA, McLeod JG, Pollard JD. Peripheral neuropathy in childhood. 2nd edition. London: Cambridge University Press; 1999. p. 1–335.

Neuropathies due to Conditions Intrinsic to Nerves

Hereditary conditions

Most hereditary neuropathies present during the first 2 decades of life.[8] On MR imaging, there may be increased T2 signal intensity and cystic changes along the nerves. The fascicular pattern may be preserved or accentuated with asymmetric fascicle enlargement.[1,9] In some forms of hereditary neuropathies (ie, hypertrophic Charcot-Marie-Tooth, Dejerine-Sottas, and Refsum disease), nerve enlargement may also be identified (see **Fig. 5**).

Neoplastic conditions

Neurofibromas (NF) and schwannomas are the 2 most common peripheral nerve tumors in children,

each accounting for approximately 5% of all soft tissue tumors.[10] The histologic hallmark of both peripheral nerve tumors is neoplastic proliferation with Schwann cell differentiation, more mature and homogeneous in schwannomas than NF. In addition, other nonneoplastic cells are present, including neurons (axons), perineurial cells, fibroblasts, mast cells, and lymphocytes.[11] Both NF and schwannomas can give rise to their malignant counterpart: malignant peripheral nerve sheath tumor (MPNST).

Neurofibroma

NF is the most common peripheral nerve sheath tumor in children.[10,12] Three types of NF have been described: localized NF, diffuse NF, and plexiform NF.[10] Localized and diffuse NF are isolated in most cases (90%) and not associated with neurofibromatosis type 1 (NF-1).[10,13] On the other hand, the plexiform type is associated with NF-1 in 90% of cases.[14,15]

Most NFs are of the localized form (90%), either cutaneous or involving a major nerve. These NFs are usually oval or fusiform masses of less than 5 cm in size at a specific peripheral nerve location. On MR imaging, the entering and exiting nerve can be identified central to the mass, particularly when larger peripheral nerves are affected. NFs are usually isointense to muscle on T1-weighted images and homogeneous with variable gadolinium enhancement. NFs are hyperintense on T2-weighted images, and up to 70% of the time have a lower T2 signal intensity center, the so-called target appearance.[10,12,16]

Diffuse NF is an uncommon lesion seen predominantly in children and young adults affecting the skin and subcutaneous tissues of the extremities, trunk, and head/neck region.[17] It has a particular histology that includes abundant S100-positive pseudomeissnerian corpuscles.[11] Morphologically, it can present as plaquelike thickening of the skin and subcutaneous tissues due to tumoral infiltration. Less commonly, it can present as an infiltrative pattern involving the subcutaneous soft tissues only, with interspersed areas of macroscopic fat. Most diffuse NFs are isointense to slightly hyperintense to muscle on T1-weighted and hyperintense on fluid-sensitive sequences compared with muscle (**Fig. 10**A, B). After intravenous contrast administration, enhancement tends to be intense (see **Fig. 10**C). In the less common infiltrative type, the presence of fat may produce internal reticulation.[17]

Plexiform NFs are typically seen in younger children, most related to NF-1 before cutaneous NF develops. Histologically, plexiform NF resembles both localized and diffuse NF.[11] The MR findings are

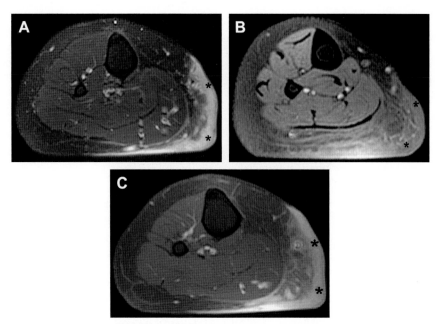

Fig. 10. Plaque-type diffuse neurofibroma of the leg in an adolescent girl. (*A*) Axial T2-weighted MR image with fat saturation shows high signal and thickening of the dermis as well as high signal and stranding of the subcutaneous soft tissues (*asterisks*) of the distal leg posterolaterally. (*B*) Fat-saturated T1-weighted MR images precontrast and (*C*) postcontrast administration show strong contrast enhancement of the biopsy-proven diffuse neurofibroma (*asterisks*).

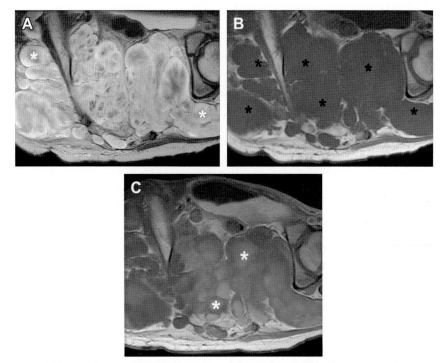

Fig. 11. A 9-year-old boy with neurofibromatosis type I. (*A*) Axial T2-weighted MR image demonstrates a large plexiform neurofibroma involving the sacral plexus extending into the gluteal regions. Note the hypointense center consistent with target sign (*asterisks*). (*B*) On axial T1-weighted MR image, the lesion (*asterisks*) is diffusely and homogeneously hypointense. (*C*) Fat-saturated T1-weighted image after intravenous gadolinium administration shows central enhancement (*asterisks*).

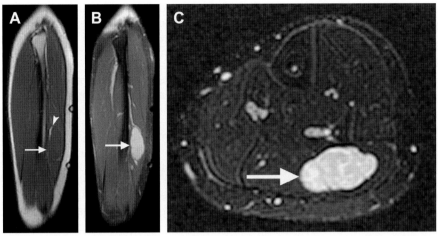

Fig. 12. Schwannoma in an adolescent girl who presented with a painful leg lump. (A) Sagittal T1-weighted MR image of the leg demonstrates a fusiform circumscribed mass (*arrow*) isointense to muscle along the course of the common peroneal nerve with the "split fat" sign (*arrowhead*). (B) On postcontrast T1-weighted MR image with fat saturation, the mass has intense homogeneous enhancement (*arrow*). (C) On axial T2-weighted MR image with fat saturation, the mass is diffusely hyperintense (*arrow*).

multinodular or fascicular masses with sharp borders resembling a "bag of worms" along a specific nerve distribution and frequently exhibiting a target T2-weighted image appearance. Extensive nodular changes along a segment of a nerve may give a "rosary"-like appearance. On T1-weighted image, the lesions can be isointense or hypointense to muscle, with central and heterogeneous gadolinium enhancement (**Fig. 11**).[10,12,18]

Schwannoma

Schwannomas are seen more frequently in the second decade of life. Most schwannomas are solitary, slow-growing lesions of <5 cm in size.

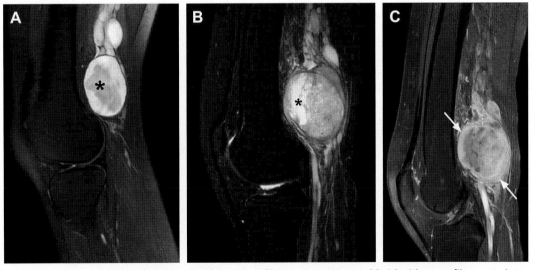

Fig. 13. Malignant transformation of a plexiform neurofibroma in a 15-year-old girl with neurofibromatosis type I who presented with pain. Surgical biopsy confirmed the malignant transformation. (A) Sagittal T2-weighted MR image with fat saturation demonstrates a hyperintense mass with central hypointensity, the so-called target sign (*asterisk*), involving the peroneal nerve. Note the nerve entering the mass superiorly. (B) On a sagittal T2-weighted MR image with fat saturation obtained 8 months after the previous MR study (A) when the patient presents with pain, the mass has increased in size, displays central cystic changes (*asterisk*) and surrounding soft tissue edema. (C) Fat contrast-enhanced T1-weighted MR image with fat saturation shows reversal of the enhancement pattern (now peripheral rather than central) (*arrows*).

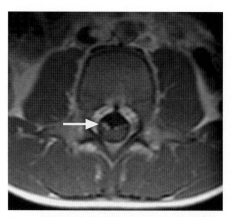

Fig. 14. Guillain-Barré syndrome in an 8-year-old boy who presented with progressive lower extremity weakness. Axial contrast-enhanced T1-weighted MR image with fat saturation at the level of the lumbar spine demonstrates enhancement and mild thickening of the ventral spinal nerves (*arrow*).

Approximately 5% of schwannomas are associated with NF-1, particularly if multiple.[10] They are composed histologically of compacted cellular spindles (Antoni A) or loose hypocellular myxoid tissue (Antoni B).[16] Schwannomas are encapsulated, involving one nerve fascicle, resulting in the frequent eccentric location in relation to the nerve. On MR, the lesions are hypointense on T1-weighted image with substantial homogeneous enhancement after gadolinium administration (**Fig. 12**A, B). On T2-weighted image, the lesions are of higher signal intensity than adjacent muscle, with or without heterogeneity of the parenchyma (see **Fig. 12**C). The target sign, more commonly seen in plexiform NFs, can be present but in less than 50% of cases.[10,16] The splaying of fat at the edges of the mass (split fat sign) (see **Fig. 12**A)

can be observed in both schwannomas and NF, and although suggestive, it is not specific to nerve sheath tumors.[10] Cystic changes are much more common in schwannomas compared with NF.[16]

Malignant peripheral nerve sheath tumors

MPNST are markedly aggressive tumors, accounting for 5% to 10% of soft tissue sarcomas.[10] The typical age range of initial clinical presentation is between 20 and 50 years. In the setting of NF-1 (50% of cases), it can be seen earlier (10–20 years), with a male predominance (80%).[10,12] Although they can arise de novo or after radiation therapy, most MPNSTs arise from plexiform neurofibromas involving major nerves (**Fig. 13**A).[19] The development of pain, severe motor weakness, and rapid mass growth may suggest malignant transformation clinically. Perilesional edema, cystic component, peripheral enhancement, and larger lesions (>5 cm) may help to differentiate MPNST from other nerve sheath tumors with 90% specificity and 61% sensitivity if 2 of these 4 criteria are met (see **Fig. 13**B, C).[20] In NF-1 patients younger than 30 years old, the burden of plexiform neurofibromas has been proven to be substantially greater among patients with MPNST compared with control patients with NF-1 without MPNST.[21]

Infectious and/or inflammatory conditions

The proposed mechanisms by which infection causes neuropathy include direct nerve involvement, immunologic response, vasculitis, and post-treatment-related.[22] Of the infection-related neuropathies, Guillain-Barré syndrome (GBS) is worth mentioning. GBS is not a direct infectious neuritis itself but an immune response to an infection (*Campylobacter jejuni*, CMV, EBV, *Mycoplasma pneumoniae*) or an antigenic challenge by a vaccine

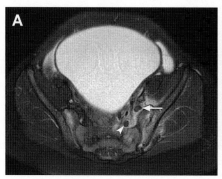
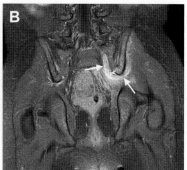

Fig. 15. Pyogenic neuritis in a 5-year-old boy with left pyriform pyomyositis who presented with sciatica and fever. (*A*) Axial T2-weighted MR image with fat saturation shows marked enlargement of a left sacral root (*arrowhead*) and of the proximal sciatic nerve (*arrow*) surrounded by soft tissue edema, indicating adjacent inflammation. (*B*) Coronal T1-weighted MR image with fat saturation after contrast administration better depicts the longitudinal extent of the abnormally enhancing left sciatic nerve (*arrows*) as it passes under the sacrosciatic notch. Note the enlargement and accentuated fascicular pattern of the nerve (*arrows*).

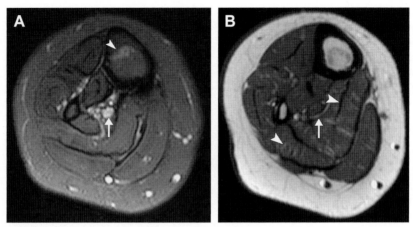

Fig. 16. An adolescent boy with a history of extraskeletal Ewing sarcoma status postradiation therapy. (*A*) Axial T2-weighted MR image with fat saturation below the knee shows an enlarged and hyperintense tibial nerve with enlargement of the individual fascicles (*arrow*). Postradiation bone marrow changes are also evident (*arrowhead*) at this level. (*B*) Axial T1-weighted MR image shows an enlarged tibial nerve (*arrow*) and fatty atrophy of the posterior compartment muscles of the leg, resulting in a striated appearance (*arrowheads*).

(flu, rabies). It is a clinical diagnosis that usually requires imaging to exclude other diagnoses rather than for confirmation.[23] Although MR imaging findings can be normal in affected pediatric patients, thickening of the intradural-extramedullary spinal roots or the cranial nerves with variable enhancement has been described.[23–25] Enhancement of the spinal roots is due to loss of the blood-nerve barrier, whereas nerve thickening is related to inflammation with loss of tissue support due to the absence of the epi-perineurium.[23,25] These changes also tend to affect the ventral more frequently than the dorsal roots, possibly due to higher P2 antigen in the anterior roots (**Fig. 14**).[25]

Chronic inflammatory demyelinating polyradiculoneuropathy presents clinically similar to GBS and can be differentiated only according to the course of the disease (ie, progressive or relapsing disease). Chronic inflammatory demyelinating polyradiculoneuropathy imaging findings can also mimic the hypertrophic hereditary neuropathies.[26] Acute pyogenic neuritis is uncommon and is usually related to direct extension from a nearby infection (**Fig. 15**).[9]

Traumatic conditions

Traumatic injuries are frequent and affect the upper extremities more commonly. In children, the frequency of underlying causes is different than in adults, with obstetric injuries (46.7%) and iatrogenic lesions (17%) being more common.[27] Iatrogenic causes include surgical procedures, radiation therapy (**Fig. 16**), and injections, the latter affecting the sciatic nerve more commonly.[27] Overall, trauma

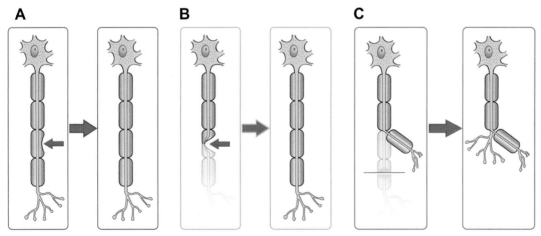

Fig. 17. Degrees of nerve injury by Seddon. (*A*) Neurapraxia (2 images on the left), (*B*) axonotmesis (2 middle images), and (*C*) neurotmesis (2 images on the right).

is the most common cause of mononeuropathy, most of the time leading to a neuroma. In 1943, Seddon described 3 basic types of traumatic peripheral nerve injuries, including (1) neurapraxia; (2) axonotmesis; and (3) neurotmesis, which are still used to assist in determining the prognosis and the treatment strategy.[28,29]

The term neurapraxia, also called conduction block, is used to indicate a mild degree of neural insult resulting in the blockage of impulse conduction across the affected segment (**Fig. 17**). It implies disruption of the myelin sheet; however, it is reversible. Muscle wasting does not occur because of the rapid reinnervation.[28,29]

Axonotmesis, a more severe type of injury than neurapraxia, occurs when only the axon is physically disrupted with preservation of the enveloping endoneurial and other supporting connective tissue structures, such as perineurium and epineurium (see **Fig. 17**). Substantial compression and traction are typical underlying causes. When the axon is disrupted, Wallerian degeneration occurs. A preserved endoneurium means that, once the remnants of the degenerated nerve have been removed, the regenerating axon simply has to follow its original course to the appropriate end organ. An excellent prognosis can be expected when neural damage results only in axonotmesis.[28–30]

Neurotmesis, the most severe of the traumatic injuries, is the complete disruption of the axon and all supportive connective tissue structures, which are no longer in continuity (see **Fig. 17**). It results in neuroma formation and has a poor prognosis for complete functional recovery. Surgical reapproximation might be needed, and it does not guarantee proper endoneurial tube alignment, but it at least improves the chances that axonal growth will occur across the injury site.[28,29]

On histology, traumatic neuromas characteristically have a tangle of multidirectional regenerating axons, with Schwann cells, endoneurial cells, and perineurial cells in a dense collagenous matrix with surrounding fibroblasts.[10] There are 2 types of posttraumatic neuromas depending on the location of the injury within the nerve. The fusiform neuroma may be related to stretching, blunt trauma, or chronic friction, producing a lesion that is encased within the intact nerve trunk. These lesions are usually well-defined on MR imaging with fusiform enlargement of the nerve, intermediate T1-weighted image signal (**Fig. 18**), and higher T2-weighted image signal than the normal parent nerve.[10] On axial MR images, a ringlike fascicular pattern is seen best on T2-weighted images, in keeping with the neural origin. A terminal or lateral neuroma, on the other hand, is usually related to partial or complete avulsion or transection

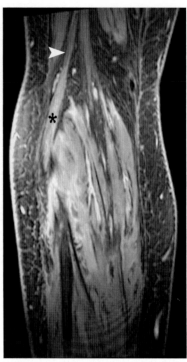

Fig. 18. Reconstructed enhanced coronal T1-weighted MR image with fat saturation of the leg of an 11-year-old girl with a history of severe compartment syndrome demonstrates focal bulbous thickening with abnormal enhancement (*asterisk*) of the common peroneal nerve after prolonged compression by the fibular head. The more proximal nerve has a normal appearance (*arrowhead*).

(including surgical transection) of a nerve (see **Fig. 4**A). On imaging, an entering nerve ending in a bulbous enlargement is seen. It can be well-defined or ill-defined (from multidirectional axonal proliferation), with a signal similar to the fusiform type. In children, bone fractures may be responsible for nerve injuries as well (see **Fig. 6**).

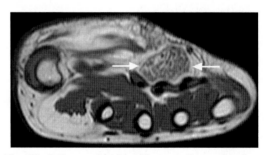

Fig. 19. A 6-year-old girl with macrodystrophia lipomatosa. Axial T1-weighted MR image of the wrist demonstrates enlargement of the median nerve with fat infiltrating and surrounding the nerve fascicles, pathognomonic for a neural fibrolipoma (*arrows*).

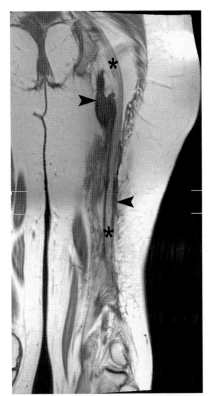

Fig. 20. A 13-year old girl with a history of fibromatosis of the thigh with prior surgical resection. Coronal reconstructed T1-weighted MR image of the thigh shows residual hypointense tumor (*arrowheads*) partially encasing the sciatic nerve (*asterisks*).

Neuropathies due to Conditions Extrinsic to Nerves

Neural tumor

A neural fibrolipoma, also known as fibrolipomatous nerve hamartoma, is a rare benign tumor that results in fibroadipose neural infiltration. It is due to an overgrowth of the underlying fibroadipose tissue along a nerve trunk. It most commonly affects the median nerve (85%) and, in up to 67% of cases, it can be associated with macrodystrophia lipomatosa (**Fig. 19**).[10]

Soft tissue tumors

Soft tissue tumors may infiltrate peripheral nerves and, in children, 2 tumors should be mentioned: fibromatosis and lipoblastoma due to their potentially infiltrative growth pattern. Deep fibromatosis, particularly of the extra-abdominal type, more commonly seen in younger children,[31] is histologically benign but may be locally aggressive, as it infiltrates the surrounding soft tissues, including nerves (**Fig. 20**). Amputation of the affected limb is sometimes required due to a loss of function and pain or significant nerve or bone involvement.[32] Lipoblastoma is usually seen in children during the first year of life.[33] Localized lipoblastoma is the most common (80%) and well circumscribed. The diffuse type or lipoblastomatosis (30%) is infiltrative and can involve nerves (**Fig. 21**). Even though the latter type may infiltrate the neurovascular bundle, most lipoblastomas eventually differentiate into lipomas; hence, efforts to spare the nerve during surgery must be made.[34] In very young children, lipoblastomas may not have a fatty signal due to mixoid tissue predominance.[33]

Osseous tumors

Osteochondromas are common benign bone tumors in children. They are more frequently solitary but can be inherited as a polyostotic, familial, autosomal-dominant disease. Although osteochondromas are usually diagnosed on plain radiographs when characteristic osseous outgrowths on the surface of the bone with the typical corticomedullary continuity are seen, MR imaging

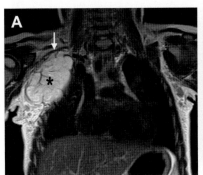
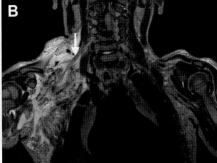

Fig. 21. A 3-year old boy with a lipoblastoma. (*A*) Coronal T2-weighted MR image with fat saturation shows the large lipoblastoma (*asterisk*) encasing and stretching a right brachial plexus trunk (*arrow*). (*B*) Coronal T2-weighted MR image after resection clearly depicts the spared right brachial plexus trunk (*arrow*). There is thickening and stranding of the adjacent soft tissues.

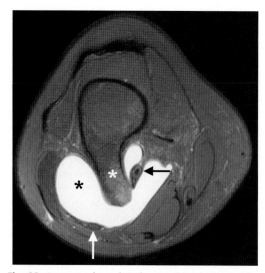

Fig. 22. Large pedunculated osteochondroma arising from the posterolateral aspect of the distal femoral metaphysis (*white asterisk*) in a 10-year-old boy who presented with foot weakness. There is a large pseudobursa (*black asterisk*) overlying this large pedunculated osteochondroma. The osteochondroma also splits the neurovascular bundle (*black arrow*), causing posterior displacement and flattening of the tibial nerve (*white arrow*).

can help in their evaluation when symptomatic after fracturing or by causing mechanical irritation and compression of the adjacent structures, such as muscle, soft tissues, and nerves. MR neurography may help delineate the relationship of the nerve with the osteochondroma for preoperative planning to decrease the risk of iatrogenic nerve injury. Compression of peripheral nerves can occur in up

to 8.1% of patients, most commonly of the peroneal nerve (**Fig. 22**).[35]

Vascular malformations

Vascular malformations are common in pediatric patients, especially the slow-flow type (ie, venous and lymphatic). A frequent therapeutic approach is percutaneous sclerotherapy. When evaluating an MR imaging study of a slow-flow vascular malformation especially of the venous type, close inspection of the neighboring nerves should be performed to assess for neural infiltration. Nerve involvement is suggested by focal nerve enlargement, high T2 signal, and in cases of venous malformations, contrast enhancement of the nerve itself (**Fig. 23**).[36] The possible mechanisms of neuropathy associated with embolo/sclerotherapy are as follows: (1) extravasation and diffusion of the sclerosing agent around a nerve trunk; (2) obstruction of the vasa nervorum; and (3) severe soft tissue edema associated with compartment syndrome and subsequent nerve injury.[37] Nerve infiltration by the lesion may be a contraindication for sclerotherapy, especially in cases of venous malformations, because the commonly used agents (eg, Sotradecol and absolute alcohol) are neurotoxic.[37] Acute or delayed neural dysfunction, sometimes irreversible, have been described during sclerotherapy of head and neck vascular malformations and may be related to the proximity to or involvement of the nerve by the malformation.[38,39] Even in cases of lymphatic malformations, caution must be applied when the lesion is in close proximity or intimately associated with a major nerve trunk because iatrogenic extravasation of doxycycline during sclerotherapy can damage the nerve.[40]

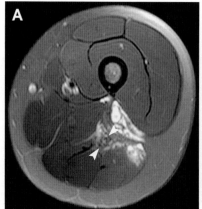
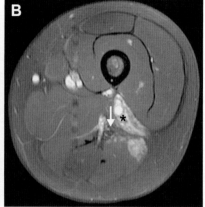

Fig. 23. An 11-year-old boy with a venous malformation of the thigh. (*A*) Axial T2-weighted MR image with fat saturation at the level of the mid thigh shows the enlargement of the sciatic nerve with focal hyperintensities (*arrowheads*) due to infiltration by the venous malformation. (*B*) Axial T1-weighted MR image with fat saturation after intravenous contrast shows some of the varicosities of the venous malformation (*asterisk*) partially encasing the sciatic nerve (*arrow*) and infiltrating it. This finding precluded the option of percutaneous sclerotherapy.

SUMMARY

Various underlying pathologic conditions can affect the peripheral nerves of children and, unfortunately, the difficulties of evaluating peripheral nerves are heightened in children due to their smaller size and rarity of the potential pathologies relative to adults. Careful imaging planning between the radiologist and the referring physician is important before an MR neurography to maximize the yield of the examination and keep the imaging time to a minimum. The findings of peripheral nerve pathologic condition include direct findings in the nerve and indirect findings in the denervated muscles. MR imaging, which is a noninvasive imaging modality and not associated with ionizing radiation, is an excellent imaging tool for detecting both direct and indirect findings associated with peripheral nerve pathology, particularly in the pediatric population. Clear understanding of clinical indications, MR imaging technique, and MR imaging findings of both normal and abnormal peripheral nerves in the pediatric population can lead to early diagnosis and optimal patient care.

REFERENCES

1. Maravilla KR, Bowen BC. Imaging of peripheral nervous system: evaluation of peripheral neuropathy and plexopathy. AJNR Am J Neuroradiol 1998;19: 1011–23.

2. Edelstein WA, Glover GH, Hardy CJ, et al. The intrinsic signal-to-noise ratio in NMR imaging. Magn Reson Med 1986;3:504–618.

3. Filler AG, Maravilla KR, Tsuruda JS. MR neurography and muscle MR imaging for image diagnosis of disorders affecting the peripheral nerves and musculature. Neurol Clin 2004;22:643–82.

4. Dailey A, Tsuruda J, Goodkin R, et al. Magnetic resonance neurography of peripheral nerve degeneration and regeneration. Lancet 1997;350(9086): 1221–2.

5. Grant GA, Goodkin R, Maravilla KR, et al. Neurography: diagnostic utility in the surgical treatment of peripheral nerve disorders. Neuroimaging Clin N Am 2004;14:115–33.

6. Chappell KE, Robson MD, Stonebridge-Foster A, et al. Magic angle effects in MR neurography. AJNR Am J Neuroradiol 2004;25:431–40.

7. Fleckenstein JL, Watumull D, Conner KE, et al. Denervated skeletal muscle imaging. Radiology 1993;187:213–8.

8. Ouvrier RA, McLeod JG, Pollard JD. Peripheral neuropathy in childhood. 2nd edition. London: Cambridge University Press; 1999. p. 1–335.

9. Thawait SK, Chaudhry V, Thawait GK, et al. High-resolution MR neurography of diffuse peripheral nerve lesions. AJNR Am J Neuroradiol 2011;32: 1365–72.

10. Murphey M, Smith S, Smith S, et al. Imaging of musculoskeletal neurogenic tumors: radiologic-pathologic correlation. Radiographics 1999;19: 1253–80.

11. Rodriguez F, Folpe A, Giannini C. Pathology of peripheral nerve sheath tumors: diagnostic overview and update on selected diagnostic problems. Acta Neuropathol 2012;123:295–319.

12. Laffan E, Ngan B, Navarro O. Pediatric soft-tissue tumors and pseudo-tumors: MR imaging features with pathologic correlation: part 2. Tumors of fibroblastic/myofibroblastic, so-called fibrohistiocytic, muscular, lymphomatous, neurogenic, hair matrix, and uncertain origin. Radiographics 2009;29:e36.

13. Huang G, Huang C, Lee H. Diffuse neurofibromas of the arm: MR characteristics. AJR Am J Roentgenol 2005;184:1711–2.

14. Lin V, Daniel S, Forte S. Is a plexiform neurofibromas pathognomonic of neurofibromatosis type 1? Laryngoscope 2004;114:1410–4.

15. Aloi FG, Massobrio R. Solitary plexiform neurofibromas. Dermatologica 1998;179:84–6.

16. Beaman F, Kransdorf M, Menke D. Schwannoma: radiologic-pathologic correlation. Radiographics 2004;24:1477–81.

17. Hassell D, Bancroft L, Kransdorf M, et al. Imaging appearance of diffuse neurofibromas. AJR Am J Roentgenol 2008;190:582–8.

18. Wilkinson L, Manson D, Smith C. Best cases from the AFIP: plexiform neurofibroma of the bladder. Radiographics 2004;24:S237–42.

19. Hrehorovich P, Franke H, Maximin S, et al. Malignant peripheral nerve sheath tumor. Radiographics 2003; 23:790–4.

20. Wasa J, Nishida Y, Tsukushi S, et al. MRI features in the differentiation of malignant peripheral nerve sheath tumors and neurofibromas. AJR Am J Roentgenol 2010;194:1568–74.

21. Mautner V, Asuagbor F, Dombi E, et al. Assessment of benign tumor burden by whole-body MRI in patients with neurofibromatosis 1. Neuro Oncol 2008; 10:593–8.

22. De Freitas MR. Infectious neuropathy. Curr Opin Neurol 2007;20:548–52.

23. Byun W, Park W, Park B. Guillain-Barré Syndrome: MR imaging findings of the spine in eight patients. Radiology 1998;208:137–41.

24. Zuccoli G, Panigrahy A, Bailey A. Redefining the Guillain-Barré spectrum in children: neuroimaging findings of cranial nerve involvement. AJNR Am J Neuroradiol 2011;32:639–42.

25. Berciano J. Thickening and contrast enhancement of spinal roots on MR imaging in Guillain-Barré

syndrome: thoughts on pathologic background. AJNR Am J Neuroradiol 2011;32:E179.

26. Duarte J, Cruz Martinez A, Rodriguez A. Hypertrophy of multiple cranial nerves and spinal roots in chronic inflammatory demyelinating neuropathy. J Neurol Neurosurg Psychiatry 1999;67:685–7.

27. Uzun N, Tanriverdi T, Savrun FK, et al. Traumatic peripheral nerve injuries: demographic and electrophysiologic findings of 802 patients from a developing country. J Clin Neuromuscul Dis 2006;7:97–103.

28. Seddon HJ. Three types of nerve injuries. Brain 1943;66:237.

29. Noble J, Munro CA, Prasad VS. Analysis of upper and lower extremity peripheral nerve injuries in a population of patients with multiple injuries. J Trauma 1998;45:116–22.

30. Flores AJ, Lavernia CJ, Owens PW. Anatomy and physiology of peripheral nerve injury and repair. Am J Orthop (Belle Mead NJ) 2000;29:167–73.

31. Kingston CA, Owens CM, Jeanes A. Imaging of desmoids fibromatosis in pediatric patients. AJR Am J Roentgenol 2002;178:191–9.

32. Lewis J, Boland P, Leung D. The enigma of desmoids tumors. Ann Surg 1999;229:866–73.

33. Murphey M, Carroll J, Flemming D, et al. From the archives of the AFIP: benign musculoskeletal lipomatous lesions. Radiographics 2004;24:1433–66.

34. Pham N, Poirier B, Fuller S, et al. Pediatric lipoblastoma in the head and neck: a systematic review of 48 reported cases. Int J Pediatr Otorhinolaryngol 2010;74:723–8.

35. Bottner F, Rodl R, Kordish I, et al. Surgical treatment of symptomatic osteochondroma: a three to eight year follow up study. J Bone Joint Surg Br 2003; 85:1161–5.

36. Van Gompel J, Griessenauer C, Scheithauer G, et al. Vascular malformations, rare causes of sciatic neuropathy: a case series. Neurosurgery 2010;67: 1133–42.

37. Lee KB, Kim DI, Oh SK, et al. Incidence of soft tissue injury and neuropathy after embolo/sclerotherapy for congenital vascular malformations. J Vasc Surg 2008;48:1286–91.

38. Cahill AM, Nijs E, Ballah D, et al. Percutaneous sclerotherapy in neonatal and infant head and neck lymphatic malformations: a single center experience. J Pediatr Surg 2011;46:2083–95.

39. Berenguer B, Burrows PE, Zurakowski D, et al. Sclerotherapy of craniofacial venous malformations: complications and results. Plast Reconstr Surg 1999;104:1–11.

40. Kirse DJ, Stern SJ, Suen JY, et al. Neurotoxic effects of doxycycline sclerotherapy. Otolaryngol Head Neck Surg 1998;118:356–62.

Cartilage Imaging in Children
Current Indications, Magnetic Resonance Imaging Techniques, and Imaging Findings

Victor M. Ho-Fung, MD*, Diego Jaramillo, MD, MPH

KEYWORDS

- Articular cartilage • Epiphyseal cartilage • Physeal cartilage • MRI morphologic cartilage imaging
- MRI functional cartilage imaging

KEY POINTS

- Structural differences in the matrix and cellularity of the 3 types of hyaline cartilage (articular, physeal, and epiphyseal) in children determine their morphology and signal characteristics on magnetic resonance (MR) imaging.
- There are 2 main approaches to cartilage MR imaging: morphologic and biochemical evaluation.
- T2-weighted images are particularly helpful in pediatric patients for the morphologic evaluation of the different types of hyaline cartilage and the depiction of physiologic changes related to skeletal maturation.
- Biochemical MR imaging techniques (delayed gadolinium-enhanced MR imaging of cartilage, T2, and T1rho mapping, among others) allow the quantitative evaluation of cartilage matrix composition for early detection and monitoring of degenerative changes.

INTRODUCTION

The imaging evaluation of cartilage in children plays a crucial role in the assessment of musculoskeletal pathology. The developing skeleton of children is unique because of the presence of physeal and epiphyseal cartilage in addition to articular cartilage. Current indications for both morphologic and biochemical cartilage imaging in children and adolescents are expanding as new therapy techniques for cartilage repair emerge. In infants, complications of the treatment in complicated developmental dysplasia of the hip (ie, epiphyseal femoral head avascular necrosis) can be detected with magnetic resonance (MR) imaging before permanent damage ensues. In young children with Legg-Calvé-Perthes disease, the determination of the extent of physeal and epiphyseal involvement and of the pattern of reperfusion helps establish the prognosis. In older children and adolescents, increasing participation in organized sports has caused a concomitant increased in sports injuries.[1] Both acute and chronic osteochondral injuries and physeal injuries are part of the spectrum in sports injuries in the pediatric population. At all ages, the evaluation of articular cartilage abnormalities helps establish the potential for the development of osteoarthritis. In addition, inflammatory and infectious arthritis account for an additional source of cartilage-related morbidity. Effective imaging techniques are required for the management of patients in these diverse groups of conditions in children and adolescents. Because of its high spatial resolution, excellent tissue contrast, and more recently developed biochemical cartilage sequences, MR imaging provides both morphologic and structural information necessary for the early and accurate

Perelman School of Medicine, The Children's Hospital of Philadelphia, University of Pennsylvania, 34th Street and Civic Center Boulevard, Philadelphia, PA 19104, USA
* Corresponding author.
E-mail address: hov@email.chop.edu

Radiol Clin N Am 51 (2013) 689–702
http://dx.doi.org/10.1016/j.rcl.2013.04.003
0033-8389/13/$ – see front matter © 2013 Elsevier Inc. All rights reserved.

radiologic.theclinics.com

diagnosis, monitoring of disease progression, and response to medical and surgical therapy for cartilage injuries in pediatric patients.

CURRENT INDICATIONS

In children, MR imaging in acute musculoskeletal injury is most commonly performed in the knee. The most common injuries following trauma to the immature knee are chondral.[2] Lateral patellar dislocation remains one of the main causes of chondral and osteochondral injuries in children. The incidence of chondral and osteochondral injuries can be as high as 38% for the inferomedial patellar cartilage, 38% for the lateral femoral condyle, and osteochondral fragments can be seen in approximately 42%.[3] The mechanism of injury is the transient lateral patellar translation and impaction of the medial aspect of the patella into the lateral femoral condyle causing the characteristic pattern of injury (**Fig. 1**).

After the identification of a primary injury, such as meniscal or anterior cruciate ligament tears or lateral patellar dislocation, it is crucial to perform a close inspection of the articular cartilage and the underlying subchondral region for subtle osteochondral injuries. These injuries can be found at sites of impaction or bony edema both in the acute phase and the follow-up evaluation. The evolution of an apparently minor injury can degenerate into more severe changes for which the referring clinician may be required to modify the course of therapy.

Successful communication with the clinicians taking care of patients requires a consistent language for the description of chondral injuries. The arthroscopic classification of cartilage injuries in the knee using the Outerbridge classification categorizes lesions according to the depth of cartilage loss. A validated MR imaging classification emulating this concept is the modified Outerbridge classification, which is used for

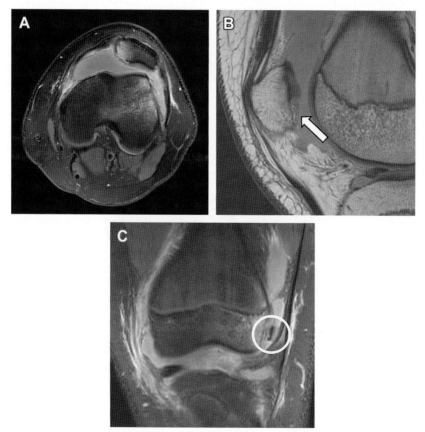

Fig. 1. A 16-year-old boy with acute left knee injury following fall playing basketball. (*A*) Axial fat-suppressed proton-density MR image shows bone marrow edema pattern with kissing contusions of the medial patella and lateral femoral condyle consistent with transient lateral patellar dislocation. (*B*) Sagittal proton-density MR image shows chondral defect (grade IV) (*arrow*) of the lower patella. (*C*) Coronal fat-suppressed T2 MR image shows intra-articular osteochondral fragment (*circle*) at the lateral femoral region from donor site in the lower patella.

preoperative evaluation (**Figs. 2** and **3, Table 1**). This classification system is predominantly used for the knee, but it is appropriate for any other articular surface in the body.

There have been remarkable advances in cartilage repair procedures in the last decade. Orthopedic surgeons now have multiple procedures for the treatment of articular cartilage lesions, including osteochondral autografting, microfracture techniques, and autologous chondrocyte implantation. In the postoperative setting, the MR evaluation of cartilage repair tissue (MOCART) classification has been recently proposed (**Box 1**).[4] This classification is a comprehensive classification using multiple parameters: degree of defect filling, integration to border zone, surface of repair tissue, structure of repair tissue, signal intensity of repair tissue, subchondral lamina, subchondral bone, adhesions, and synovitis. Some of these parameters have been subsequently validated and demonstrated good correlation with clinical outcome scores in postsurgical patients with repaired cartilage tissue.[5] In general, the signal intensity of the cartilage repair tissue should normalize; the cartilage defect should be filled in completely with a smooth, congruent articular surface; and the hyperintense bone marrow signal along with joint effusion should resolve (**Fig. 4**).[6]

Autologous osteochondral autografting or mosaicplasty (multiple plugs) involves the removal of small cylindrical osteochondral plugs from the non–weight-bearing portion of the joint and transfer to the chondral lesion site at the weight-bearing portion of the articular surface.[7] The osteochondral plug should be perpendicular to the articular surface for optimal results and the transferred cartilage cap should be flush to the adjacent native articular surface (**Fig. 5**).

The surgical techniques involving bone marrow stimulation attempting to expose pluripotential stem cells in the subchondral bone into the chondral lesion include microfracture technique, drilling, and abrasion arthroplasty. There is formation of a fibrin clot at the microfracture site, with formation of reparative fibrocartilaginous tissue in these procedures.[8,9] The presence of subchondral cyst or persistent extensive perigraft marrow hyperintensity/edema may reflect poor osseous incorporation and potential graft instability.[10]

Autologous chondrocyte implantation is a 2-step procedure in which chondrocytes are harvested from a non–weight-bearing region, subsequently replicated in vitro, and then injected into the chondral defect in the weight-bearing region and covered with a periosteal flap.[11]

IMAGING TECHNIQUES: STRUCTURAL/BIOCHEMICAL/FUNCTIONAL APPROACH

Cartilage repair and pharmacologic therapies are areas of major clinical interest and research, particularly for the prevention and treatment of osteoarthritis. There are MR imaging techniques for cartilage matrix assessment, including delayed gadolinium-enhanced MR imaging of cartilage (dGEMRIC), T2 mapping, and T1rho mapping

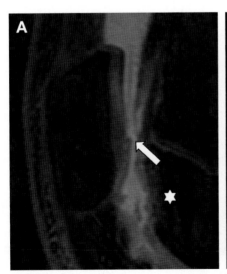
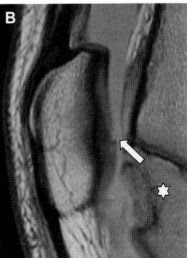

Fig. 2. A 12-year-old boy with history of lateral patellar dislocation. (*A*) Sagittal double echo steady state and (*B*) sagittal proton-density MR images demonstrate superficial fissuring of the articular cartilage in the patella consistent with a grade I chondral injury (*arrow*). Also focal osteochondral defect in the anterior aspect of the lateral femoral condyle (*asterisk*).

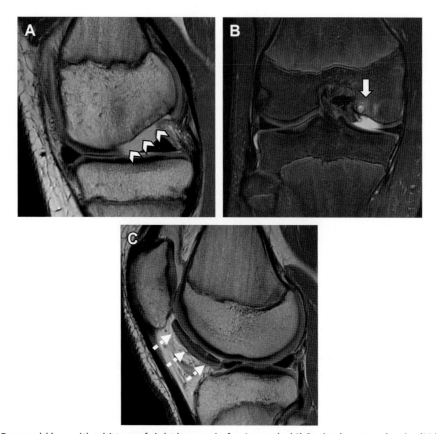

Fig. 3. A 15-year-old boy with a history of right knee pain for 1 month. (*A*) Sagittal proton-density (PD) MR image shows large osteochondral defect (*arrowheads*) in the medial femoral condyle (grade IV). (*B*) Coronal fat-suppressed T2-weighted MR image shows subchondral cystic changes and bone marrow edema signal intensity (*solid arrow*). (*C*) Sagittal PD MR image shows osteochondral fragment (*interrupted arrowheads*) anterior to the lateral femoral condyle.

techniques in the forefront for guidance and monitoring of these therapies (**Table 2**).[12,13] The main objective behind the advancement of these MR techniques is the early identification of potentially reversible cartilage damage, which is a topic of great importance when treating young children and the potential morbidity and incapacitating symptoms of osteoarthritis as young adults.

Table 1	
Modified Outerbridge classification	
0	Intact articular cartilage
1	Articular cartilage thickening with abnormal signal
2	Superficial ulceration or fissuring
3	Deep ulceration or fissuring
4	Full-thickness chondral injury with bruising of subchondral bone
5	Osteochondral injury with separation of osteochondral fragment

The structural evaluation of T2 relaxation of the cartilage reflects the interaction of water and matrix. This interaction seems to be primarily related to the collagen content of the tissue. The loss of collagen increases the amount of free water; the greater the volume of free water, the longer the relaxation time.[12] With higher concentration of macromolecules to bind water, T2 relaxation is shorter.

If the macromolecules of the matrix begin to break down, the increased free water results in prolongation of T2 relaxation. T2 can be measured by a turbo spin echo sequence obtained with multiple echo times. A map is generated in which the T2 relaxation time of each pixel is coded by a color (**Fig. 6**). The technique is available commercially and can be implemented with greater ease than any other of the structural techniques. T2 maps are specific but not sensitive to cartilage degeneration, which may be because glycosaminoglycan (GAG) loss precedes collagen loss in osteoarthritis and T2 maps reflect more collagen mapping, particularly evaluating for differences in visual appearance of the maps, has been used to evaluate early cartilage damage in hip dysplasia.[17]

T1rho or spin lock imaging is a technique that is sensitive to chemical exchanges by molecules, such as proteoglycans.[18] Multiple biochemical studies have shown that a prolongation of T1rho is primarily associated with GAG loss.[19] The collagen content, however, does seem to modify T1rho times. This technique relies on delivering a long radiofrequency pulse that serves to lock the spins and prevents T2 decay and in subsequently measuring the decay in transverse magnetization that is independent of T2 effects. Unfortunately the technique is not commercially available and still requires postprocessing.[19]

dGEMRIC is a technique that specifically looks at GAGs. The GAGs are negatively charged, and the fixed charge density of cartilage is closely related to the GAG concentration. Gadopentetate dimeglumine^{2-} (Gd-DTPA^{2-}) has a negative charge and

than GAG abnormalities.[14] In pediatrics, T2 mapping has been used to evaluate juvenile inflammatory arthritis in children.[15,16] It has been demonstrated that T2 relaxation times are higher in children with juvenile inflammatory arthritis, correlating with structural collagen breakdown. T2

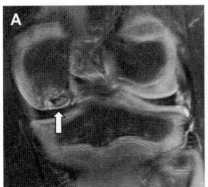
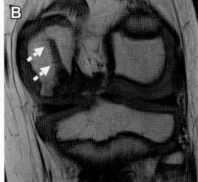
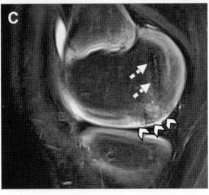

Fig. 4. An 8-year-old boy with left knee medial osteochondritis dissecans (OCD) with persistent pain. (A) Preoperative coronal fat-suppressed proton-density MR images shows OCD lesion (*solid arrow*) within the lateral aspect of the medial femoral condyle. One-year follow-up evaluation. (B) Postoperative coronal T1-weigthted MR image shows fixation of the osteochondral fragment with bioabsorbable screw track (*interrupted arrows*). (C) Sagittal fat-suppressed T2-weighted MR image shows bioabsorbable screw track (*interrupted arrows*) without underlying bone marrow edema or cystic changes. There is mild superficial irregularity of the articular cartilage at the surgical site (*arrowhead*) but grossly normalized signal intensity and no gaps relative to the adjacent normal cartilage.

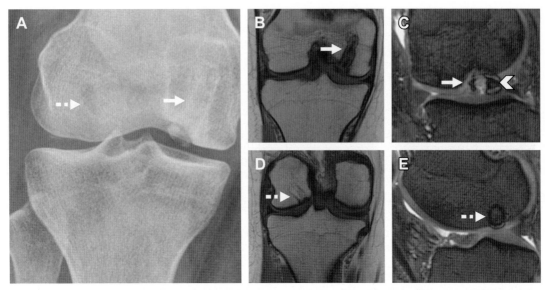

Fig. 5. A 15-year-old boy with history of unstable medial osteochondritis dissecans and 1-year follow-up after autologous bone graft surgery. (*A*) Frontal radiograph shows small lucency at donor site for osteochondral plug (*interrupted arrows*) and well-corticated bioabsorbable screw track (*solid arrow*). Coronal proton-density (PD) MR image (*B*) demonstrates the bioabsorbable screw track (*solid arrow*), and sagittal fat-suppressed T2-weighted MR image (*C*) demonstrates almost complete filling of the articular cartilage with adequate thickness and homogeneous signal intensity similar to native cartilage in the medial femoral condyle. Low signal intensity corresponding to bony components (*arrowhead*) of the osteochondral plug and perpendicular orientation to the articular surface are noted. Coronal PD MR image (*D*) and sagittal fat-suppressed T2-weighted MR image (*E*) demonstrate the donor site at the non–weight-bearing portion of the lateral intercondylar notch. No bony edema is noted within the surgical sites.

is repelled by GAGs in the cartilage. When there is a breakdown of GAGs, cartilage loses its negative charge. Given time to penetrate into cartilage, Gd-DTPA^{2-} is distributed in higher concentrations in areas of low glycosaminoglycan content and in lower concentrations in areas rich in glycosaminoglycans.[20] Creating a T1 map reflects the concentrations of Gd-DTPA^{2-} in the cartilage. An area of GAG loss will allow more Gd-DTPA^{2-} into its matrix and a shorter T1 relaxation time. The clinical

Table 2
Advanced MR imaging techniques for evaluation of cartilage composition

MR Imaging Technique	Cartilage Component Evaluated	Advantages	Disadvantages
T2 mapping	Collagen orientation and water content	Robust clinical software and easy implementation in routine clinical protocols Fast acquisition time	Detection of early cartilage degeneration, particularly glycosaminoglycan depletion, remains inconclusive
dGEMRIC	Glycosaminoglycans	Robust clinical software and easy implementation in routine clinical protocols High image resolution and indirect arthrographic effect	Requires intravenous contrast administration and increased time before imaging to allow diffusion of contrast into cartilage
T1rho	Glycosaminoglycans and collagen	Early detection of prostaglandin depletion	Not readily available in daily clinical use High radiofrequency power and specific absorption rate limits

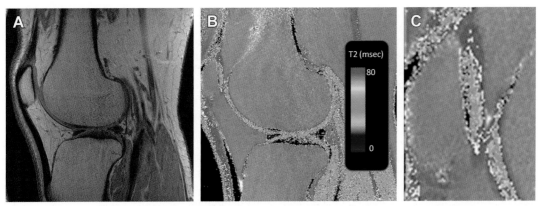

Fig. 6. A 19-year-old boy with normal articular cartilage. (A) Sagittal proton-density–weighted MR image shows intact articular cartilage of the patella and femur. (B) Sagittal T2 map shows normal homogeneous low values through the articular surface of the distal femur and patella. (C) Magnified view of the patellar and trochlear cartilage T2 map with progressive increase in T2 values from deep to superficial cartilage layers, which is an expected finding based on the anisotropy of collagen fibers running perpendicular to cortical bone in the deep layer of cartilage.

success of the dGEMRIC technique relies in the attention to detail. Gd-DTPA^{2-} is injected intravenously 60 to 90 minutes before imaging for adequate diffusion of the contrast into the joint and to achieve equilibrium with the cartilage. The patient is then requested to exercise lightly (ambulation in the authors' protocol) to facilitate the distribution of the contrast. T1 maps of the affected joint can be generated by using short tau inversion recovery (STIR) images with variable inversion times, fast spin echo images with variable repetition times, or more recently, gradient echoes with variable flip angles. Currently commercially available programs allow the generation of 3-dimensional (3D) gradient echo–based T1 maps. dGEMRIC has been used to evaluate degenerative changes associated with hip dysplasia (Fig. 7).[21] Elevated T1 values related to GAG loss were found in patients with hip dysplasia and pain even without loss of thickness of the cartilage. The authors have also applied dGEMRIC for the qualitative assessment of articular cartilage in the

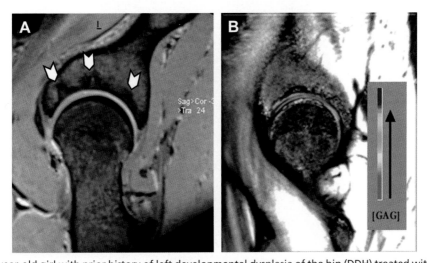

Fig. 7. A 9-year-old girl with prior history of left developmental dysplasia of the hip (DDH) treated with spica casting and new onset of pain. Normal T1 maps (dGEMRIC). (A) Sagittal fat-suppressed radial reconstruction T1-weighted MR image shows normal spherical contour of the femoral head with congruent alignment to the acetabular roof. The articular cartilage appears morphologically normal. There are mild focal sclerotic changes (arrowheads) within the subchondral region of the acetabulum reflecting minor chronic changes of treated DDH. (B) Sagittal post-gadolinium T1 map (dGEMRIC) shows normal homogeneous T1 values (blue, green) consistent with intact cartilage.

femoral head of patients with chronic sequela of Legg-Calve-Perthes or avascular necrosis disease and new onset of pain after years of stable chronic morphologic changes (**Fig. 8**).

Diffusion-weighted images (DWI) probe the structure of cartilage by looking at the patterns of diffusion of water within the tissue.[22] Most diffusion techniques use echo-planar images. The challenge with echo-planar imaging is that susceptibility artifacts arise at the interface between bone and cartilage. Therefore, DWI of cartilage may benefit from using techniques to decrease susceptibility. Line scan diffusion imaging, single-shot fast spin echo techniques, periodically rotated overlapping parallel lines with enhanced reconstruction-echo-planar imaging (PROPELLER-EPI), and steady state precession sequence imaging can be used for the evaluation of cartilage.[23] In epiphyseal and physeal cartilage, water is organized around macromolecules and it is likely that tissue disruption will affect the diffusion of water as measured by this technique (**Fig. 9**).[24,25] Diffusion tensor imaging (DTI) maps may reflect both the macromolecular environment and the direction of motion of water protons, which in turn reflects the alignment of the collagenous fiber network.[26] DWI and DTI are promising techniques to visualize cartilage ultrastructure.[27]

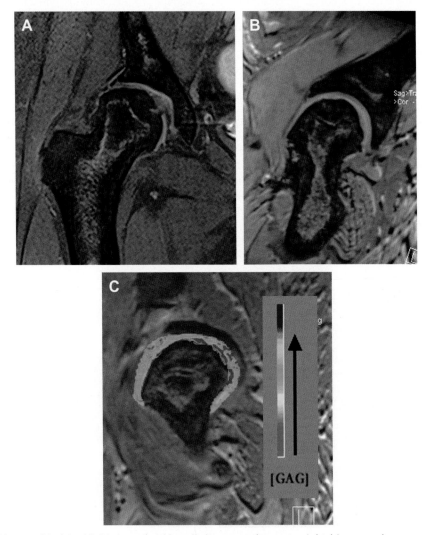

Fig. 8. A 12-year-old girl with history of sickle cell disease and remote right hip avascular necrosis now with increasing right hip pain. (*A*) Coronal fat-suppressed T1-weighted and (*B*) sagittal fat-suppressed radial reconstruction T1-weighted MR images show irregularity and flattening of the femoral head contour. Abnormal bone marrow signal intensity characteristic of bone infarcts are present through the iliac bone and the femoral head and neck region. There is thinning of the underlying cartilage within the anterior and posterior articular regions. (*C*) Sagittal postgadolinium T1 map (dGEMRIC) shows heterogeneous regions of lower T1 values (*red and yellow*) corresponding to these anatomic sites and consistent with cartilage degeneration.

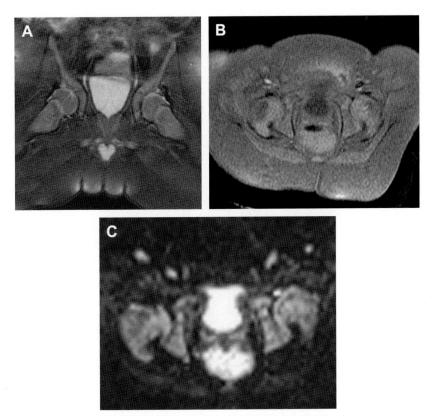

Fig. 9. An 11-month-old girl with left developmental dysplasia of the hip with closed reduction and spica cast placement. Postoperative MR image. (A) Coronal fat-suppressed T2-weighted MR image shows adequate reduction of the left hip with subtle smaller size of the left femoral head relative to the right. (B) Axial postcontrast fat-suppressed T1-weighted MR image shows bilateral homogeneous enhancement with speckled appearance of the anatomically located femoral head epiphysis. (C) Axial diffusion-weighted MR image shows normal epiphyseal signal intensity.

NORMAL ANATOMY

The imaging of cartilage in children differs from that in adults because physeal and epiphyseal cartilage are present. Physeal and epiphyseal cartilage are structurally and biochemically different than articular cartilage. However, the 3 types of cartilage have the same matrix comprised of collagen and GAGs.[28] The collagen provides stability, tensile strength, and resistance to shear forces. GAGs provide water-absorbent properties allowing cartilage to resist compressive forces and return to its original shape after dissipation of these forces.

The main role of articular cartilage is to provide almost frictionless movement for the joint surfaces.[29] Articular cartilage does not contain nerves, lymphatics, or vascularity. The nutrition to the superficial layers of the articular cartilage is thought to originate from the synovial fluid, and the deep layers are probably nourished from subchondral bone. The lack of vascularity has been proposed as one of the main reasons for the inherent lack of reparative capacity of the articular cartilage. Approximately 70% of the articular cartilage weight is water, and the remaining components are a matrix of collagen and proteoglycans with very few cells (less than 2% volume).[30–32] Five well-defined histologic zones are present in the articular cartilage (**Box 2**). The density of chondrocytes is highest close to subchondral bone and decreases toward the articular surface. In children, chondrocyte replication is present in all zones of the cartilage; but with skeletal maturity, replication is only present in the radial or deep zone of the cartilage. This physiologic change in proliferative capacity can represent one of the underlying reasons for the superior healing capacity of pediatric cartilage compared with adult cartilage, which is a relevant observation in pediatric patients with osteochondritis dissecans.

Both physeal and epiphyseal cartilage are responsible for the longitudinal growth in long bones. The arrangement of collagen fibers in the example, vascular canals are prominent in diseases that result in inflamed synovium, such as juvenile idiopathic arthritis, and when infection invades the epiphyseal cartilage. They are attenuated when there is ischemia of the cartilage, such as during excessive abduction in spica casts for the treatment of developmental dysplasia of the hip, and during epiphyseal ischemia related to septic arthritis in large joints, such as the hip and shoulder.

MR IMAGING APPEARANCE OF THE CARTILAGE: MORPHOLOGIC EVALUATION

Before skeletal maturation, structural, functional, and maturational differences between the 3 types of cartilage in the ends of the long bones determine their morphology and signal characteristics on MR imaging (**Table 3**). Familiarity with these physiologic processes related to growth and development is important for successful diagnostic interpretation of MR imaging in children.[33]

On T1-weighted (T1-W) images, all 3 hyaline cartilage is of intermediate signal intensity; therefore, this sequence is not particularly helpful for differentiation among each type of immature hyaline cartilage. However, there is good contrast with fibrocartilaginous structures (menisci and labral fibrocartilaginous tissue of the knee, hip, or glenoid), which are of low signal intensity.

Water-sensitive sequences, namely, STIR and spin-echo T2-weighted (T2-W) images, are extremely useful for differentiation among the 3 types of hyaline cartilage in the developing skeleton. The epiphyseal cartilage is of low signal intensity, whereas the physeal and articular cartilage are of high signal intensity on T2-W images (**Fig. 10**). Lengthening the echo time (TE) will decrease the signal from the epiphyseal cartilage and further accentuate the contrast between the

physis and epiphysis is more uniform than in the articular cartilage. Also, water is less tightly bound in physeal cartilage. In contradistinction to articular cartilage, physeal cartilage is very cellular. In particular, the hypertrophic zone of the physis demonstrates 75% of the volume made up by cells. The vascularity of the physeal and epiphyseal cartilage is also different than the avascular articular cartilage. The epiphyseal cartilage is a vascularized structure. The physeal cartilage is only vascular during the first 18 months of life and then becomes avascular. These changes also determine the pathologic changes seen at different stages of skeletal maturation. For

MR Imaging Sequence	Articular Cartilage	Physeal Cartilage	Epiphyseal Cartilage	Fibrocartilage (Menisci/Labra)
T1-weighted	Intermediate SI	Intermediate SI	Intermediate SI	Low SI
STIR or T2-weighted with fat suppression	High SI	High SI	Low SI	Low SI
Intermediate PD-weighted	High SI	High SI	High SI	Low SI
GRE with fat suppression	Intermediate to high SI	High SI	Intermediate to high SI	Low to intermediate SI

Table 3
MR imaging signal characteristics of hyaline cartilage

Abbreviations: GRE, gradient recalled echo; PD, proton density; SI, signal intensity.

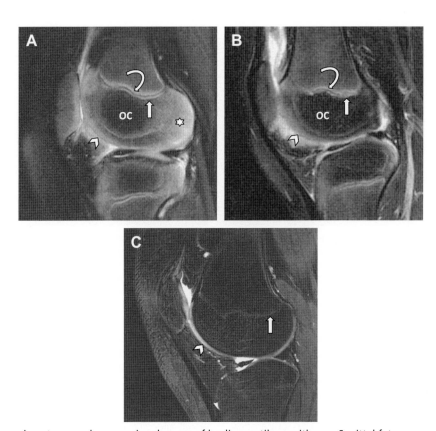

Fig. 10. Normal anatomy and progressive changes of hyaline cartilage with age. Sagittal fat-suppressed fast spin echo T2-W MR images in different patients. (*A*) A 2-year-old girl. Distal femoral physis is hyperintense (*solid arrow*). Zone of provisional calcification is a thin hypointense line (*curved solid arrow*) with smooth contour at this age. The nonossified epiphyseal cartilage of the posterior femoral condyle demonstrates heterogeneous signal intensity (*asterisk*), a normal variant. The secondary ossification center (OC) is the ossified portion of the distal femoral epiphysis. The articular cartilage demonstrates homogeneous high signal intensity (*arrowhead*) relative to less organized nonossified epiphyseal cartilage. (*B*) A 5-year-old girl. Distal femoral physis remains hyperintense (*solid arrow*). Zone of provisional calcification remains as a thin hypointense line (*curved solid arrow*) but appears more undulated and irregular in contour. The articular cartilage demonstrates homogeneous high signal intensity (*arrowhead*) relative to less organized nonossified epiphyseal cartilage that appears progressively smaller with age. (*C*) A 15-year-old girl. Distal femoral physis (*solid arrow*) is barely perceptible as a physeal scar in keeping with complete skeletal maturation. Other structures are not longer visualized as discrete structures (zone of provisional calcification, secondary ossification center of the epiphysis). The articular cartilage remains homogeneous with high signal intensity (*arrowhead*). Note the complete fat suppression of yellow marrow in the distal femoral and proximal tibial metadiaphysis.

epiphyseal and physeal cartilage. On the contrary, shortening of TE (creating proton density/intermediate-weighted sequences) causes less contrast between these regions of cartilage. Water-sensitive sequences are also helpful for identification of physiologic changes related to skeletal maturation, including the presence of preossification centers in the epiphyseal cartilage, characterized by areas of increased signal intensity on water-sensitive sequences representing the hypertrophic changes on the epiphyseal cartilage just before its transformation into bone (**Fig. 11**). Typical locations for these preossification centers include the trochlea of the distal humerus and the posterior aspect of the

nonossified epiphyseal cartilage of the distal femoral condyle.[34] An additional maturation process seen of water-sensitive sequences is noted with the progression of standing and walking in toddler infants, causing a decrease in the signal intensity of epiphyseal cartilage along the weight-bearing portions of the distal femoral condyles, a process that probably is related to the displacement of water within the epiphyseal cartilage caused by increased axial loading and weight bearing (**Fig. 12**).[33,35] On the metaphyseal side of the physis and paralleling it, a thin band of very low signal intensity corresponds to the zone of provisional calcification, usually evident on all pulse sequences. A continuous low-signal-intensity line

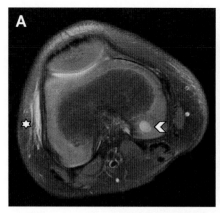
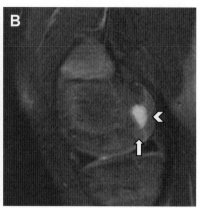

Fig. 11. A 4-year-old boy lateral knee pain. (*A*) Axial fat-suppressed proton-density and (*B*) sagittal fat-suppressed T2-W MR images show well-circumscribed rounded hyperintense structure (*arrowhead*) within the posterior non–weighted-bearing portion of the nonossified medial epiphyseal cartilage (*arrow*). There is absence of bony edema or adjacent articular cartilage changes. Findings are consistent with preossification changes in the posterior distal femoral condyle, unrelated to patient's symptoms. Only mild subcutaneous soft tissue edema was noted along the lateral knee region (*asterisk*).

reflects healthy endochondral ossification. Discontinuity of the high physeal signal intensity on water-sensitive sequences implies cartilage disruption and an accompanying interruption of the adjacent low-signal-intensity zone of provisional calcification indicates resultant abnormal endochondral ossification. The normal physis also undergoes change with skeletal maturity; it becomes thinner, less conspicuous, and more undulating.

On gradient recalled echo (GRE) imaging, all forms of hyaline cartilage are uniformly intermediate or high signal intensity. A particular advantage of GRE

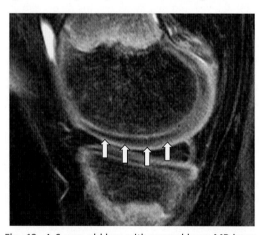

Fig. 12. A 6-year-old boy with normal knee MR imaging. Sagittal fat-suppressed T2-W MR image shows homogeneous decrease in signal intensity in the weight-bearing portion of the epiphyseal cartilage of the distal medial femoral condyle (*arrows*), a physiologic finding seen in young children. The decrease in signal intensity in this region is likely related to displacement of water within the epiphyseal cartilage caused by axial loading and weight bearing.

sequences is the contrast between cartilage and adjacent synovial fluid. Gradient recalled T1-W images (flip angle of 45° or greater), also called spoiled gradient echo images or fast low-angle shot images, provide excellent contrast between the high-signal-intensity cartilage and the lower-signal-intensity articular fluid. Similarly, gradient recalled T2-W images (lower flip angle of 15°–20°) provide excellent contrast between the lower-signal-intensity cartilage and higher-signal-intensity fluid. The conspicuity of the cartilage increases significantly with fat suppression on gradient recalled T1-W images; however, this sequence does not allow differentiation between regions of cartilage because all hyaline cartilage are of high signal. A double-echo steady state (DESS) sequence, particularly when used with water excitation, also provides excellent visualization of cartilaginous detail; it is a mixed T1/T2*–W sequence. With all GRE imaging, isotropic imaging allows thinner sections and, if necessary, additional multiplanar reconstructions.

The authors' current protocols for morphologic cartilage evaluation are a combination of all these sequences, with an emphasis on proton density/intermediate-weighted images and isotropic fat-saturated (FS) GRE (3D FS DESS) sequences; the former provides exquisite zonal architecture of the 3 types of cartilage and the latter offers detailed information of the thickness and integrity of the cartilage. The authors think that these sequences are complementary to each other and allow for greater diagnostic accuracy (see **Fig. 2**).

Ultra short echo time imaging (UTE) allows evaluation of structures with short T2 and T2* not seen on conventional T2-W clinical images, such as the radial and calcified zones of the articular cartilage.[36] At present, UTE is the only available tool for the assessment of the osteochondral junction, which can be an important interface for nourishment of the deep articular cartilage and probably implicated in the pathogenesis of osteoarthritis.[37] Other sequences for morphologic evaluation of cartilage include driven equilibrium Fourier transform imaging and steady state free precession imaging. Although they provide superior contrast between cartilage and adjacent joint fluid, neither one has attained generalized use. These sequences remain experimental and have not yet been well assessed in children.

SUMMARY

Advances in morphologic imaging of cartilage allow high-detail evaluation of focal abnormalities, whereas biochemical imaging reflects changes in the tissue that precede morphologic disruption. A combination of both approaches will allow early detection of pediatric patients at risk for degeneration, accurate mapping of established lesions, and assessment of postsurgical changes.

REFERENCES

1. Ho-Fung VM, Jaimes C, Jaramillo D. Magnetic resonance imaging assessment of sports-related musculoskeletal injury in children: current techniques and clinical applications. Semin Roentgenol 2012;47(2):171–81.
2. Oeppen RS, Connolly SA, Bencardino JT, et al. Acute injury of the articular cartilage and subchondral bone: a common but unrecognized lesion in the immature knee. AJR Am J Roentgenol 2004; 182(1):111–7.
3. Zaidi A, Babyn P, Astori I, et al. MRI of traumatic patellar dislocation in children. Pediatr Radiol 2006;36(11):1163–70.
4. Marlovits S, Striessnig G, Resinger CT, et al. Definition of pertinent parameters for the evaluation of articular cartilage repair tissue with high-resolution magnetic resonance imaging. Eur J Radiol 2004; 52(3):310–9.
5. Marlovits S, Singer P, Zeller P, et al. Magnetic resonance observation of cartilage repair tissue (MOCART) for the evaluation of autologous chondrocyte transplantation: determination of interobserver variability and correlation to clinical outcome after 2 years. Eur J Radiol 2006;57(1):16–23.
6. Chang G, Horng A, Glaser C. A practical guide to imaging of cartilage repair with emphasis on bone marrow changes. Semin Musculoskelet Radiol 2011;15(3):221–37.
7. Hangody L, Fules P. Autologous osteochondral mosaicplasty for the treatment of full-thickness defects of weight-bearing joints: ten years of experimental and clinical experience. J Bone Joint Surg Am 2003;85(Suppl 2):25–32.
8. Polster J, Recht M. Postoperative MR evaluation of chondral repair in the knee. Eur J Radiol 2005; 54(2):206–13.
9. Gnannt R, Chhabra A, Theodoropoulos JS, et al. MR imaging of the postoperative knee. J Magn Reson Imaging 2011;34(5):1007–21.
10. Alparslan L, Winalski CS, Boutin RD, et al. Postoperative magnetic resonance imaging of articular cartilage repair. Semin Musculoskelet Radiol 2001; 5(4):345–63.
11. Micheli LJ, Browne JE, Erggelet C, et al. Autologous chondrocyte implantation of the knee: multicenter experience and minimum 3-year follow-up. Clin J Sport Med 2001;11(4):223–8.
12. Mosher TJ, Dardzinski BJ. Cartilage MRI T2 relaxation time mapping: overview and applications. Semin Musculoskelet Radiol 2004;8(4):355–68.
13. Link TM, Stahl R, Woertler K. Cartilage imaging: motivation, techniques, current and future significance. Eur Radiol 2007;17(5):1135–46.
14. Regatte RR, Akella SV, Borthakur A, et al. Proteoglycan depletion-induced changes in transverse relaxation maps of cartilage: comparison of T2 and T1rho. Acad Radiol 2002;9(12):1388–94.
15. Dardzinski BJ, Laor T, Schmithorst VJ, et al. Mapping T2 relaxation time in the pediatric knee: feasibility with a clinical 1.5-T MR imaging system. Radiology 2002;225(1):233–9.
16. Kight AC, Dardzinski BJ, Laor T, et al. Magnetic resonance imaging evaluation of the effects of juvenile rheumatoid arthritis on distal femoral weight-bearing cartilage. Arthritis Rheum 2004;50(3):901–5.
17. Nishii T, Tanaka H, Sugano N, et al. Evaluation of cartilage matrix disorders by T2 relaxation time in patients with hip dysplasia. Osteoarthr Cartil 2008; 16(2):227–33.
18. Regatte RR, Akella SV, Lonner JH, et al. T1rho relaxation mapping in human osteoarthritis (OA) cartilage: comparison of T1rho with T2. J Magn Reson Imaging 2006;23(4):547–53.
19. Kneeland JB, Reddy R. Frontiers in musculoskeletal MRI: articular cartilage. J Magn Reson Imaging 2007;25(2):339–44.
20. Williams A, Gillis A, McKenzie C, et al. Glycosaminoglycan distribution in cartilage as determined by delayed gadolinium-enhanced MRI of cartilage (dGEMRIC): potential clinical applications. AJR Am J Roentgenol 2004;182(1):167–72.
21. Kim YJ, Jaramillo D, Millis MB, et al. Assessment of early osteoarthritis in hip dysplasia with delayed gadolinium-enhanced magnetic resonance imaging of cartilage. J Bone Joint Surg Am 2003;85(10):1987–92.
22. Van Breuseghem I. Ultrastructural MR imaging techniques of the knee articular cartilage: problems for

routine clinical application. Eur Radiol 2004;14(2): 184–92.

23. Mamisch TC, Menzel MI, Welsch GH, et al. Steady-state diffusion imaging for MR in-vivo evaluation of reparative cartilage after matrix-associated autologous chondrocyte transplantation at 3 tesla–preliminary results. Eur J Radiol 2008;65(1):72–9.

24. Filidoro L, Dietrich O, Weber J, et al. High-resolution diffusion tensor imaging of human patellar cartilage: feasibility and preliminary findings. Magn Reson Med 2005;53(5):993–8.

25. Jaramillo D, Connolly SA, Vajapeyam S, et al. Normal and ischemic epiphysis of the femur: diffusion MR imaging study in piglets. Radiology 2003; 227(3):825–32.

26. Glaser C. New techniques for cartilage imaging: T2 relaxation time and diffusion-weighted MR imaging. Radiol Clin North Am 2005;43(4):641–53, vii.

27. Potter HG, Black BR, Chong le R. New techniques in articular cartilage imaging. Clin Sports Med 2009; 28(1):77–94.

28. Jaramillo D. Cartilage imaging. Pediatr Radiol 2008; 38(Suppl 2):S256–8.

29. Buckwalter JA, Mankin HJ, Grodzinsky AJ. Articular cartilage and osteoarthritis. Instr Course Lect 2005; 54:465–80.

30. Mankin HJ, Thrasher AZ. Water content and binding in normal and osteoarthritic human cartilage. J Bone Joint Surg Am 1975;57(1):76–80.

31. Brandt KD, Doherty M, Lohmander S. Osteoarthritis. Oxford (NY): Oxford University Press; 2003.

32. Borthakur A, Reddy R. Imaging cartilage physiology. Top Magn Reson Imaging 2010;21(5): 291–6.

33. Jaramillo D, Laor T. Pediatric musculoskeletal MRI: basic principles to optimize success. Pediatr Radiol 2008;38(4):379–91.

34. Jaimes C, Jimenez M, Marin D, et al. The trochlear pre-ossification center: a normal developmental stage and potential pitfall on MR images. Pediatr Radiol 2012;42(11):1364–71.

35. Varich LJ, Laor T, Jaramillo D. Normal maturation of the distal femoral epiphyseal cartilage: age-related changes at MR imaging. Radiology 2000;214(3): 705–9.

36. Robson MD, Gatehouse PD, Bydder M, et al. Magnetic resonance: an introduction to ultrashort TE (UTE) imaging. J Comput Assist Tomogr 2003; 27(6):825–46.

37. Choi JA, Gold GE. MR imaging of articular cartilage physiology. Magn Reson Imaging Clin N Am 2011; 19(2):249–82.

Juvenile Idiopathic Arthritis
Current Practical Imaging Assessment with Emphasis on Magnetic Resonance Imaging

Ricardo Restrepo, MD[a], Edward Y. Lee, MD, MPH[b,*],
Paul S. Babyn, MD[c]

KEYWORDS

- Juvenile idiopathic arthritis • Imaging assessment • Magnetic resonance imaging • Ultrasound

KEY POINTS

- The diagnosis of juvenile idiopathic arthritis (JIA) is based on clinical and laboratory findings. However, there is evidence that ultrasonography and magnetic resonance imaging (MRI) may play an important role in detecting subclinical disease and treatment response.
- T2 relaxation mapping allows the early detection of microstructural cartilage changes before irreversible changes occur in patients with JIA.
- Whole body MRI can optimally evaluate activity and extent of disease in pediatric patients with enthesis-related arthritis as it frequently involves areas difficult to evaluate clinically.

INTRODUCTION

Juvenile idiopathic arthritis (JIA) represents not a single disease but a broad spectrum of arthritides of unknown cause occurring in patients younger than 16 years that lasts for at least 6 weeks. JIA is the most common chronic rheumatologic childhood disease and causes significant disability. The diagnosis of JIA is based on clinical and laboratory findings. However, the diagnosis of JIA mandates the exclusion of other types of arthritis.[1] Imaging plays a vital role throughout the disease process, from the time of the initial diagnosis, helping exclude other diseases, in staging once the diagnosis is made, assessing treatment response to newer and more effective medications and disease activity, as well as evaluating complications. This review focuses on the classification of JIA, the role of imaging with emphasis on magnetic resonance (MR) imaging at diagnosis, staging, and follow-up, including its challenges, and some future directions.

EPIDEMIOLOGY

JIA occurs worldwide, with regional variations believed to be caused by differences in the distribution of HLA alleles and environmental factors.[2] Among developed nations, JIA has a yearly incidence rate of 2 to 20 cases per 100,000 people and a prevalence of 16 to 150 cases per 100,000 people.[3] The incidence of chronic arthritis in childhood ranged from 0.008 to 0.026 per 1000 children and the prevalence ranged from 0.07 to 4.01 per 1000 children in a comprehensive worldwide survey from 2002.[4] The incidence of JIA is believed to vary widely in part because it is composed of a heterogeneous group of arthritides, which are diagnosed clinically.[5] The disease tends to occur

[a] Department of Radiology, Miami Children's Hospital, 3100 Southwest, 62nd Avenue, Miami, FL 33155, USA;
[b] Division of Magnetic Resonance and Thoracic Imaging, Department of Radiology and Pediatrics, Boston Children's Hospital and Harvard Medical School, 300 Longwood Avenue, Boston, MA 02115, USA;
[c] Department of Medical Imaging, Saskatoon Health Region, Royal University Hospital, University of Saskatchewan, Room 1566.1, 103 Hospital Drive, Saskatoon SK S7N 0W8, Canada
* Corresponding author.
E-mail address: Edward.Lee@childrens.harvard.edu

Radiol Clin N Am 51 (2013) 703–719
http://dx.doi.org/10.1016/j.rcl.2013.03.003
0033-8389/13/$ – see front matter © 2013 Elsevier Inc. All rights reserved.

more frequently in children of European descent, with the lowest incidence among Japanese and Filipino children.[5,6]

JIA CLASSIFICATION: THE CURRENT AND THE FUTURE

JIA is currently divided into 7 distinct subtypes (**Table 1**) based on the classification scheme established by the International League of Associations for Rheumatology (ILAR) in 2001.[1] This classification represents a work in progress, which has helped to subdivide and classify this group of chronic arthritides into more homogeneous categories based on clinical and laboratory grounds. The classification has also unified terminology amongst clinicians and researchers from Europe and North America, replacing the old classifications of juvenile chronic arthritis and juvenile rheumatoid arthritis (RA). The current classification is based on the number of joints involved, specific serologic markers, and systemic manifestations present during the first 6 months of the disease (see **Table 1**).[6,7] With the greater understanding of the disease at every level, it is slowly becoming more evident that, in children, some of these categories could be reclassified into more homogeneous groups, with some criterion modification, that more closely resemble the adult categories.[8]

Of the 7 categories of JIA, the better characterized are rheumatoid factor (RF)-positive polyarthritis and systemic JIA (sJIA). The former appears identical to its adult counterpart in all respects. On the other hand, sJIA is distinct from the other subtypes of JIA because of its predominant systemic manifestations, the lack of association with HLA genes, and its similarities to other autoinflammatory syndromes. sJIA can occur at any age in childhood and rarely in adults (adult-onset Still disease). In about 5% to 8% of children with sJIA, a life-threatening complication occurs, called macrophage activation syndrome, a form of hemophagocytic lymphohistiocytosis (**Fig. 1**).[3,8–11]

Early-onset antinuclear antibodies (ANA)-positive oligoarthritis has a clear predilection for girls younger than 6 years, strong HLA association, high risk for developing iridocyclitis, and presents with asymmetric involvement of fewer than 4 joints. Other children who are ANA positive are

Table 1
ILAR classification of JIA

Category	Definition	Frequency (%)
Oligoarthritis	Arthritis affecting up to 4 joints during the initial 6 mo	27–56
Persistent	Affects no more than 4 joints throughout the disease course	
Extended	Affects more than 4 joints after the initial 6 mo of disease	
Polyarthritis RF-negative	Arthritis affecting more than 5 joints in the first 6 mo of disease	11–28
Polyarthritis RF-positive	Arthritis affecting more than 5 joints in the first 6 mo of disease. RF test is positive at least twice 3 mo apart during the first 6 mo of disease	2–7
Psoriatic arthritis	Arthritis and psoriasis or arthritis and at least 2 of the following: dactylitis, nail pitting, family history of psoriasis in a first-degree relative	2–11
Enthesis-related arthritis	Arthritis or enthesitis with at least 2 of the following: sacroiliac tenderness of lumbosacral pain, presence of HLA-B27, onset of arthritis in a male <6 y, family history of ankylosing spondylitis, Reiter syndrome, enthesis-related arthritis, inflammatory bowel disease, or anterior uveitis in a first-degree relative	3–11
Systemic arthritis	Arthritis in 1 or more joints with or preceded by quotidian fever of at least 3 d and 1 of the following: evanescent erythematous rash, generalized adenopathy, hepatomegaly or splenomegaly, serositis	4–17
Undifferentiated arthritis	Arthritis that does not fulfill the other category criteria	11–21

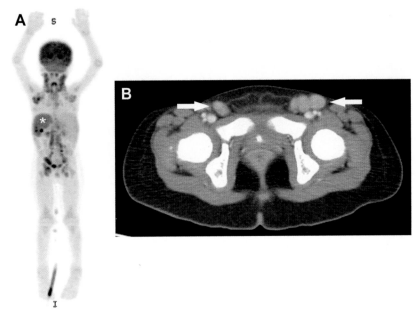

Fig. 1. sJIA in a 6-year-old girl who presented with fever of unknown origin for several weeks, initially believed to be lymphoma. (*A*) Coronal posterior positron emission tomography image shows extensive adenopathy in the retroperitoneum and pelvis as well as in both cervical, axillary, and inguinal regions. An enlarged and hypermetabolic spleen (*asterisk*) is also present. (*B*) Axial enhanced computed tomography image at the groin level shows bilateral slightly enhancing adenopathy (*arrows*).

classified into different disease categories; more precisely, persistent or extended oligoarthritis, RF-negative polyarthritis, psoriatic arthritis, and undifferentiated arthritis share these same features and likely are the same disease irrespective of the course of joint involvement or the presence of psoriatic features.[7,8,12–14] Some investigators have suggested that if reclassified together, this subgroup would represent a more homogeneous oligoarticular category with the most patients. Removing this category from the RF-negative polyarthritis, the remainder of the patients could potentially be included in an ANA-negative, symmetric polyarthritis category similar to the adult counterpart, creating an even more homogeneous classification.[7,8,12]

There is significant debate regarding the presence of psoriasis as a major classification criterion. Psoriatic arthritis in children is still a heterogeneous disease, with 2 subtypes based on the different age of onset and the underlying pathogenesis. The adolescent-onset disease shares clinical features and pathogenesis with adult-type spondyloarthropathies such as male predominance, HLA-B27 association, enthesitis, and axial skeletal involvement. The earlier-onset subtype usually manifests between 2 and 3 years of age and has similar characteristics to the ANA-positive oligoarthritis, including a female

predominance, as mentioned earlier. Based on the current ILAR classification, the presence of enthesitis is an exclusion criterion for psoriatic JIA, which precludes the grouping of the older-onset disease into a more homogeneous category similar to adult psoriatic arthritis and the other subtype into the early-onset ANA-positive oligoarthritis referred to earlier. A feature that remains unexplained is the presence of dactylitis, which is seen in both subtypes of psoriatic JIA (**Fig. 2**).[7,8,15]

Enthesis-related arthritis (ERA) shares several clinical and laboratory features with the adult spondyloarthropathy, such as enthesitis and marked increased prevalence of HLA-B27. In children, the presentation is different, with uncommon spinal involvement, and there is frequent hip arthritis (**Fig. 3**) and enthesitis. Sacroiliac (SI) joint involvement develops in some patients (**Fig. 4**) more frequently in adulthood or when assessed with MR imaging. Even though most adult patients with spondyloarthritis begin experiencing symptoms in the third and fourth decades of life, disease onset may extend well into the pediatric age range. Considering the differences in clinical presentation and removing the history of psoriasis as a classification criterion would allow ERA to be classified as spondyloarthropathy of juvenile onset, similar to the adult counterpart.[8,16]

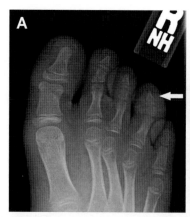
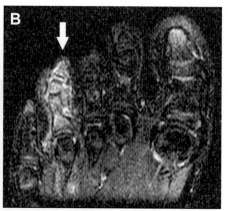

Fig. 2. Dactylitis in a 12-year-old boy with family history of psoriasis. (*A*) Radiograph of the right foot shows marked swelling of the fourth toe (*arrow*). (*B*) Axial short-tau inversion recovery image shows diffuse swelling confined to the soft tissues of the fourth toe (*arrow*) and diffuse bone marrow edema of all the phalanges, indicating osteitis and a joint effusion.

THE ROLE OF IMAGING IN JIA
Pathophysiology of JIA

Although the diagnosis of JIA is based on clinical and, to a lesser extent, on laboratory data, imaging is helpful in excluding other joint-affecting disease that may mimic JIA. Imaging may also play a role in staging, evaluating responses to therapy, and complications. To understand the role of the different imaging modalities in the evaluation of JIA, it is important to be familiar with the pathogenesis of the disease.

The hallmark of JIA is synovial inflammation clinically manifested as painful joint swelling, causing a restricted range of joint motion. Acute synovitis, which tends to progress to chronic synovitis, leads to synovial hypertrophy, resulting in soft tissue edema and joint effusion (**Fig. 5**). Subsequently, highly cellular pannus forms and spreads from the periphery to the center of the joint, leading to damage of the articular cartilage, underlying cortical bone, and the bone marrow (**Fig. 6**).[17,18] The disease process in JIA begins at the synovium, spreading to the cartilage and then into the underlying bone. Narrowing of the joint space develops early, with progression to ankylosis, although this is rare with the newer therapeutic agents (see **Fig. 4**B; **Fig. 7**). Bone erosions in JIA, unlike in adults, develop late and represent the irreversible end stage of the disease.[17–19]

Differences Between JIA and Adult RA

An accurate evaluation of joint damage, although crucial in children with JIA, is complicated by the natural ongoing skeletal growth and bone maturation. Bones in children are more cartilaginous not

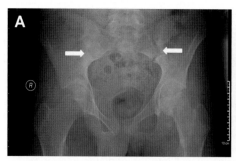
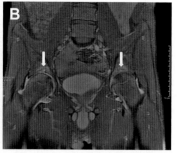

Fig. 3. A 14-year-old boy with ankylosing spondylitis. (*A*) Radiograph of the pelvis shows the more typical bilateral hip joint involvement with joint space narrowing. Although it is less commonly seen in children, this patient has erosive changes in both sacroiliac joints (*arrows*) but has no spinal involvement. (*B*) Contrast-enhanced T1-weighted MR image with fat saturation of the hips shows bilateral hip effusions with synovial enhancement, indicating synovitis. Enhancing erosions (*arrows*) in the roof of both acetabula are also present. These findings are not seen on the radiograph.

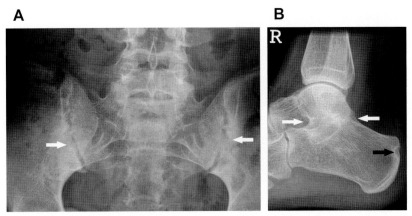

Fig. 4. A 16-year-old boy with ERA (HLA-B27 positive). (A) Radiograph of the SI joints shows mild widening, irregularity, and sclerosis of both SI joints (arrows). (B) Radiograph of the calcaneus shows a small erosion (black arrow) at the Achilles tendon insertion. Note also ankylosis (white arrows) of the entire subtalar joint.

only at the physis but at the epiphysis. In adults, articular surface cartilage is relatively avascular, protecting to a certain degree the underlying subchondral plate and cancellous bone from inflammation-driven destructive processes. Thus, bone erosions in adults are typically marginal. By contrast, in very young children, the epiphyses are vascularized and metaphyseal vessels anastomose with epiphyseal vessels through the growth plate. As a result, inflammation affecting the epiphyseal cartilage can spread to the ossification center, causing excessive growth (ie, epiphyseal

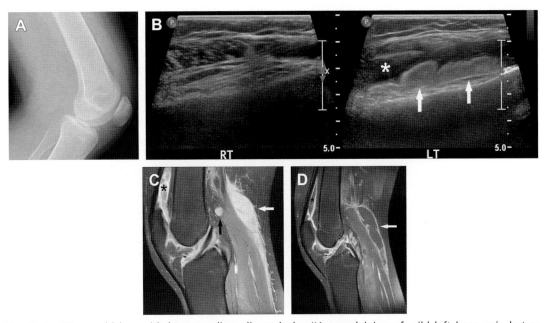

Fig. 5. An 18-year-old boy with long-standing oligoarticular JIA complaining of mild left knee pain but no swelling. (A) Radiograph of the knee shows no bone or soft tissue abnormality. (B) US image of the left knee shows marked eccentric nodular synovial hypertrophy (arrows) and a complex joint effusion (asterisk), with low-level echoes. The right knee is normal (for comparison). (C) Sagittal T2-weighted MR image with fat saturation of the knee shows a joint effusion (asterisk) with internal hypointense debris, popliteal adenopathy (black arrow), and a large popliteal cyst (white arrow). (D) Contrast-enhanced sagittal T1-weighted MR image with fat saturation of the knee shows the joint effusion (asterisk) with enhancing synovial thickening as well as the large popliteal cyst (arrow) with evidence of synovitis.

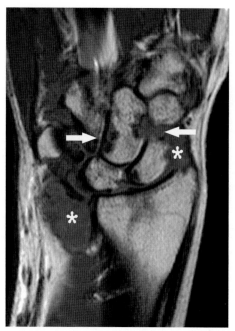

Fig. 6. A 15-year-old girl with long-standing RF-positive JIA. Coronal T1-weighted MR image of the wrist shows pannus formation (*asterisks*) and cortical and marrow erosions (*arrows*) involving several carpal bones.

worth mentioning in children with JIA: the cervical spine (**Fig. 8**) and temporomandibular joint, where growth disturbances are most likely to occur.[18–21]

Imaging JIA: Where Do We Stand?

The 3 main imaging modalities used in the evaluation of JIA are radiographs, ultrasonography (US), and MR imaging. Although all 3 modalities have advantages and disadvantages, they may complement not only each other but more importantly also the clinical examination (**Table 2**).

Conventional Radiographs

Conventional radiographs are recommended at the time of the initial diagnosis to exclude other causes of arthralgia, including fractures or tumors. Radiographs can also detect local growth disturbances seen in JIA such as epiphyseal overgrowth, early physeal fusion (**Fig. 9**), joint deformity (**Fig. 10**), ankylosis (see **Fig. 4B**), and limb length discrepancy, as well as treatment complications such as pathologic fractures.[17,18,22] The main disadvantages of radiographs are the inability to assess the soft tissues (see **Fig. 5**), indirect evaluation of cartilage thickness, and late finding of erosions. In children, because of the cartilaginous nature of the ossifying epiphysis, significant and irreversible cartilage destruction occurs before bone changes are radiographically evident.

The fact that cartilage thinning and erosions can occur early in JIA has shifted the attention of researchers away from conventional radiographs as a means of evaluating disease activity.[17,22–25]

ballooning), deformities, or destruction with epiphyseal erosions rather than marginal erosions.[19] To further complicate the matter, the clinical presentation and pattern of joint involvement differs across the subtypes of JIA; for example, progressive joint destruction is more common in the polyarticular subtype.[18] Two sites of involvement are

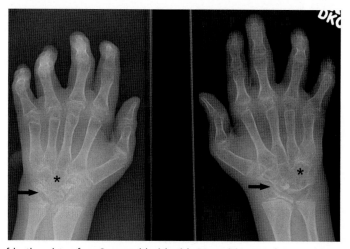

Fig. 7. Radiograph of both wrists of an 8-year-old girl with RF-positive JIA shows substantial narrowing of the intercarpal spaces, with ankylosis (*asterisks*) and erosions (*arrows*) of some of the carpal bones as well as erosions of all the metacarpophalangeal joints. Fixed flexion deformities of the first metacarpophalangeal and distal interphalangeal joints are present.

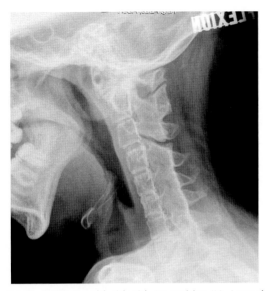

Fig. 8. A 14-year-old girl with RF-positive JIA. Lateral radiograph of the cervical spine on flexion shows ankylosis of almost every facet joint with secondary underdevelopment and squaring of the vertebral bodies from C4 to C7.

Several radiographic scoring systems have been validated and used to evaluate peripheral joint abnormalities in JIA, focusing on the hand and wrist. Although a complete discussion of these scoring systems is beyond the scope of this article, Doria and colleagues[26] found significant interreader and intrareader variability among these systems. These systems are based on adult score systems, which are not ideal for evaluating the changes occurring in the growing joint. Follow-up radiographs are not routinely used, as they are poor predictors of disease activity because of the slow development of visible and frequently irreversible radiographic findings.[26–28]

US

US has a well-established role in the evaluation of JIA (see **Table 2**). An advantage of US is the ability to evaluate soft tissues and, to a certain extent, the joint space (see **Fig. 5B**). US allows the visualization of joint effusion, synovitis (**Fig. 11**), tenosynovitis, enthesitis, synovial cysts, and adenopathy. US can differentiate between synovitis and tenosynovitis in a joint more accurately than the clinical examination, with clear classification and therapeutic implications.[29–31] This characteristic is especially important in anatomically complex joints such as the ankle joint, in which isolated tibiotalar synovitis is uncommon, whereas tenosynovitis alone is common.[30] If color Doppler is added to the technique (see **Fig. 11**), it can help

differentiate disease activity, because the synovial hyperplasia seen on gray scale may be residual and does not necessarily indicate disease activity.[17,32] US, with its real-time and multiplanar capabilities, can be used for guidance to access a joint for diagnostic or therapeutic fluid aspiration (**Fig. 12**).[17]

US has been used to evaluate the integrity of cartilage in the immature skeleton, because the high water content allows good visualization. Findings of cartilage thinning and erosion can be detected as blurring and obliteration of the normally sharp margins of the articular surface. Bone erosions on US, according to Outcome Measures in Rheumatology Clinical Trials (OMERACT), are defined as interruption of the bone profile or cortical breaks with a step-off bone defect visible in 2 perpendicular planes.[33] Age-related and sex-related standard reference values for US measurements of articular cartilage thickness for children between 7 and 16 years of age have been established in an attempt to validate the use of US in the articular cartilage evaluation.[34–36] A drawback of the use of US, including color Doppler, to evaluate cartilage is the lack of scientific studies focusing on the anatomy and sonographic appearance of healthy children needed to better understand and identify abnormal patients.[25,36]

MR Imaging

MR imaging is the only imaging modality with the ability to simultaneously assess all relevant structures in inflammatory joint disease. MR imaging is also superior to radiographs and US in evaluating the temporomandibular joint and axial skeleton. One of the main advantages of MR imaging over conventional radiographs is the ability to evaluate the soft tissues, including the cartilaginous structures (see **Fig. 5**). To evaluate synovitis, intravenous (IV) gadolinium must be administered, because synovial inflammation can be difficult to identify in the presence of a joint effusion (**Fig. 13**). In addition, IV contrast also helps assess the disease activity; in active synovitis, synovial enhancement tends to be more homogeneous and intense as opposed to the patchy and mild enhancement seen in the fibrotic inactive stage. MR images should be obtained immediately after contrast injection, because gadolinium diffuses into joint fluid, allowing the evaluation of only a single joint at a time.[17,18]

MR imaging may be helpful in differentiating types of recent-onset arthritis, especially between infectious arthritis and JIA. In JIA, low signal intensity synovial tissue on T2 with no enhancement on T1 is a supporting diagnostic finding (**Fig. 14**),

Table 2
Imaging modalities for evaluating JIA

	Advantages	Disadvantages
Radiographs	Readily available Low cost Overall picture of disease Shows growth disturbances and bone density Validated scoring methods Synchronous evaluation of multiple joints	Radiation exposure Indirect cartilage assessment Poor soft tissue assessment Poor detection of early changes Late detection of erosions Projectional superimposition
US	Readily available High patient acceptability Non invasive, no sedation No radiation exposure Easy to reproduce Synchronous evaluation of multiple joints Excellent evaluating soft tissues Direct evaluation of cartilage and erosions	Operator dependent Reliability is machine dependent for follow-up Time consuming Limited evaluation of certain joints such axial skeleton Usefulness is limited with patient age because of ossified bones Inability to evaluate the entire joint Ongoing validation standards
MR imaging	Excellent evaluation of soft tissues, cartilage, and bone Detection of early changes Multiplanar capabilities Morphologic and physiologic evaluation of cartilage Evaluates the entire joint Ability to evaluate axial skeleton and difficult joints such as temporomandibular joint No radiation Easy to reproduce	High cost Require IV contrast May need sedation Least available technique worldwide Long examination time Evaluation of only 1 or 2 joints at the same time Ongoing validation standards Sensitivity maybe affected by normal variants

especially with a lack of significant periarticular soft tissue edema. On the other hand, significant periarticular soft tissue edema, bone marrow edema, and decreased epiphyseal enhancement after gadolinium administration are more frequently seen in infectious arthritis.[37] The presence of rice bodies in children is also highly suggestive of JIA and can be accurately evaluated on MR imaging. Rice bodies are more conspicuous on fluid-sensitive sequences, being hypointense compared with the surrounding hyperintense fluid, and display no gadolinium enhancement (**Fig. 15**).[17,18,38] A gradient echo sequence should be routinely included as part of the MR protocol to identify hemosiderin, seen as blooming artifacts, a finding suggestive of pigmented villonodular synovitis (**Fig. 16**).[39]

A unique advantage of MR imaging is the ability to discriminate between articular and epiphyseal cartilage at the different stages of the developing joint. This ability allows MR imaging to detect bone erosions earlier than US or conventional radiographs, especially in patients with shorter disease duration (**Fig. 17**), making MR imaging the best modality to identify erosions. A three-dimensional (3D) image acquisition using T1 gradient sequence is useful in the detection of erosions, because it allows the generation of multiplanar reconstructions, which adds diagnostic confidence.[25]

MR imaging also has the unique capability to identify areas of bone marrow edema that may predate future erosions, sometimes called preerosive osteitis (**Fig. 18**). This finding has been validated in adult patients with RA but no information exists on the prognostic value of this finding in JIA. Furthermore, focal areas of apparent bone marrow edema have been seen in healthy children, and thus longitudinal studies are required to clarify their significance.[40]

Two recent MR imaging techniques are worth mentioning: contrast-enhanced MR imaging (DCE-MRI) and T2 relaxation mapping. DCE-MRI enables the quantitative assessment of joint

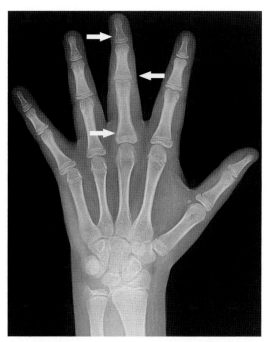

Fig. 9. A 12-year-old girl with polyarticular JIA and premature fusion of the phalangeal physes. Radiograph of the left hand shows diffuse soft tissue edema to the middle finger and early fusion (*arrows*) of the physes of the third metacarpal and phalanges.

inflammation by analyzing the timing of signal changes after IV gadolinium administration, because synovial thickening is not necessarily related to the degree of inflammation.[41–43] The earlier the enhancement, the more active the disease, reflecting the local tissue vascularity and

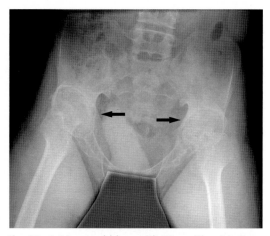

Fig. 10. A 14-year-old boy with RF-positive JIA. Frontal radiograph of the hips in this patient with limited range of hip motion shows ballooning and deformity of the femoral heads, significant bilateral hip joint space narrowing, and protrusion acetabula (*arrows*).

capillary permeability. This method provides a more accurate assessment of the disease activity, because improvement in synovial thickening may lag behind dynamic evaluation of the enhancement parameters.[41–43]

DCE-MRI uses a 3D T1gradient echo sequence before and after the administration of gadolinium. Several data sets of images are acquired every 5 seconds after contrast injection for 3 minutes. Then, the precontrast image is subtracted from all subsequent images and the data are analyzed using software. DCE-MRI shows promise as a reliable and accurate tool for quantitative assessment of synovial inflammation and disease activity.[41–43]

T2 relaxation time mapping provides a physiologic evaluation of the articular cartilage. The biochemical properties of cartilage are strongly influenced by the content and structure of collagen and proteoglycans, which differ within the normal structure of the cartilage. The orientation and alignment of collagen fibrils vary according to the depth. One of the earliest physiologic changes in cartilage degeneration is increased permeability of the matrix, which leads to increased content and motion of water, creating stress on the cartilage and subsequent morphologic changes. The transverse relaxation time (T2) is constant for a given tissue at a given MR field strength, unless altered by tissue damage or a contrast agent.[44,45] The transverse relaxation time is also sensitive to slow-moving protons and is a function of the water and collagen content and orientation of the highly ordered anisotropic arrangement of collagen fibrils in the extracellular matrix.[44] In patients with JIA, higher relaxation times have been found when compared with healthy individuals, allowing the ideal early detection of microstructural changes in cartilage before irreversible changes occur that would allow earlier and more aggressive therapeutic interventions (**Fig. 19**).[46,47]

Whole-body MR imaging has recently being integrated in the workup of adult patients with spondyloarthropathies, including psoriasis. Whole-body MR imaging not only evaluates the disease activity but also the extent, because this subtype of arthritis can and frequently does involve areas that are not readily accessible to clinical examination. The assessment of active enthesitis is also difficult clinically and inconclusive, especially in complex joints such as the ankle.[48–51] State-of-the-art MR scanners using phase array coils, enable imaging of the entire patient from head to toe without the need of patient repositioning. In children with ERA, Rachlis and colleagues[52] found that whole-body MR imaging can contribute important diagnostic information and confidence for detecting early involvement and extent of disease. In this

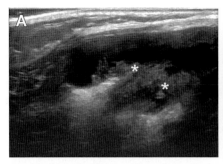
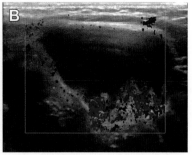

Fig. 11. A 3-year-old girl with ANA-positive oligoarticular JIA. (*A*) Grayscale US image of the knee joint shows marked eccentric synovial proliferation (*asterisks*) and a joint effusion. (*B*) Color Doppler US image shows increased color signal, indicating marked synovial hyperemia.

study of 23 children with ERA, whole-body MR imaging identified the characteristic lesions produced by the disease and was found to be superior to clinical examination in arthritis involving the hips, SI joints, and spine. For enthesis, clinical examination overestimated disease activity in the periphery, making this modality an important tool to evaluate entheseal disease. In addition to coronal T1-weighted and short-tau inversion recovery (STIR) sequences of the entire body, sagittal images of the spine and ankles, axial images of the pelvis, and paracoronal images of the SI joints should be part of the protocol to assess areas that are clinically difficult to evaluate.[52] Whole-body MR imaging is evolving into an established and sensitive imaging modality for the diagnostic workup of children with ERA and psoriatic arthritis, with the advantages of providing a comprehensive single evaluation of the entire body in a reasonable time without IV contrast or radiation.

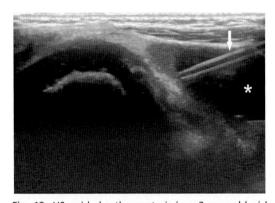

Fig. 12. US-guided arthrocentesis in a 2-year-old girl with arthralgia and joint swelling of both knees for 6 months. The patient is ANA-positive and has iridocyclitis. US image shows the sheath of the angiocatheter (*arrow*) inside the joint effusion (*asterisk*). A specimen was obtained for analysis, and corticosteroids were injected. The final diagnosis was oligoarticular JIA.

Future Imaging Perspectives and Their Challenges

The current method to assess clinical remission in JIA is based on Wallace criteria, which are composed of clinical and laboratory variables.[53,54] By directly imaging synovitis, US with color Doppler and contrast-enhanced MR imaging may have the advantage in assessing response to treatment over clinical and laboratory variables, which are indirect markers of synovial inflammation not necessarily at the primary site of disease. Histologic evidence of synovial inflammation has been found in asymptomatic joints in children with JIA.[55]

In the past few years, multiple studies have confirmed that clinical and laboratory criteria are not sensitive enough to detect subclinical synovitis, as detected by US and MR imaging.[30,56–64] US and MR imaging have been increasingly used as outcome measures in clinical trials on adult RA and even in clinical practice. Despite the abundant evidence of the value of these imaging modalities in monitoring therapeutic response and detecting subclinical synovitis in RA, this has not been fully validated yet in JIA.[56–61,63,64]

To use US or MR imaging as valid modalities for assessment of synovitis, the OMERACT filter specifies that an outcome measure must be accurate, feasible, and discriminatory.[64,65] Collado and colleagues[64] performed a systematic review of the literature before February 2011 to evaluate the validity of US as an imaging tool for the diagnosis and management of synovitis in JIA. Based on the 20 studies identified using US to assess synovitis in JIA, the investigators found that US had a higher sensitivity than clinical examinations in detecting synovitis, with potential implications in the classification of patients in a different JIA category. However, despite the increasing use of US to evaluate JIA in the clinical setting, the real validity of US in the diagnosis and follow-up of JIA was not yet available.

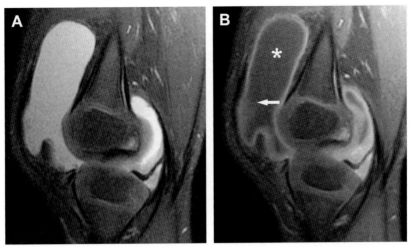

Fig. 13. A 3-year-old girl with oligoarticular JIA. (*A*) Sagittal T2-weighted MR image with fat saturation of the knee shows a large joint effusion. No synovial thickening is noted. (*B*) T1-weighted MR image after gadolinium makes the diffuse and conspicuous synovitis (*arrow*), allowing the differentiation between synovial thickening and joint effusion (*asterisk*).

An US definition of synovitis in children is necessary to develop a valid synovitis scoring system for the follow-up of patients with JIA.[64] Moreover, color Doppler signal in the growing skeleton has been described as a physiologic finding in the well-vascularized epiphyseal cartilage and synovium, adding to the need for a US definition of synovitis in children. More research about the clinical significance and prognostic value of this finding is required, because the presence of active disease on US/color Doppler has not predicted subsequent synovitis flares.[66]

Regarding MR imaging, validated MR imaging scores to assess structural damage and disease activity in children with JIA are available.[67] Furthermore, this recent MR imaging study has proved

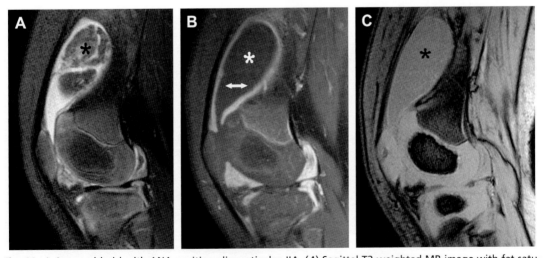

Fig. 14. A 4-year-old girl with ANA-positive oligoarticular JIA. (*A*) Sagittal T2-weighted MR image with fat saturation of the knee shows a large joint effusion (*asterisk*) in the suprapatellar compartment containing hypointense material. (*B*) Sagittal contrast-enhanced T1-weighted MR image shows significant synovial enhancement (*double-headed arrow*), indicating synovitis. However, the internal T2 hypointensities show no enhancement (*asterisk*). (*C*) Sagittal gradient echo sequence MR image shows the large joint effusion (*asterisk*) without blooming artifact to suggest hemosiderin.

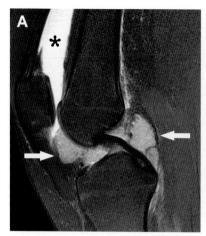
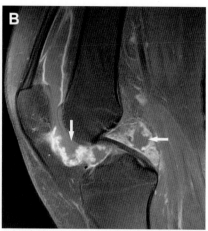

Fig. 15. A 17-year-old girl with long-standing oligoarticular JIA. (*A*) Sagittal T2-weighted MR image with fat saturation of the knee shows a large suprapatellar effusion (*asterisk*) and intermediate (cartilage) signal material (*arrows*) in the region of the intercondylar region, consistent with rice bodies. (*B*) Sagittal contrast-enhanced T1-weighted MR image of the knee shows irregular and diffuse synovial thickening and enhancement. However, the tiny hypointensities (*arrows*) corresponding to rice bodies in the intercondylar region show no enhancement.

promising in the evaluation of therapeutic response based on synovial inflammation scores.[67] A clear concern is that the lack of data from age-matched healthy controls represents a limiting factor when imaging children with JIA. Data of the US and MR appearance of the synovium in healthy children are necessary to elucidate the prognostic significance of subclinical synovitis in JIA and to provide a consistent standard of imaging remission. Likewise, the high prevalence of bony depressions, apparent bone marrow edema, and joint effusion recently described in healthy children emphasizes the need to include age-matched healthy controls in US and MR imaging

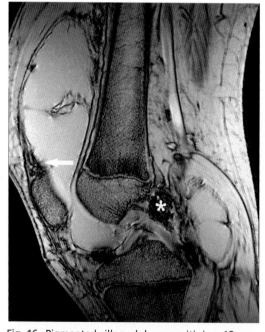

Fig. 16. Pigmented villonodular synovitis in a 13-year-old boy who presented with knee pain and swelling for several months. Sagittal gradient echo MR image shows a large joint effusion with hypointensities outlining the synovium (*arrow*) and more confluent in the intercondylar notch, corresponding to hemosiderin deposition (*asterisk*).

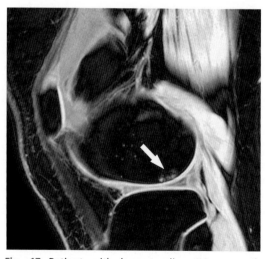

Fig. 17. Patient with long-standing JIA, currently asymptomatic. Sagittal gradient echo sequence MR image of the knee shows diffuse articular cartilage thinning and more localized erosive changes (*arrow*) posteriorly. The radiograph showed no abnormality.

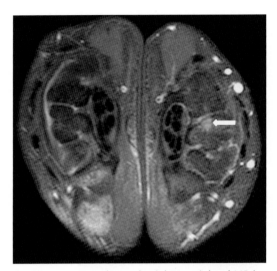

Fig. 18. Contrast-enhanced axial T1-weighted MR image with fat saturation of both wrists in the praying position in a 9-year-old girl with the recent diagnosis of JIA, showing a small focus (*arrow*) of bone marrow enhancement in the right capitate, which indicates preerosive osteitis.

studies.[67–69] The course and outcome of JIA cannot be predicted by baseline features. However, control of disease activity in the first 6 months of disease has been proven to improve long-term prognosis.[70–75]

In the past decade, there has been important progress in the management of JIA, which includes more aggressive and earlier interventions as well as the development of new therapeutic agents and combination treatment strategies. This situation has created the need for more sensitive methods to monitor the disease activity and to identify patients at risk for early erosive changes.[25]

The wrist joint is an attractive potential site that can be used as a sentinel joint in the evaluation of JIA; if the bilateral joints are imaged simultaneously, more information can be gathered for research. The wrist joint is affected in approximately 60% of patients with JIA and is second in frequency of involvement only to the knee joint.[57,76,77] The wrist along with the hip are the joints most vulnerable to changes seen on radiographs in patients with JIA.[76,77] The development of wrist disease has been associated with a higher risk of progressive disease, lower likelihood of a short-term therapy response, and a poorer functional outcome, making the wrist an attractive alternative for developing a scoring system in the near future.[57,76,77] There are not only age-matched and sex-matched standards for the wrist but studies evaluating the prevalence and location of normal variants such as bony depressions (a potential source of errors) are already available (**Fig. 20**).[68,69,78] The wrist is a unique joint for MR imaging, because both joints can be evaluated simultaneously. Bilateral MR imaging of the wrists using the praying position is feasible and tolerated well by patients (**Fig. 21**). Having comparative images of the contralateral side adds confidence to the interpretation, helps clarify normal variants without adding additional time or cost, and diffusion of gadolinium into the joint is no longer a limiting factor (see **Fig. 18**).[79] When imaging the

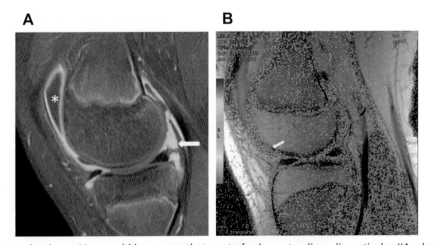

Fig. 19. T2 mapping in an 11-year-old boy on methotrexate for long-standing oligoarticular JIA who presented with mild knee swelling but no pain. (*A*) Sagittal contrast-enhanced T1-weighted MR image with fat saturation shows a small joint effusion (*asterisk*) and synovitis (*arrow*). (*B*) T2 mapping MR image shows more red and yellow (*arrow*) in the cartilage of the posterior femoral condyle, indicating abnormal T2 relaxation times and early cartilage compromise.

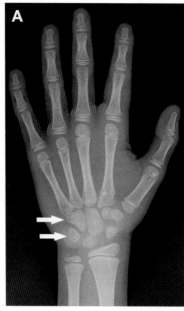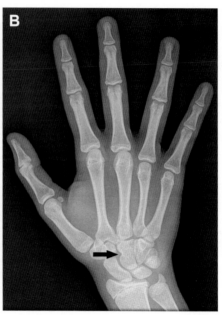

Fig. 20. Bone age radiographs in 2 children with short stature (otherwise asymptomatic). (A) Radiograph of the left hand shows lucencies (*arrows*) in the medial margin of the hamate and pisiform, representing normal variants but that could potentially be confused with erosions. (B) Radiograph of the hand shows a smooth indentation (*arrow*) along the lateral margin of the capitate, a common place for a normal developmental variant around the wrist.

wrists, attention to technical factors is important to maximize spatial and contrast resolution. The smallest phase array coil should be used, allowing both wrists to fit in the coil and the field of view should be limited to the wrist (ie, including just proximal to the radiocarpal and ulnocarpal joints to the proximal metacarpal area). Inclusion of both the hand and wrist when evaluating for fine detail such as joint space narrowing or erosions yields suboptimal images (**Fig. 22**).

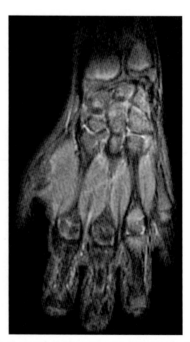

Fig. 22. Coronal STIR sequence MR image that includes the entire hand and wrist obtained using a flexible coil. Note the lack of spatial resolution and the signal loss at the end of the coil, which precludes adequate evaluation of detail.

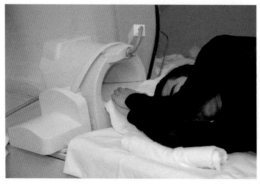

Fig. 21. Patient positioning inside the magnet. Both hands are imaged using an 8-channel knee coil.

SUMMARY

In recent years, a greater understanding of the pathogenesis and evolution of JIA has created room for a potential new classification with more homogeneous groups; however, consensus in its application is still needed. Imaging is routinely used at the initial diagnosis of JIA, with mounting evidence of its potential to accurately stage and evaluate disease activity. With new medications offering more aggressive and effective treatments, monitoring response to treatment becomes increasingly important. Therefore, the use of more sensitive imaging modalities such as US and more importantly MR imaging is gaining favor, because the clinical and laboratory parameters are less reliable. The time has come to consider the incorporation of imaging in the scoring and evaluation of disease activity in JIA. Validation studies focusing on normal standards are a critical step in this promising process.

REFERENCES

1. Petty RE, Southwood TR, Manners P, et al. International League of Associations for Rheumatology classification of juvenile idiopathic arthritis: second revision, Edmonton, 2001. J Rheumatol 2004;31: 390-2.
2. Murray K, Thompson SD, Glass DN. Pathogenesis of juvenile chronic arthritis: genetic and environmental factors. Arch Dis Child 1997;77: 530-4.
3. Ravelli A, Martini A. Juvenile idiopathic arthritis. Lancet 2007;369:767-78.
4. Manners PJ, Bower C. Worldwide prevalence of juvenile arthritis. Why does it vary so much? J Rheumatol 2002;29:1520-30.
5. Saurenmann K, Rose JB, Tyrell P, et al. Epidemiology of juvenile idiopathic arthritis in a multiethnic cohort: ethnicity as a risk factor. Arthritis Rheum 2007;56:1974-84.
6. Espinosa M, Gottlieb BS. Juvenile idiopathic arthritis. Pediatr Rev 2012;33:303-12.
7. Martini A. Are the number of joints involved or the presence of psoriasis still useful tools to identify homogeneous disease entities in juvenile idiopathic arthritis? J Rheumatol 2003;30:1900-3.
8. Martini A. It is time to rethink juvenile idiopathic arthritis classification and nomenclature. Ann Rheum Dis 2012;71(9):1437-9.
9. Prakken B, Albani S, Martini A. Juvenile idiopathic arthritis. Lancet 2011;377:2138-49.
10. Masters SL, Simon A, Aksentijevich I, et al. Horror autoinflammaticus: the molecular pathophysiology of autoinflammatory disease. Annu Rev Immunol 2009;27:621-68.
11. Jordan A, McDonagh JE. Juvenile idiopathic arthritis: the paediatric perspective. Pediatr Radiol 2006;36:734-42.
12. Ravelli A, Varnier GC, Oliveira S, et al. Antinuclear antibody positive patients should be grouped as a separate category in the classification of juvenile idiopathic arthritis. Arthritis Rheum 2011;63: 267-75.
13. Martini A, Lovell D. Juvenile idiopathic arthritis: state of the art and future perspectives. Ann Rheum Dis 2010;69:1260-3.
14. Ravelli A, Felici E, Magni-Manzoni S, et al. Patients with antinuclear antibody-positive juvenile idiopathic arthritis constitute a homogeneous subgroup irrespective of the course of joint disease. Arthritis Rheum 2005;52:826-32.
15. Stoll ML, Punaro M. Psoriatic juvenile idiopathic arthritis: a tale of two subgroups. Curr Opin Rheumatol 2011;23:1-7.
16. Colbert R. Classification of juvenile spondyloarthritis: enthesis related arthritis and beyond. Nat Rev Rheumatol 2010;6(8):477-85.
17. Restrepo R, Lee EY. Epidemiology, pathogenesis and imaging of arthritis in children. Orthop Clin North Am 2012;43(2):213-25.
18. Johnson K. Imaging of juvenile idiopathic arthritis. Pediatr Radiol 2006;36:743-58.
19. Breton S, Jousse-Joulin S, Finel E, et al. Imaging approach for evaluating peripheral joint abnormalities in juvenile idiopathic arthritis. Semin Arthritis Rheum 2012;41:698-711.
20. Karmazyn B, Bowyer SL, Schmidt KM, et al. US findings of metacarpophalangeal joints in children with idiopathic juvenile arthritis. Pediatr Radiol 2007;37:475-82.
21. Pedersen TK, Jensen JJ, Melsen B, et al. Resorption of the temporomandibular condylar bone according to subtypes of juvenile chronic arthritis. J Rheumatol 2001;28:2109-15.
22. Azouz EM. Juvenile idiopathic arthritis: how can the radiologist help the clinician? Pediatr Radiol 2008; 38(Suppl 3):S403-8.
23. Mason T, Reed AM, Nelson AM, et al. Frequency of abnormal hand and wrist radiographs at the time of diagnosis of polyarticular juvenile rheumatoid arthritis. J Rheumatol 2002;29:2214-8.
24. Selvaag AM, Flatø B, Dale K, et al. Radiographic and clinical outcome in early juvenile rheumatoid arthritis and juvenile spondyloarthropathy: a 3 year prospective study. J Rheumatol 2006;33:1382-91.
25. Malattia C, Damasio MB, Magnaguagno F, et al. Magnetic resonance imaging, ultrasonography and conventional radiography in the assessment of bone erosions in juvenile idiopathic arthritis. Arthritis Rheum 2008;59:1764-72.
26. Doria AS, Babyn PS, Feldman B. A critical appraisal of radiographic scoring systems for

assessment of juvenile idiopathic arthritis. Pediatr Radiol 2006;36:759–72.

27. Doria AS, de Castro CC, Kiss MH, et al. Inter and intrareader variability in the interpretation of two radiographic classification systems for juvenile rheumatoid arthritis. Pediatr Radiol 2003;33:673–81.

28. Johnson K. Commentary on "inter and intrareader variability in the interpretation of two radiographic classification systems for juvenile rheumatoid arthritis". Pediatr Radiol 2003;33:671–2.

29. Pascoli L, Wright S, McAllister C, et al. Prospective evaluation of clinical and ultrasound findings in ankle disease in juvenile idiopathic arthritis: importance of ankle ultrasound. J Rheumatol 2010;37: 2409–14.

30. Rooney ME, McAllister C, Burns JFT. Ankle disease in juvenile idiopathic arthritis: ultrasound findings in clinically swollen ankles. J Rheumatol 2009;36: 1725–9.

31. Laurel L, Court-Payen M, Nielsen S, et al. Ultrasonography and color Doppler in juvenile idiopathic arthritis: diagnosis and follow up of ultrasound-guided steroid injections in the ankle region. A descriptive interventional study. Pediatr Rheumatol Online J 2011;9:4.

32. Larmer S, Sebag GH. MRI and ultrasound in children with juvenile idiopathic arthritis. Eur J Radiol 2000;33:85–93.

33. Grassi W, Filipucci E, Farina A, et al. Ultrasonography in the evaluation of bone erosions. Ann Rheum Dis 2001;60:98–103.

34. Spannow AH, Stenboeg E, Pfeiffer-Jensen M, et al. Ultrasound and MRI measurements of joint cartilage in healthy children: a validation study. Ultraschall Med 2011;32:s1110–6.

35. Spannow AH, Pfeiffer-Jensen M, Andersen NT, et al. Ultrasonographic measurements of joint cartilage thickness in healthy children: age and sex related standard reference values. J Rheumatol 2010;37:2595–601.

36. Larche MJ, Roth J. Toward standardized ultrasound measurements of cartilage thickness in children [editorial]. J Rheumatol 2010;37:12.

37. Kirkhus E, Flato B, Riise O, et al. Differences in MRI findings between subgroups of recent onset childhood arthritis. Pediatr Radiol 2011;41:432–40.

38. Chung C, Coley BD, Martin LC. Rice bodies in juvenile rheumatoid arthritis. AJR Am J Roentgenol 1998;170:698–700.

39. Hughes TH, Sartoris DJ, Schweitzer ME. Pigmented villonodular synovitis: MRI characteristics. Skeletal Radiol 1995;24:7–12.

40. Magni-Manzoni S, Malattia C, Lanni S, et al. Advances and challenges in imaging in juvenile idiopathic arthritis. Nat Rev Rheumatol 2012;8:329–36.

41. Graham TB, Laor T, Dardzinski BJ. Quantitative magnetic resonance imaging of the hands and wrists of children with juvenile idiopathic arthritis. J Rheumatol 2005;32:1811–20.

42. Malattia C, Damasio MB, Basso C, et al. Dynamic contrast-enhanced magnetic resonance imaging in the assessment of disease activity in patients with juvenile idiopathic arthritis. Rheumatology 2010;49:178–85.

43. Workie DW, Dardzinski BJ, Graham TB, et al. Quantification of dynamic contrast-enhanced MR imaging of the knee in children with juvenile rheumatoid arthritis based on a pharmacokinetic modeling. Magn Reson Imaging 2004;22:1201–10.

44. Gold GE, Chen CA, Koo S, et al. Recent advances in MRI of articular cartilage. AJR Am J Roentgenol 2009;193:628–38.

45. Choi J, Gold G. MR imaging of articular cartilage physiology. Magn Reson Imaging Clin North Am 2011;19:249–82.

46. Kim HK, Laor T, Graham TB. T2 relaxation time changes in distal femoral articular cartilage in children with juvenile idiopathic arthritis: a 3-year longitudinal study. AJR Am J Roentgenol 2010;195: 1021–5.

47. Knight AC, Dardzinski BJ, Laor T, et al. Magnetic resonance imaging evaluation of the effects of juvenile rheumatoid arthritis on distal femoral weight-bearing cartilage. Arthritis Rheum 2004;50:901–5.

48. Weckbach S, Schewe S, Michaely HJ, et al. Whole-body MR imaging in psoriatic arthritis: additional value for therapeutic decision making. Eur J Radiol 2011;77:149–55.

49. Weber U, Hodler J, Kubik RA, et al. Sensitivity and specificity of spinal inflammatory lesions assessed by whole-body magnetic resonance imaging in patients with ankylosing spondylitis or recent-onset inflammatory back pain. Arthritis Rheum 2009;61: 900–8.

50. Weber U, Maksymowych WP, Jurik AG, et al. Validation of whole body against conventional magnetic resonance imaging for scoring acuter inflammatory lesions in the sacroiliac joints of patients with spondyloarthritis. Arthritis Rheum 2009; 61:893–9.

51. Weber U, Hodler J, Jurik AG, et al. Assessment of active spinal inflammatory changes in patients with axial spondyloarthritis: validation of whole body MRI against conventional MRI. Ann Rheum Dis 2010;69:648–53.

52. Rachlis AC, Babyn PS, Lobo-Mueller E, et al. Whole body magnetic resonance imaging in juvenile spondyloarthritis: will it prove vital information compared to clinical exam alone? [abstract]. Arthritis Rheum 2011;63(Suppl 10):749.

53. Wallace CA, Ruperto N, Giannini E. Preliminary criteria for clinical remission for select categories of juvenile idiopathic arthritis. J Rheumatol 2004; 31:2290–4.

54. Wallace CA, Giannini EH, Huang B, et al. American College of Rheumatology provisional criteria for defining clinical inactive disease in select categories of juvenile idiopathic arthritis. Arthritis Care Res (Hoboken) 2011;63:929–36.

55. Kraan MC, Patel DD, Haringman JJ, et al. The development of clinical signs of rheumatoid synovial inflammation is associated with increased synthesis of the chemokine CXCL8 (interleukin-8). Arthritis Res 2001;3:65–71.

56. Helders PJ, van der Net J, Nieuwenhuis MK. Splinting the juvenile arthritis wrist: a clinical observation. Arthritis Rheum 2002;47:99–103.

57. Oen K. Long-term outcomes and predictors of outcomes for patients with juvenile idiopathic arthritis. Best Pract Res Clin Rheumatol 2002;16:347–60.

58. Janow G, Panghaal V, Trinh A, et al. Detection of active disease in juvenile idiopathic arthritis: sensitivity and specificity of the physical examination vs ultrasound. J Rheumatol 2011;38:2671–4.

59. Haslam KE, McCann LJ, Wyatt S, et al. The detection of subclinical synovitis by ultrasound in oligoarticular juvenile idiopathic arthritis: a pilot study. Rheumatology 2010;49:123–7.

60. Malattia C, Consolaro A, Pederzoli S, et al. MRI versus conventional measures of disease activity and structural damage in evaluating treatment efficacy in juvenile idiopathic arthritis. Ann Rheum Dis 2013;72(3):363–8.

61. Gardner-Medwin JM, Killeen OG, Ryder CA, et al. Magnetic resonance imaging identifies features in clinically unaffected knees predicting extension of arthritis in children with monoarthritis. J Rheumatol 2006;33(11):2337–43.

62. Hoger M. Silent arthritis in JIA children with clinically inactive disease detected by MRI [abstract]. Ann Rheum Dis 2011;70(Suppl 3):90.

63. Brown A, Hirsch R, Laor T, et al. Do patients with juvenile idiopathic arthritis in clinical remission have evidence of persistent inflammation on 3-T magnetic resonance imaging? Arthritis Care Res 2012;64:1846–54.

64. Collado P, Jousse-Joulin S, Alcalde M, et al. Is ultrasound a validated imaging tool for the diagnosis and management of synovitis in juvenile idiopathic arthritis? A systematic literature review. Arthritis Care Res 2012;64:1011–9.

65. Boers M, Brooks P, Strand CV, et al. The OMERACT filter for outcome measures in rheumatology [editorial]. J Rheumatol 1998;25:198–9.

66. Magni-Manzoni S, Scire CA, Ravelli A, et al. Ultrasound-detected synovial abnormalities are frequent in clinically inactive juvenile idiopathic arthritis, but do not predict a flare of synovitis. Ann Rheum Dis 2013;72:223–8.

67. Malattia C, Damasio MD, Pistorio A, et al. Development and preliminary validation of a pediatric-targeted MRI score system for the assessment of disease activity and damage in juvenile idiopathic arthritis. Ann Rheum Dis 2011;70:440–6.

68. Muller LS, Avenarius D, Damasio B, et al. The pediatric wrist revisited: redefining MR findings in healthy children. Ann Rheum Dis 2011;70:605–10.

69. Avenarius D, Muller LS, Eldevik P, et al. The pediatric wrist revisited-findings of bony depressions in healthy children on radiographs compared to MRI. Pediatr Radiol 2012;42:791–8.

70. Wallace CA, Huang B, Bandeira M, et al. Patterns of clinical remission in selected categories of juvenile idiopathic arthritis. Arthritis Rheum 2005;52:3554–62.

71. Minden K. Adult outcomes of patients with juvenile idiopathic arthritis. Horm Res 2009;72(Suppl 1):20–5.

72. Magnani A, Pistori A, Mangi-Manzoni S, et al. Achievement of a state of inactive disease at least once in the first 5 years predicts better outcome of patients with polyarticular juvenile idiopathic arthritis. J Rheumatol 2009;36:628–34.

73. Marzan KA, Shaham B. Early juvenile idiopathic arthritis. Rheum Dis Clin North Am 2012;38:355–72.

74. Fantini F, Gerloni V, Gattinara M, et al. Remission in juvenile chronic arthritis: a cohort study of 683 consecutive cases with a mean of 10 year follow up. J Rheumatol 2003;30:579–84.

75. Flato B, Hoffmann-Vold AM, Reiff A, et al. Long-term outcome and prognostic factors in enthesis related arthritis: a case control study. Arthritis Rheum 2006;54:3573–82.

76. Magni-Manzoni S, Rosi F, Pistorio A, et al. Prognostic factors for radiographic progression, radiographic damage and disability in juvenile idiopathic arthritis. Arthritis Rheum 2003;48:3509–17.

77. Al-Matar MJ, Petty RE, Tucker LB, et al. The early pattern of joint involvement predict disease progression in children with oligoarticular (pauciarticular) juvenile idiopathic arthritis. Arthritis Rheum 2002;46:2708–15.

78. Shabshin N, Schweitzer ME. Age dependent T2 changes of bone marrow in pediatric wrist MRI. Skeletal Radiol 2009;38:1163–8.

79. Demertzis J, Rubin DA. MR imaging assessment of inflammatory, crystalline-induced and infectious arthritides. Magn Reson Imaging Clin North Am 2011;19:339–63.

Magnetic Resonance Imaging of Pediatric Muscular Disorders
Recent Advances and Clinical Applications

Hee Kyung Kim, MD[a],*, Diana M. Lindquist, PhD[b],
Suraj D. Serai, MS, PhD[a], Yogesh K. Mariappan, PhD[c],
Lily L. Wang, MBBS, MPH[a], Arnold C. Merrow, MD[a],
Kiaran P. McGee, PhD[c], Richard L. Ehman, MD[c],
Tal Laor, MD[d]

KEYWORDS

- Magnetic resonance imaging • Skeletal muscle • T2 relaxation time • Diffusion-weighted imaging
- Dixon imaging • Diffusion tensor imaging • Magnetic resonance spectroscopy
- Magnetic resonance elastography

KEY POINTS

- Recent advances in magnetic resonance (MR) imaging techniques, particularly quantitative measurements, are just beginning to be utilized in the assessment of normal muscle and various muscle abnormalities.
- Most investigations are performed in adults. However, the spectrum of muscle disorders in children might be a fertile area for future application.
- Further investigation of these quantitative MR imaging techniques may aid in understanding the pathophysiology of various muscle disorders in children, and offer new opportunities for establishing diagnoses and directing therapies.

INTRODUCTION

Historically, magnetic resonance (MR) imaging techniques used to evaluate muscle disorders in children have included T1-weighted images (T1WI) and water-sensitive sequences, such as short-tau inversion recovery (STIR) or T2-weighted images (T2WI), with or without fat suppression. These techniques have been limited primarily to the evaluation of gross morphologic changes of the muscles.[1] Recent developments in advanced MR techniques and postprocessing software have expanded the use of MR imaging to include quantitative analysis.[2–4] These advances allow for the objective analysis of composition,[4–7] architecture,[8,9] mechanical properties,[10] and function down to a microscopic level in normal and pathologic skeletal muscles in the pediatric population.[11,12]

This article reviews T1WI and water-sensitive sequences as examples of qualitative or semiquantitative imaging tools used to subjectively analyze the morphology and compositional

Disclosures: Grant Support: RSNA Research Scholar Grant (H.K. Kim); None (D.M. Lindquist, S.D. Serai, L.L. Wang, T. Laor); Grant Support: NIH EB07593, NIH EB 001981 (Y.K. Mariappan, K.P. McGee, R.L. Ehman); Author and content manager for Amirsys, Inc (A.C. Merrow).
 a Department of Radiology, Cincinnati Children's Hospital Medical Center, 3333 Burnet Avenue, MLC 5031, Cincinnati, OH 45229, USA; b Department of Radiology, Imaging Research Center, Cincinnati Children's Hospital Medical Center, 3333 Burnet Avenue, MLC 5031, Cincinnati, OH 45229, USA; c Department of Radiology, Center for Advanced Imaging Research, Mayo Clinic, 200 First St SW, Rochester, MN 55905, USA; d Department of Radiology, Cincinnati Children's Hospital Medical Center, University of Cincinnati College of Medicine, 3333 Burnet Avenue, MLC 5031, Cincinnati, OH 45229, USA
* Corresponding author.
E-mail address: hee.kim@cchmc.org

Radiol Clin N Am 51 (2013) 721–742
http://dx.doi.org/10.1016/j.rcl.2013.03.002
0033-8389/13/$ – see front matter

Table 1
MR parameters of quantitative MR imaging

	TR/TE	Matrix	Echo Train Length	Section Thickness	Section Gap (mm)	Field of View (cm)	Acquisition Time (min)	Pretreatment
T2 relaxation time mapping (pelvic and thigh MR)	1500/8, 16, 24,..., 128 ms	512 × 512	16	5 mm	10–50	32–46	5–7	Forgo excessive exercise for 12 h before MR examination
Dixon (pelvis and thigh MR)	For 3 T: 3.5/1.15 (TE1)/2.3 (TE2) For 1.5 T: 7/2.3 (TE1)/4.6 (TE2)	220 × 196	1	1.5–3 mm	0	32–46	2–3	
DW imaging	3000/27.5	192 × 128	1	6 mm	9	Depends on the size of the ROI	2–5	
DT imaging	6514/72	76 × 76	b-value = 500	2–3 mm	0	18–24	4	
MR elastography	100/19.6 (100 Hz motion)	256 × 64	1	5–10 mm	0	24–36	1–2	
PRESS MR spectroscopy	3000/20	Spectral width 2000 Hz, number of points 1024, 32–138 averages	NA	2 cm/side	NA	NA	5	

Abbreviations: DT, diffusion tensor; DW, diffusion-weighted; NA, no data available; PRESS, point-resolved spectroscopy; ROI, region of interest; TE, echo time; TR, repetition time.

Table 2
Summary of quantitative MR imaging interpretation

Quantitative Images		
T2 map	Decay of MR signal from altered environmental water binding	Increased inflammation: T2 relaxation time prolonged Increased fatty infiltration: T2 relaxation time prolonged
Dixon	Fat quantification using in-phase and opposed-phase imaging	Increased fatty infiltration; increased fat fraction (fat/ fat + water)
DW imaging	Random motion of water molecule	Increased cellularity in neoplasm: ADC value decreased Increased inflammation: ADC value increased Increased fatty infiltration: ADC value decreased
DT imaging	Muscle fiber tracking	Increased muscle injury: FA value decreased Increased muscle injury: MD increased
MR elastography	Mechanical properties measuring shear stiffness	Increased stiffness with increased disease
MR spectroscopy	Chemical information	Increased fatty infiltration; Increased lipid peak

Abbreviations: ADC, apparent diffusion coefficient; FA, fractional anisotropy; MD, mean diffusivity.

changes of muscle. Quantitative MR imaging techniques, such as T2 relaxation time mapping, Dixon imaging, diffusion-weighted (DW) imaging, diffusion tensor (DT) imaging, MR elastography, and MR spectroscopy are also reviewed, along with their physiologic basis and clinical applications (**Tables 1** and **2**).

SEMIQUANTITATIVE MR IMAGING TECHNIQUES

T1WI is a basic MR imaging sequence that can detect the hyperintense signal characteristic of fat. STIR sequences and T2WI sequences with fat suppression primarily are used to detect muscle disorders that result in hyperintense signal associated with increased water content. These qualitative or semiquantitative MR imaging sequences have been applied to identify anatomic abnormalities such as absent, aberrant, or accessory muscles (**Fig. 1**),[13] changes in tissue composition such as fatty infiltration (**Fig. 2**)[14] or increased water content (**Fig. 3**),[2] and masses (**Fig. 4**) or mass-like lesions (**Fig. 5**).[15]

Semiquantitative MR techniques have been used to subjectively grade compositional changes in muscle.[14] For example, the degree of fatty infiltration on T1WI has been graded from 0 to 4 as follows: grade 0, homogeneous low T1 signal of the muscle; grade 1, minimal fatty infiltration; grade 2, mild fatty infiltration with patchy areas of

fatty infiltration affecting less than 30% of the muscle mass; grade 3, moderate fatty infiltration with 30% to 60% of muscle mass involved and preservation of the demarcation between muscle and subcutaneous fat; and grade 4, severe fatty infiltration with more than 60% of muscle mass

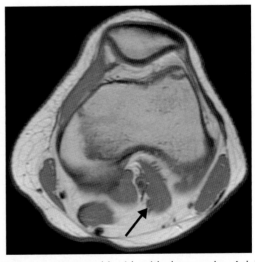

Fig. 1. A 15-year-old girl with knee pain. Axial intermediate-weighted MR image demonstrates accessory band (third head) (*arrow*) of the lateral head of the gastrocnemius muscle. Although this is seen in asymptomatic patients, it can cause mass effect on popliteal vessels in patients with popliteal entrapment syndrome.

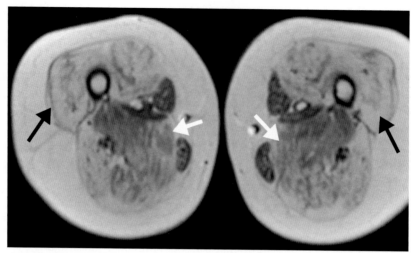

Fig. 2. An 11-year-old boy with Duchenne muscular dystrophy (DMD). Axial T1-weighted MR image shows extensive fatty infiltration of the majority of the thigh muscles bilaterally. Note that while the degree of involvement varies by muscle, individual muscle severity is relatively symmetric between the thighs (adductor magnus, *white arrows*; vastus lateralis, *black arrows*).

involved and loss of the muscle–subcutaneous fat interface (**Fig. 6**).[14,16,17]

The degree of water signal intensity in muscle, often reflecting edema or inflammation, has been graded on STIR or T2WI with fat suppression from 0 to 3 as follows: grade 0, homogeneous low T2 signal; grade 1, minimal interfascicular edema; grade 2, minimal interfascicular and/or intrafascicular edema; and grade 3, moderate interfascicular and/or intrafascicular edema.[16,17]

QUANTITATIVE MR IMAGING TECHNIQUES
T2 Relaxation Time Mapping

T2 relaxation time mapping (T2 mapping) is an MR imaging measurement of the time constant of decay of the nuclear MR signal, and has been used widely in the evaluation of articular cartilage.[16,18] In the magnetic field the hydrogen nuclei are excited, causing them to oscillate and generate a detectable magnetic signal. Immediately after excitation, the nuclei start to dephase while there is concurrent signal decay. Decay of the magnetic resonance signal is called T2 relaxation or transverse relaxation.[19] T2 relaxation time is defined as the time for the signal to reach 37% ($1/e$) of its initial signal after generation by tipping the longitudinal magnetization toward the transverse magnetic plane (**Fig. 7**A).[20] T2 relaxation time can be affected by a variety of factors.[21] Physiologic or pathologic macromolecular environmental changes of skeletal muscle can affect

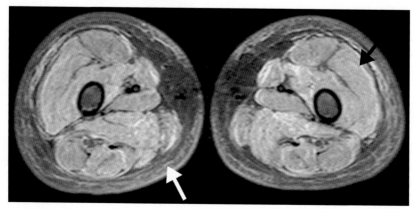

Fig. 3. A 7-year-old boy with juvenile dermatomyositis. Axial short-tau inversion recovery MR image shows a symmetric pattern of diffusely increased fluid signal intensity throughout all visualized thigh muscles (*black arrow*) consistent with muscle edema. Edema of the subcutaneous fat (*white arrow*) is also seen bilaterally, which is associated with a worse prognosis.

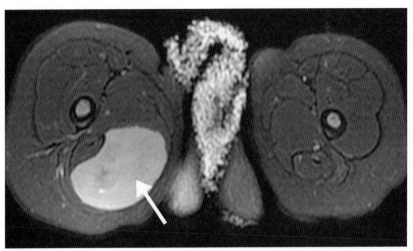

Fig. 4. A 22-month-old girl with thigh mass. Axial fat-saturated (FS) T2-weighted MR image shows a well-circumscribed mass (*arrow*) in the posteromedial musculature of the proximal right thigh with nearly homogeneous high T2 signal intensity (though not as bright as fluid). No surrounding muscle or soft-tissue edema is seen. Surgical pathology confirmed the diagnosis of rhabdomyosarcoma.

T2 relaxation times by alterations of water binding to neighboring molecules.[2,14,22] The main disease processes of the skeletal muscles, namely inflammation/edema and fatty infiltration, both affect T2 relaxation times. In addition, T2 relaxation times are longer when measured with lower field strengths than when measured with higher field strengths.[23,24]

A T2 map is generated by sampling multiple echo times (TE) and plotting the TE against the natural log of the signal intensity (see **Fig. 7**B). T2 relaxation time is calculated by using a least-square curve fitting algorithm.[25] The spatial compartmentalization of water in the intracellular and extracellular spaces of muscle contributes different components to the T2 relaxation time. Intracellular water, which comprises 80% of the water signal of muscle, contributes a fast component on the order of 20 to 40 milliseconds.[21] Extracellular water, which comprises 10% of the water signal of muscle, contributes a slow component with a T2 relaxation time between 150 and 400 milliseconds.[21] A small remainder of the T2 signal from muscle (less than 10%) is determined by the hydrogen shell of macromolecules, which contributes a very fast component, less than 5 milliseconds.[26] Owing to this multiexponential decay, the use of a sequence that includes multiple echo acquisitions at very short echo spacing, on the order of less than 1 millisecond, is ideal for more accurate analysis of skeletal muscles.[27] However, in light of technical limitations of current clinical MR scanning systems, monoexponential decay of the muscles is generally observed.[2,16,22,27]

T2 relaxation time mapping can be used to quantify muscle edema and inflammation in a variety of skeletal muscle disorders that affect children. The most commonly encountered pediatric myopathies are related to hereditary muscular dystrophies and nonhereditary autoimmune diseases, both of which typically affect numerous

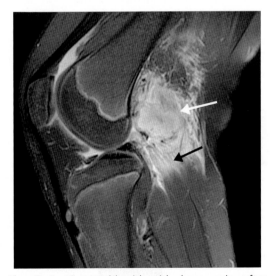

Fig. 5. A 12-year-old girl with knee pain after dancing. Sagittal FS T2-weighted MR image shows a round heterogeneous mass (*white arrow*) in the proximal muscle fibers of the gastrocnemius lateral head, with intense surrounding muscle edema (*black arrow*) and less pronounced surrounding fat edema. Given the intramuscular location, intense surrounding edema, and lower T2 signal intensity rim, myositis ossificans was suggested. Subsequent radiographs confirmed the typical peripheral to central calcification pattern seen with this entity.

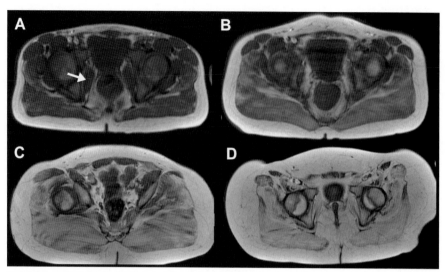

Fig. 6. Grading of fatty infiltration of the pelvic muscles on T1WI. (*A*) Grade 0, homogeneous low T1 signal of the iliacus muscle (*arrow*); grade 1, minimal fatty infiltration of the gluteus maximus muscles bilaterally. (*B*) Grade 2, mild fatty infiltration with patchy areas of fatty infiltration (affecting <30% of the muscle mass) of the gluteus maximus muscle. (*C*) Grade 3, moderate fatty infiltration (30%–60% of muscle mass involvement with preserved demarcation between muscle and subcutaneous fat) of the gluteus maximus muscle. (*D*) Grade 4, severe fatty infiltration with (>60% of muscle mass involvement with loss of the muscle-subcutaneous fat interface).

muscle groups symmetrically. Juvenile dermatomyositis (JDM), the most common idiopathic myositis, typically presents with proximal, symmetric muscle weakness and a characteristic violaceous rash. The disease can be self-limited or chronic with systemic morbidity. MR imaging shows characteristic symmetric muscle edema (see **Fig. 3**). Concurrent fascial and subcutaneous involvement frequently is seen, with the latter conferring a worse and more chronic prognosis.[28] Dystrophic calcifications ultimately may develop within the affected muscles (**Fig. 8**).[28,29] Maillard and colleagues[2] described significantly increased T2 relaxation times of muscle in children with

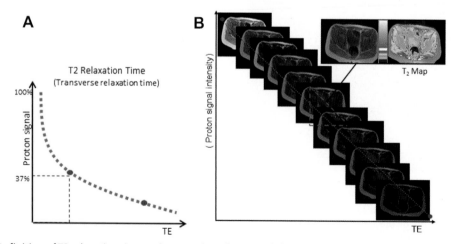

Fig. 7. Definition of T2 relaxation time and generation of T2 map. (*A*) T2 relaxation time is the time required for the signal to reach 37% (1/e) of its initial signal after generation by tipping the longitudinal magnetization toward the transverse magnetic plane. (*B*) Generation of T2 map. T2 map is generated by sampling multiple echo times by using multiecho sequences and plotting the echo time (TE) versus the natural log of the signal intensity. T2 relaxation time is calculated by using a least-square curve fitting algorithm. Gray-scale map is converted to color-coded map, and each color represents a different range of T2 relaxation time. (*Modified from* BJ Dardzinski, PhD, Philadelphia, PA.)

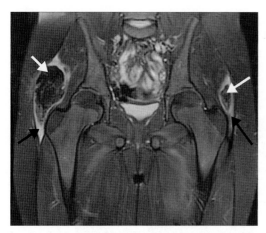

Fig. 8. An 8-year-old girl with juvenile dermato-myositis with dystrophic calcification. Coronal FS T2-weighted MR image shows low signal intensity masses (*white arrows*) in the lateral aspects of the gluteus maximus muscles bilaterally, with surrounding muscle edema (*black arrows*). The masses correspond to dystrophic calcifications.

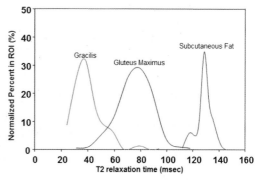

Fig. 9. Histogram obtained from pelvic muscles of an 8-year-old boy with DMD. Placement of region of interest (ROI) produces the distribution of the T2 relaxation times of the ROI. As each muscle has a different volume, pixel volumes are normalized and a histogram is made for each ROI. This histogram demonstrates distribution of T2 relaxation times of the subcutaneous fat (*right*, longest), gluteus maximus muscle (*middle*), and gracilis muscle (*left*, shortest).

active disease in a comparison with healthy controls and patients with inactive disease.

T2 relaxation time mapping can also be used to quantitate fatty infiltration in children with a variety of muscular dystrophies. Duchenne muscular dystrophy (DMD), an X-linked disorder found in boys, is the most common progressive muscular dystrophy of children. DMD is caused by mutations in the gene that encodes dystrophin, a protein essential to normal muscle function. Muscle fiber damage results from a destabilized sarcolemma, with subsequent muscle necrosis and eventual fatty replacement (see **Fig. 2**). This disease typically is diagnosed around 5 years of age as symmetric and progressive muscle weakness, classically involving the thighs. Death usually occurs by the third to fourth decades. MR imaging can show muscle edema secondary to inflammation, but the hallmark of MR imaging in DMD is the gradual and symmetric fatty replacement of select muscle groups.[14]

Prior studies have described T2 mapping in children with DMD, showing increased T2 relaxation times consequent to this fatty infiltration (**Figs. 9** and **10**).[14,22] T2 relaxation times have good correlation with fatty infiltration grading assessed qualitatively on T1WI and with clinical functional motor scores in DMD patients.[14] T2 mapping also can be used to quantify the small amount of physiologic fat in normal skeletal muscles of healthy children and enable the complete segregation of boys with DMD from healthy boys, even when the difference in fatty infiltration is not easily appreciated on T1WI (see **Fig. 10**).[5,30,31]

Acquiring T2 mapping data without and with fat-suppression techniques allows for the separation of concurrent fatty infiltration from edema and/or inflammation in boys with DMD.[6] Application of this quantitative and objective MR imaging method can be extended to a longitudinal study to determine the treatment response in diseases of skeletal muscle.[14]

T2 relaxation times may be affected by muscle activity. Muscle contraction requires energy consumption and produces by-product osmolites such as sodium, phosphate, and lactate. Increased osmolality causes water influx into the muscles, which in turn results in increased intracellular water. This increase in water content increases T2 relaxation times.[32] Therefore, it is important when using T2 mapping to evaluate skeletal muscle that subjects should be asked to refrain from excessive ambulation and exercise for at least 12 hours before MR imaging.[19]

T2 mapping has great potential to demonstrate nonuniform involvement of muscles in a variety of normal and pathologic states,[19] such as localized nerve injury. Improvements in spatial resolution in T2 mapping techniques are still needed, to enable mapping of territories as small as individual motor units.

Dixon Imaging

Dixon imaging is an MR imaging technique used to measure fat fractions and obtain homogeneous fat-suppressed images when other conventional techniques fail because of inhomogeneities of the magnetic field.[33–35] In Dixon imaging, first proposed and developed by Thomas Dixon, modified

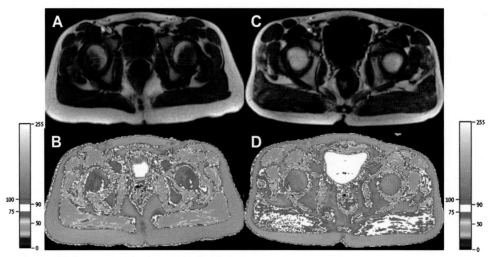

Fig. 10. T2 mapping in a 7-year-old healthy boy (*left*) and a boy with DMD (*right*). T1-weighted MR image demonstrates minimal degree of fatty infiltration of gluteus maximus muscles in the healthy boy (*A*) and the boy with DMD (*C*). Both boys were graded as grade 1 fatty infiltration on T1-weighted MR images. T2 relaxation time mapping, however, demonstrates a significant difference between the two boys. T2 map demonstrates increased T2 relaxation times within the gluteus maximus muscles in the boy with DMD (*D*) in comparison with those of the healthy boy (*B*).

dual spin-echo sequences are used such that the first echo image is acquired when water and fat protons are in phase with each other, and the next echo image is acquired when water and fat are in opposed phases. Both echoes are acquired in a single repetition time. The in-phase and opposed-phase TE are based on the chemical shift between the precessing water and lipid protons and, hence, are field-strength dependent (**Fig. 11**).[36] On a typical 3-T MR scanner the first echo is acquired at approximately 1.2 milliseconds, which is the TE for an opposed-phase image, and the second in-phase echo is acquired at a TE of 2.4 milliseconds, in contrast to a 1.5-T scanner where the opposed-phase TE is approximately 2.3 milliseconds and the in-phase TE 4.6 milliseconds.

With the Dixon technique, the net signal from a voxel is determined by the water and fat

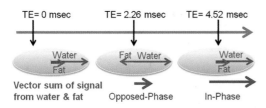

Fig. 11. Dixon imaging with in-phase and opposed-phase. The in-phase and opposed-phase acquisition times or echo times (TE) are based on chemical shift time between the precessing water and lipid protons. At 1.5 T, the opposed-phase TE is approximately 2.26 milliseconds and the in-phase TE is 4.52 milliseconds.

composition of the tissue; if the voxel contains only water or fat, its net signal for the 2 acquisitions will be the same, because the signal from one component will be zero. By contrast, a voxel containing both water and fat will have different signals from the two acquisitions (**Fig. 12**). Using this information, the in-phase and opposed-phase images are then added or subtracted to generate a water-only or a fat-only image (see **Fig. 12**).[37,38]

In the presence of magnetic-field inhomogeneity (eg, adjacent to surgical hardware or locations such as the neck, breast, or ankle where there are convoluted soft tissue–air interfaces), the fat resonance frequency typically varies over the entire image volume. Such circumstances result in poor fat suppression with conventional frequency-selective fat-suppression techniques. The water-only image obtained through the Dixon technique can be used in such scenarios when fat suppression is desired for clinical indications (**Fig. 13**).[33,38,39] Dixon imaging is also a successful technique with which to obtain uniform fat-saturation images at higher field strengths.[40,41]

A quantitative fat-fraction value can also be calculated from the generated water-only and fat-only images by taking a ratio of fat signal intensity versus the sum of the water and fat signal intensities.[3] The fat-fraction value can be plotted as a map on a pixel-by-pixel basis or by drawing a region of interest (ROI). The fat fraction is equal to the ratio of the signal intensity from the fat-only image to the sum of the signal intensity on

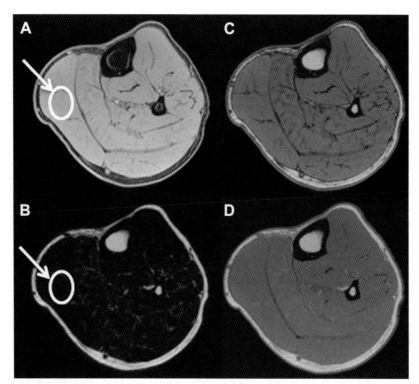

Fig. 12. An example of (A) water, (B) fat, (C) opposed-phase, and (D) in-phase images of the calf in a healthy subject. The benefit of Dixon imaging is that multiple image contrasts can be acquired in single scan: water, fat, in-phase, and opposed-phase images. In addition, muscle fat fraction can be calculated by drawing an ROI (*arrow*) on the water and fat images (fat fraction = signal intensity on fat image/signal intensity on fat image + signal intensity on water image). The fat fraction for this subject was calculated to be 5%.

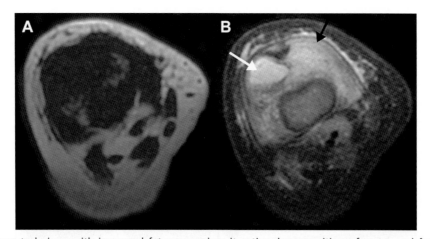

Fig. 13. Dixon technique with improved fat suppression: iterative decomposition of water and fat with echo asymmetry and least-squares estimation (IDEAL). (A) Axial T2-weighted MR image of the right knee with conventional fat suppression and (B) Dixon applied water imaging in a patient with septic arthritis and osteomyelitis. (A) Fat suppression is nonuniform owing to an inhomogeneous magnetic field created by a large field of view (covering both lower extremities from hip to ankle), as well as flexion of the knee, yielding images with minimal water signal. (B) The initially obscured but highly significant findings of joint fluid (*white arrow*) and muscle edema (*black arrow*) (representing septic arthritis and myositis in this case, respectively) are clearly visualized with the Dixon technique.

the fat-only image and the signal intensity of the water-only image (see **Fig. 12**).

The muscle fat-fraction measurement by Dixon imaging is noninvasive, objective, and highly reproducible. Gaeta and colleagues[7] report that the muscle fat-fraction value acquired using MR imaging correlates well with histopathology results in patients with neuromuscular disorders. Other reports show that the fat-fraction value obtained with the Dixon technique is accurate in the assessment of disease severity in patients with DMD[42] and correlates with muscle histology.[43] Therefore, the quantitative fat-fraction measurement obtained with MR imaging may be a useful biomarker in quantifying fatty infiltration as a predictor of disease progression and therapeutic response.

Diffusion-Weighted Imaging

DW imaging is sensitive to the effects of water diffusion on MR signal intensity.[44] The cellular membrane integrity affects the transcellular, intracellular, and extracellular motion of water molecules (**Fig. 14**). In an unrestricted environment, water moves freely (free Brownian motion) (see **Fig. 14A**). In biological tissue, however, cellular membranes restrict the motion of water molecules. Thus the apparent diffusion coefficient (ADC) of tissue water reflects cellular membrane integrity and microcirculation (perfusion) (see **Fig. 14B**). In DW imaging, there is a dephasing of spins and subsequent rephasing by gradients placed generally on either side of a refocusing pulse. While stationary molecules are rephased at the end of the sequence, molecules in motion are incompletely rephased, which results in loss of signal (signal attenuation) (**Fig. 15**).[45] DW sequences can be generated using spin-echo DW imaging,[46] echo planar imaging,[47] and steady-state free precession sequences.[48] The ADC of water is calculated by plotting the signal intensity of the tissue against the applied diffusion gradient strength (b-value). Diffusion attenuation depends on the b-value for contrast, with higher b-values leading to greater sensitivity to diffusion and greater attenuation of the signal. A higher ADC means a longer mean free path length of the water molecules, a steeper slope of the plot, and less cellularity (**Fig. 16**).

ADC values have been used as markers of tissue cellularity in oncologic imaging,[49] with ADC values less than 1.5×10^{-3} mm^2/s reflecting high cellularity (>150 cells per high-power field).[50] However, Humphries and colleagues[50] showed that ADC values are not able to differentiate benign from malignant neoplasms. DW imaging can also be used to evaluate the cellularity of skeletal muscle neoplasms in children (**Fig. 17**).

Normal skeletal muscle has a biexponential attenuation pattern. ADC estimates obtained with b-values from 0 to 50 s/mm^2 reflect a combination of diffusion and perfusion, whereas ADC estimates using b-values of 50 to 750 s/mm^2 reflect true diffusion. Therefore, the ADC of skeletal muscles should be obtained using b-values of at least 100 s/mm^2.

A   **B**

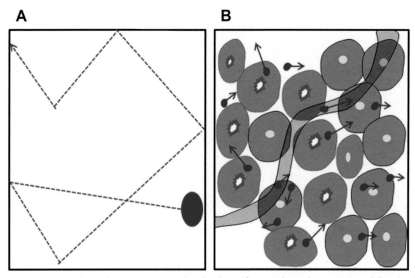

Fig. 14. (*A*) In the uninhibited condition, water molecules have free and random motion. (*B*) In biological tissue, the motion of water molecules is limited by interaction with cellular components; cellular membrane integrity and cellularity. ([*B*] *Adapted from* Koh DM, Collins DJ. Diffusion-weighted MRI in the body: applications and challenges in oncology. AJR Am J Roentgenol 2007;188(6):1622–23; with permission.)

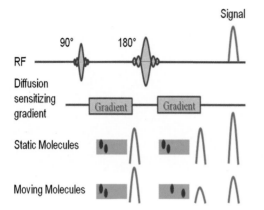

edema from radiation or inflammation, there is an increase in free mean path length of the water molecules, which results in an increase in ADC value[45]; this situation is similar to cytotoxic edema of the brain, which also increases the ADC.

Diffusion Tensor Imaging

DT imaging measures the anisotropy of water diffusion, and is used widely in brain imaging to show the orientation and integrity of white matter tracts.[51,52] The underlying principle of DT imaging is that the water diffusion will be greater along the orientation of the fibers than in another direction. Estimates of the diffusion anisotropy can be generated from DW imaging data and the corresponding calculated maps.

To minimize magnetic field inhomogeneity, reduce noise, and optimize the coil-filling factor, DT imaging is preferentially performed using the smallest-volume coils.[53] DT imaging data sets are generated by adding at least 6 diffusion gradient directions to a typical DW imaging sequence and by using 2 b-values (**Fig. 19**), usually b = 0 and b = 500 to 1000 s/mm^2.[54] A DT value is calculated from the DW imaging data for each voxel in the dataset. The fractional anisotropy (FA), a measure of how "directional" the water diffusion is, and the mean diffusivity, or average length of diffusion along the selected directions, are calculated from the tensor images. The mathematical calculations for the tensor values are described in detail by Le Bihan and colleagues.[54–56] FA is the most widely used tensor value and represents the anisotropy index of water molecules. For easy visualization, the FA maps are color-coded in red, green, and blue. A color code is assigned to each of the x, y, and z orientations (**Fig. 20**). A numerical FA value can be obtained from the FA map on a pixel-by-pixel basis, or an ROI can be drawn on the map to compute a cumulative number. The FA values in a normal and an abnormal population can be compared. Fiber tracking is a method that shows simplified directional tensor information by connecting similarly oriented neighboring vectors to follow a trajectory.[57–59] This technique can help identify location, size, and shape of specific fiber tracks of interest.

DT imaging can be applied to skeletal muscle imaging to probe muscle architecture and define structural details, such as in the evaluation of skeletal muscle injury.[8,9,60–63] Muscle injury from trauma or neuropathy will affect the integrity of muscle microstructure and, hence, change the DT imaging parameters. These microstructural changes are reflected by changes in FA and often precede gross morphologic or anatomic changes

Fig. 15. Diffusion-weighted (DW) imaging sequences. Initially, diffusion sequences cause dephasing of spins and subsequent rephasing by an opposite gradient. While static molecules are rephased at the end of the sequences, molecules in motion are less uniformly rephased than more static molecules, resulting in and loss of signal (signal attenuation) and being out of plane. (*Adapted from* Koh DM, Collins DJ. Diffusion-weighted MRI in the body: applications and challenges in oncology. AJR Am J Roentgenol 2007;188(6):1623; with permission.)

The application of DW imaging to evaluate systemic skeletal muscle disorders has been used only in scientific studies.[4] ADC values of normal skeletal muscle are significantly higher than those of subcutaneous fat (**Fig. 18**).[4] Muscle edema from radiation therapy and muscle inflammation associated with adjacent osteomyelitis both lead to an increase in extracellular water content. In cytotoxic

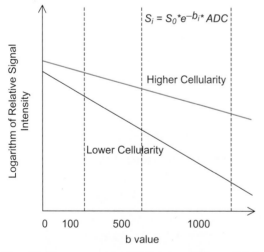

Fig. 16. The apparent diffusion coefficient (ADC) value is calculated by using a plot of log of signal intensity versus the diffusion strength (b-value) of the tissue; higher ADC means greater mean free path length of the water molecules, steeper slope of a plot, and less cellularity.

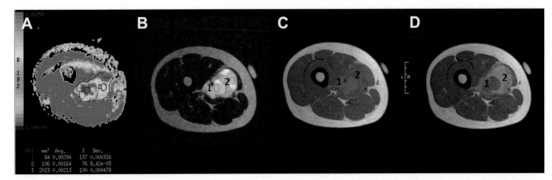

Fig. 17. An 18-year-old boy with spindle-cell sarcoma of the right thigh. (*A*) ADC map demonstrates high ADC values (>1.5 × 10^{-3} mm²/s): mean value of entire tumor, 2.13 × 10^{-3} mm²/s (ROI 3); central necrosis (ROI 1), 2.94 × 10^{-3} mm²/s; relatively high cellular area, 1.64 × 10^{-3} mm²/s (ROI 2). Corresponding high cellular area (ROI 2) demonstrates solid component on (*B*) T2-weighted MR image with fat suppression, and more contrast enhancement than area of necrosis (ROI 1) on (*C*) precontrast and (*D*) postcontrast T1-weighted MR images.

of the muscles, thus enabling early detection of skeletal muscle disease.[64] The quantitative nature of DT imaging can play a very important role as a noninvasive surrogate marker in monitoring the therapeutic response in muscle injuries. For skeletal muscle applications, b-values of 0 and 500 are typically used with 7 or more directions.

MR Elastography Imaging

MR elastography is a phase-contrast MR imaging–based elasticity imaging technique that can calculate the shear stiffness of soft tissues by imaging the propagation of externally induced shear waves. MR elastography currently is used clinically in the evaluation of hepatic fibrosis.[65] The technique essentially involves 3 steps:

1. *Generation of shear waves.* External mechanical driver systems controlled by the MR pulse sequence generate continuous harmonic shear waves in the frequency range of 50 to 300 Hz.[66]
2. *Imaging the propagation of shear waves.* This critical step defines MR elastography, and is accomplished by the inclusion of motion-encoding gradients (MEG) in conventional pulse sequences, which encode the propagating shear wave information into the phase of the MR images.[67] The phase of harmonically vibrating tissue is directly proportional to its displacement. The schematic of a typical gradient-recalled echo MR elastography pulse sequence with a bipolar MEG pair (of duration 3.33 milliseconds corresponding to 300 Hz

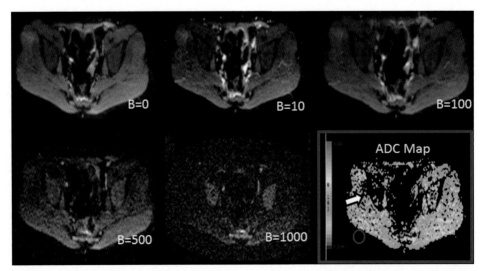

Fig. 18. DW image obtained using 5 different B values (B = 0, 10, 100, 500, and 1000). ADC map demonstrates very low ADC value of the bone (*arrow*) and subcutaneous fat (*circle*). Black color on the scale corresponds to the lowest ADC value. The skeletal muscles show higher ADC values than for bone and subcutaneous fat.

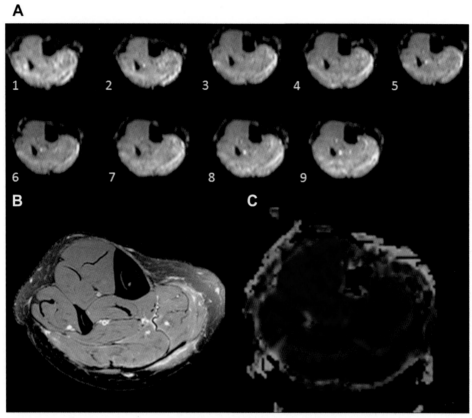

Fig. 19. Diffusion tensor (DT) imaging sequences. DT images using a single-shot spin-echo planar imaging pulse sequence (9 directions; b-value: 500 s/mm^2). (*A*) 1, image along z-axis; 2–9, images with different gradient directions. (*B*) High-resolution T2-weighted MR image with fat suppression. Baseline image used for contour overlay. (*C*) Fractional anisotropy map.

motion) in the slice-selection gradient, along with the schematic of 300 Hz motion, is shown in **Fig. 21A**.

Motion occurring in any direction and on the order of hundreds of nanometers can be successfully visualized with this technique by manipulating the position and the amplitude of the MEG. An MR image thus obtained contains both the background phase and the propagating wave information, which is typically separated by collecting 2 images with opposite MEG polarities and calculating a phase-difference image. This phase-difference image has only

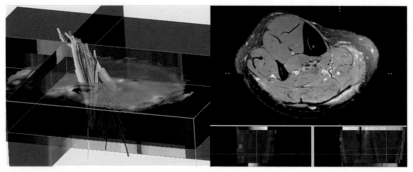

Fig. 20. Human calf muscle tractography: Fiber tracts were calculated using DTI Studio (Johns Hopkins Medical Institute, Baltimore, MD). An ROI was placed on the tibialis posterior muscle to generate fiber tracking. The different colors represent different directions of the fibers.

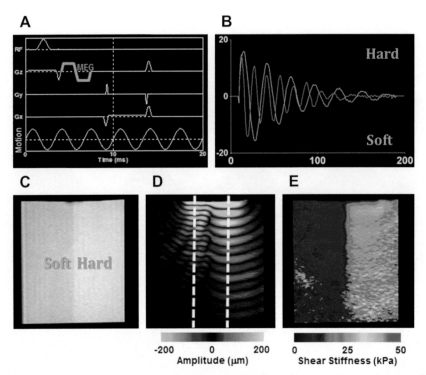

Fig. 21. MR elastography on a 2-layer phantom. (*A*) MR elastography pulse sequence; motion-encoding gradient (MEG) is indicated. (*B*) Line-profile analysis of the shear wave data shown in (*D*). (*C*) Magnitude image, (*D*) wave, and (*E*) stiffness image of a 2-layer phantom. The longer shear wavelength in the harder region is visible both in (*B*) and (*D*). (*Courtesy of* Jennifer L. Kugel, BS, Mayo Clinic, Rochester, MN.)

the motion information and is referred to as a wave image (**Fig. 21**B,D). The 2 regions, hard and soft, are indicated in the magnitude image, and the longer shear wavelength in the harder region is easily visible (see **Fig. 21**B–D).

3. *Calculation of shear stiffness maps.* Mathematical inversion algorithms[68] are used to produce quantitative maps of shear stiffness from the wave. The operating equation is $\mu = \rho V_s^2$ (where μ is shear stiffness, ρ physical density, and V_s wave speed). The wave speed within the phantom is calculated as the product of the motion frequency and the spatial shear wavelength ($V_s = f\lambda$) measured manually from the wave profile (see **Fig. 21**B). Two line profiles extracted from the wave data (indicated in **Fig. 21**D) in a direction perpendicular to the wave propagation are presented, and the change in shear wavelength is easily visible. From these profiles, the shear wavelengths were calculated to be 0.93 cm and 1.68 cm, resulting in shear stiffness values of 7.91 kPa and 21.62 kPa for the soft and hard layers, respectively. **Fig. 21**E shows the shear stiffness map of this isotropic phantom obtained with local standard frequency estimation technique.

It is well known that the Young modulus of muscle is almost directly proportional to its tension, and earlier MR elastography applications focused on observing the muscle tension.[69,70] Representative data from an in vivo MR elastography experiment performed at a frequency of 100 Hz on a calf muscle is shown in **Fig. 22**. On a sagittal magnitude image of the slice of interest, the position of the electromechanical driver used to induce shear waves is shown (indicated by the arrow in **Fig. 22**A). Wave data were obtained from MR elastography experiments performed with the muscle at its relaxed state and when exerting a force of 5, 10, and 15 N on a custom-built leg press (**Fig. 22**B–E). From these data and the wave profiles, the gradual increase in the shear wavelength and, hence, the shear stiffness (7.9, 25.6, 49.4, and 81 kPa, respectively) with the increasing force is visible (**Fig. 22**F).

Because of the power, flexibility, and clinical potential of MR elastography, this is an active area of research where many groups have successfully implemented and assessed the shear stiffness of various healthy and pathologic muscles. Skeletal muscles undergo significant changes in their mechanical properties during both normal physiologic functioning and

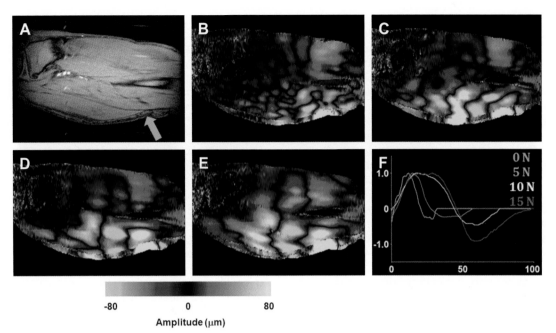

Fig. 22. MR elastography on a calf muscle. (*A*) Magnitude image. Shear wave data with the muscle exhibiting (*B*) 0, (*C*) 5, (*D*) 10, and (*E*) 15 N force. (*F*) A line profile of a single shear wave obtained from these 4 data; the gradual increase in shear wavelength is easily visible. (*Courtesy of* Thomas C. Hulshizer, BS, Mayo Clinic, Rochester, MN.)

pathologic disease processes. Noninvasive in vivo quantification of these properties can thus potentially have a substantial impact on the diagnosis, monitoring, and management of many muscular disorders. For instance, it has been found that there is a difference in the stiffness of muscles with and without neuromuscular disease.[10] The MR elastography–derived stiffness of gastrocnemius, soleus, and tibialis anterior muscles have been reported to be significantly higher in patients with poliomyelitis, flaccid paraplegia, and spastic paraplegia.[10] Similarly, the shear stiffness of the trapezius muscle was higher in patients with myofascial pain compared with healthy volunteers and even the unaffected contralateral trapezius.[71] It has also been reported that the stiffness of the vastus medialis increases at a faster rate after treatment in hyperthyroid patients with Graves disease in comparison with healthy volunteers. The results from a study investigating the soleus muscle of patients with hypogonadism indicate that the stiffness values were different before and after therapy, indicating the potential of MR elastography as a therapy-monitoring tool.[72] The results from another study indicate that MR elastography can be directly extended to pediatric subjects and that the muscle stiffness is correlated with age.[73] The same group has also reported that the differences in muscle architecture between the pediatric muscle and adult muscle can be assessed

through the measurement of MR elastography shear wave propagation angle.[74]

In addition to the calculation of shear stiffness, MR elastography can also measure other useful mechanical properties. For example, shear wave attenuation coefficients of the vastus medialis for patients with hyperthyroid myopathy and myositis were found to be larger than those of their normal healthy counterparts.[75] It has also been reported that MR elastography displacement information could be used to examine the connectivity of adjacent tissues,[76] the slipperiness of tissue interfaces,[77] and the functional analysis of flexor muscle compartments.[78] One of the main limitations of MR elastography of the muscle is that the stiffness is still assessed with a manual technique, which could show subjective variation, but ongoing work in this domain may address this issue in the near future.[79]

Thus the assessment of stiffness of both adult and pediatric muscles by MR elastography, although not yet in clinical use, has the potential to improve the diagnosis and prognosis of many skeletal muscle disorders.

MR Spectroscopy

MR spectroscopy provides information about the chemical composition of tissue rather than its anatomic structure. The most commonly studied nucleus for muscle MR spectroscopy is phosphorus-31 (^{31}P). In addition to ^{31}P, carbon-13 (^{13}C) and proton (^{1}H) studies have been done, each of which provides unique information about muscle composition and metabolism. Although multinuclear systems are increasingly available, most are still proton-only. ^{13}C studies require additional resources.[80]

Before beginning the MR spectroscopy study, it is essential to choose the proper coil. Surface coils have high sensitivity, but their B1 fields are inhomogeneous. Surface coils have the advantage that they can be positioned nearly anywhere. Volume coils have better B1 homogeneity, but their use may restrict the anatomy studied or limit how well the subject is positioned in the scanner. For example, if the vastus lateralis muscle is under investigation, a volume coil could be used, but getting both the coil and the thigh centered in the magnet would be difficult. A surface coil would be a better choice for this muscle, whereas a volume coil would suffice for any muscle in the lower leg. The choice of coils is a greater concern for proton studies; for ^{31}P, most investigators are limited to a vendor-supplied surface coil.

When setting up the study, the patient should be positioned such that the area of interest is as close to the center of the bore as possible. Voxels should be as large as possible, but placed and sized such that no subcutaneous fat is included. The muscle fascia should be avoided.[81] For localized spectroscopy using the PRESS (Point-RESolved Spectroscopy) sequence, echo time needs to be optimized. In general, a short TE is better for measuring lipids because they tend to have relatively short transverse relaxation times. The repetition time should be relatively long (2000–3000 milliseconds) to minimize saturation effects. Although TE is not relevant for a simple pulse-and-acquire sequence, such as is commonly used for dynamic ^{31}P MR spectroscopy, the repetition time should still be long. The number of excitations or averages depends on the parameter of interest and the type of acquisition, static or dynamic. Static MR spectroscopy provides a snapshot of the metabolite levels at a particular time. Dynamic MR spectroscopy measures metabolite signal intensities following some kind of intervention, such as during an exercise challenge (for ^{31}P MR spectroscopy), and is of use when the rates of change for various metabolites are of interest. In general, for static measurements of most metabolite peaks, 64 to 128 averages should suffice. For dynamic studies, the number of averages should be the minimum that provides a signal-to-noise ratio of at least 2. For unlocalized ^{31}P MR spectroscopy of muscle, 4 to 8 averages should be adequate, particularly for dynamic scans whereby temporal resolution is important.

Unlike conventional MR imaging, the information in an MR spectroscopy experiment is contained in the peaks of the spectrum, each of which occurs at a specific, generally invariant, position. For example, the water peak occurs at 4.7 ppm, whereas the lipid peak occurs at 1.3 ppm. The term "ppm" refers to the shift of the resonant frequency of the peak with respect to the absolute frequency of some reference compound.[82] The areas under the peaks are related to the concentrations of the compounds generating the peaks, which is generally the parameter of interest.

Several software packages are available for analysis of the spectral data. The software used to identify and analyze these peaks should minimally allow for measurement of peak height and area. Most vendors supply rudimentary spectral-analysis software with the scanner that will provide this information. If more quantitative information is required, software packages such as LCModel[83] or jMRUI[84] may be used to extract estimates of metabolite concentration.

Proton MR spectroscopy

Proton MR spectroscopy studies of muscle show resonances from fat, water, creatine (Cr), and trimethylammonium-containing compounds (TMA). Significant interest in proton MR spectroscopy of muscle began with the work of Boesch and colleagues,[81,85,86] who realized that proton MR spectra from muscle depended on the orientation of the muscle fibers with respect to the main magnetic field. When the muscle fibers are parallel with the main magnetic field, the major lipid resonance, around 1.3 to 1.5 ppm, splits into two distinct peaks. The peak at 1.28 ppm is assigned to intramyocellular lipids (IMCL) and the other is assigned to extramyocellular lipids (EMCL).[85] The IMCL signal originates from droplets in the muscle cells, whereas the EMCL signal originates from "bulk" fat. The IMCL signal is insensitive to the orientation of the muscle with the field, whereas the EMCL signal, which arises from lipid stored parallel to the muscle fibers, is extremely sensitive to muscle orientation. A representative water-suppressed spectrum showing Cr, TMA, IMCL, and EMCL is shown in **Fig. 23**. To assess the intramyocellular and extramyocellular lipids (IMCL or EMCL), the fibers of the muscle of interest should be as close to parallel with the bore as possible. Thus, muscles such as vastus lateralis, semitendinosus, tibialis anterior, and gastrocnemius, in which the fibers

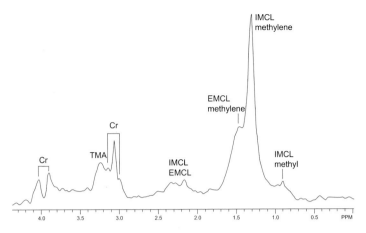

Fig. 23. Water-suppressed spectrum from the thigh of a normal subject showing the main resonances. Cr, creatine; EMCL, extramyocellular lipid; IMCL, intramyocellular lipid; TMA, trimethylammonium-containing compounds.

tend to run the length of the leg, are well suited for IMCL/EMCL measurements.

Studies of proton MR spectroscopy applied to inherited metabolic muscle disease are rare. Bongers and colleagues[87] published an early case report comparing healthy volunteers with 3 patients with muscle disease myopathy, myositis, and muscle injury from radiation, and found alterations in lipid and TMA signals with disease. A comparison study of patients with DMD and spinal muscular atrophy and normal volunteers found that both patient groups had lower TMA/water and TMA/Cr ratios than the controls, but Cr/water ratios were normal.[11] In a follow-up study, of 8 DMD patients compared with 8 healthy controls, DMD patients had lower TMA/water, Cr/water, and TMA/Cr than controls, and muscle function negatively correlated with the TMA/Cr ratio.[12] Studies of IMCL/EMCL have been restricted to diabetes, insulin resistance, and lipid metabolism, mostly performed in adult populations. Spectra from a DMD patient and normal volunteer (Fig. 24) clearly show the increased lipid content in the DMD patient, which reflects the fatty infiltration of the muscle.

Phosphorus MR spectroscopy

In contrast to proton MR spectroscopy, phosphorus MR spectroscopy has long been used to study muscle metabolism because ^{31}P MR spectroscopy can detect signals from phosphocreatine (PCr), adenosine triphosphate (ATP), and inorganic phosphate (Pi), all of which are involved in energy metabolism via the creatine kinase reaction:

$$PCr + ADP \rightarrow ATP + Pi$$

where *ADP* is adenosine diphosphate.

Other visible peaks include those from phosphomonoesters and phosphodiesters. In addition, estimates of tissue pH can be derived from the phosphorus MR spectroscopy measurement.[88] Because unlocalized ^{31}P MR spectroscopy data can be acquired quickly, the method is well suited to dynamic exercise studies from which the depletion and recovery rates of PCr can be calculated to provide additional information about mitochondrial function or health.[89] An example of such a

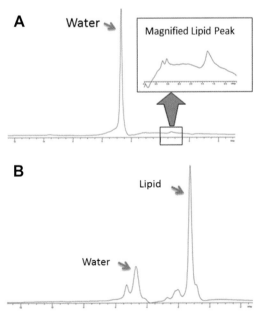

Fig. 24. (*A*) Spectrum from a normal subject showing primarily the water peak. Inset shows lipid region at increased scale; the Cr and TMA peaks are barely visible. (*B*) Non–water-suppressed spectrum from a DMD patient showing elevated lipid signal.

dynamic scan from a healthy volunteer is shown in **Fig. 25**.

In a study of sarcoglycan-deficient limb-girdle muscular dystrophy, the disease group had normal levels of the phosphorus metabolites and normal muscle oxidative metabolism in the calf, but elevated tissue pH.[90] Fat infiltration correlated inversely with pH and directly with PCr/ATP.[90] Another study comparing patients with Becker muscular dystrophy (BMD) or Friedreich ataxia (FRDA) with normal subjects found that patients with FRDA depleted PCr levels to a lesser extent than either BMD patients or normal controls.[91] Despite not depleting their PCr reserves, FRDA patients recovered PCr more slowly than controls.[91] BMD patients also recovered more slowly than controls, similar to FRDA patients, suggesting mitochondrial dysfunction in both groups.[91] The investigators did not report whether the groups

differed in baseline PCr or Pi levels. Park and colleagues[92] reported lower levels of ATP and PCr in the muscles of patients with juvenile dermatomyositis than in controls. Pi/PCr ratios and ADP levels were elevated, suggesting defective oxidative phosphorylation in the mitochondria of these patients.[92]

DMD is probably the disease most widely studied with ^{31}P MR spectroscopy.[93–95] One of the first reports using ^{31}P MR spectroscopy in DMD patients found decreased PCr/ATP and PCr/Pi ratios in subjects with DMD in comparison with normal controls.[93] Spectra from DMD patients consistently showed a phosphodiester peak not seen in control spectra.[93] DMD patients also had significantly higher tissue pH.[93] Younkin and colleagues[94] later confirmed these results and also found significant age-related changes in the phosphorus metabolites. The decreased PCr/ATP and

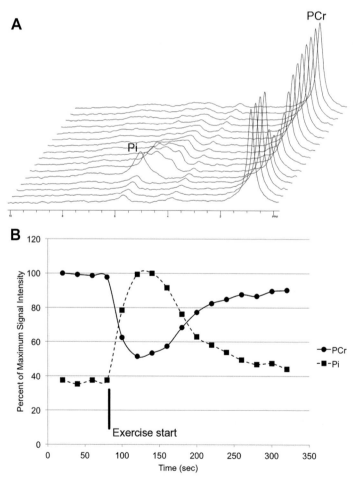

Fig. 25. (*A*) Series of spectra acquired from the tibialis anterior before, during, and after plantar flexion of the foot. Time increases along the axis running toward the back. The increase in inorganic phosphate (Pi) and decrease in phosphocreatine (PCr) are clearly visible. (*B*) Signal intensities over time for Pi and PCr extracted from the spectra in (*A*).

PCr/Pi ratios have been confirmed in multiple studies.[95–97] A combined ^{1}H and ^{31}P MR spectroscopy study found that whereas the ^{1}H MR spectroscopy studies provided measures correlated to functional score (primarily fat content), the ^{31}P MR spectroscopy, despite showing abnormalities between subjects and controls, did not correlate with functional score.[97] However, this study had a relatively small sample size and did not examine the effects of exercise on PCr, which might be expected to be a better representation of functional ability than static measurements.[97]

SUMMARY

Recent advances in MR imaging techniques, particularly quantitative measurements, are just beginning to be used in the assessment of normal muscle and various muscle abnormalities. To date, most investigations have been performed in adults. However, the spectrum of muscle disorders in children might be a fertile area for future application. This article reviews a variety of advanced MR imaging techniques that go beyond the most commonly used conventional, subjective, semiquantitative methods. Further investigation of these quantitative MR imaging techniques may aid in understanding the pathophysiology of various muscle disorders in children, and offer new opportunities for establishing diagnoses and directing therapies.

REFERENCES

1. May DA, Disler DG, Jones EA, et al. Abnormal signal intensity in skeletal muscle at MR imaging: patterns, pearls, and pitfalls. Radiographics 2000; 20(Spec No):S295–315.

2. Maillard SM, Jones R, Owens C, et al. Quantitative assessment of MRI T2 relaxation time of thigh muscles in juvenile dermatomyositis. Rheumatology (Oxford) 2004;43(5):603–8.

3. Liu P, Hwang JT. Quick calculation for sample size while controlling false discovery rate with application to microarray analysis. Bioinformatics 2007; 23(6):739–46.

4. Baur A, Reiser MF. Diffusion-weighted imaging of the musculoskeletal system in humans. Skeletal Radiol 2000;29(10):555–62.

5. Kim HK, Wang LL, Merrow AC, et al. Compounding factors affecting fat and water content of skeletal muscles in healthy children; objective measures using T2 relaxation time mapping (T2 Map). Chicago: Radiological Society of North America; 2011.

6. Arpan I, Forbes SC, Lott DJ, et al. T(2) mapping provides multiple approaches for the characterization of muscle involvement in neuromuscular diseases: a cross-sectional study of lower leg muscles in 5-15-year-old boys with Duchenne muscular dystrophy. NMR Biomed 2012;26(3):320–8.

7. Gaeta M, Mileto A, Mazzeo A, et al. MRI findings, patterns of disease distribution, and muscle fat fraction calculation in five patients with Charcot-Marie-Tooth type 2 F disease. Skeletal Radiol 2012;41(5):515–24.

8. Zaraiskaya T, Kumbhare D, Noseworthy MD. Diffusion tensor imaging in evaluation of human skeletal muscle injury. J Magn Reson Imaging 2006;24(2): 402–8.

9. Sinha S, Sinha U, Edgerton VR. In vivo diffusion tensor imaging of the human calf muscle. J Magn Reson Imaging 2006;24(1):182–90.

10. Basford JR, Jenkyn TR, An KN, et al. Evaluation of healthy and diseased muscle with magnetic resonance elastography. Arch Phys Med Rehabil 2002;83(11):1530–6.

11. Hsieh TJ, Wang CK, Chuang HY, et al. In vivo proton magnetic resonance spectroscopy assessment for muscle metabolism in neuromuscular diseases. J Pediatr 2007;151(3):319–21.

12. Hsieh TJ, Jaw TS, Chuang HY, et al. Muscle metabolism in Duchenne muscular dystrophy assessed by in vivo proton magnetic resonance spectroscopy. J Comput Assist Tomogr 2009;33(1):150–4.

13. Kim HK, Laor T, Racadio JM. MR imaging assessment of the lateral head of the gastrocnemius muscle: prevalence of segmental anomalous origins in children and young adults. Pediatr Radiol 2008; 38(12):1300–5.

14. Kim HK, Laor T, Horn PS, et al. T2 mapping in Duchenne muscular dystrophy: distribution of disease activity and correlation with clinical assessments. Radiology 2010;255(3):899–908.

15. Bordalo-Rodrigues M, Rosenberg ZS. MR imaging of the proximal rectus femoris musculotendinous unit. Magn Reson Imaging Clin N Am 2005;13(4): 717–25.

16. Kim HK, Laor T, Graham TB, et al. T2 relaxation time changes in distal femoral articular cartilage in children with juvenile idiopathic arthritis: a 3-year longitudinal study. AJR Am J Roentgenol 2010;195(4):1021–5.

17. Mercuri E, Pichiecchio A, Allsop J, et al. Muscle MRI in inherited neuromuscular disorders: past, present, and future. J Magn Reson Imaging 2007; 25(2):433–40.

18. Dardzinski BJ, Laor T, Schmithorst VJ, et al. Mapping T2 relaxation time in the pediatric knee: feasibility with a clinical 1.5-T MR imaging system. Radiology 2002;225(1):233–9.

19. Patten C, Meyer RA, Fleckenstein JL. T2 mapping of muscle. Semin Musculoskelet Radiol 2003;7(4): 297–305.

20. Mugler JP III. Basic principles. In: Edelman RR, Hesselink JR, Zlatkin MB, et al, editors. Clinical magnetic resonance imaging. 3rd edition. Philadelphia: Saunders Elsevier; 2006. p. 23–57.

21. Gambarota G, Cairns BE, Berde CB, et al. Osmotic effects on the T2 relaxation decay of in vivo muscle. Magn Reson Med 2001;46(3):592–9.

22. Huang Y, Majumdar S, Genant HK, et al. Quantitative MR relaxometry study of muscle composition and function in Duchenne muscular dystrophy. J Magn Reson Imaging 1994;4(1):59–64.

23. Gold GE, Han E, Stainsby J, et al. Musculoskeletal MRI at 3.0 T: relaxation times and image contrast. AJR Am J Roentgenol 2004;183(2):343–51.

24. Jordan CD, Saranathan M, Bangerter NK, et al. Musculoskeletal MRI at 3.0T and 7.0T: a comparison of relaxation times and image contrast. Eur J Radiol 2013;82(5):734–9.

25. Stanisz GJ, Odrobina EE, Pun J, et al. T1, T2 relaxation and magnetization transfer in tissue at 3T. Magn Reson Med 2005;54(3):507–12.

26. Hazlewood CF, Chang DC, Nichols BL, et al. Nuclear magnetic resonance transverse relaxation times of water protons in skeletal muscle. Biophys J 1974;14(8):583–606.

27. Saab G, Thompson RT, Marsh GD. Multicomponent T2 relaxation of in vivo skeletal muscle. Magn Reson Med 1999;42(1):150–7.

28. Ladd PE, Emery KH, Salisbury SR, et al. Juvenile dermatomyositis: correlation of MRI at presentation with clinical outcome. AJR Am J Roentgenol 2011;197(1):W153–8.

29. Johnson K, Davis PJ, Foster JK, et al. Imaging of muscle disorders in children. Pediatr Radiol 2006;36(10):1005–18.

30. Wang LL, Kim HK, Merrow AC, et al. MR imaging of the skeletal muscles in boys with Duchenne muscular dystrophy (DMD): part 1. Can fatty infiltration and inflammation of the gluteus maximus muscle be used as indicators of clinical assessment in boys with DMD? San Francisco (CA): Society for Pediatric Radiology Meeting; 2012.

31. Johnston JH, Kim HK, Merrow AC, et al. MR imaging of the skeletal muscles in boys with Duchenne muscular dystrophy (DMD): part 2. T2 Relaxation time mapping (T2 map) as a noninvasive biomarker to determine pathologic fatty infiltration: comparison between boys with Duchenne muscular dystrophy (DMD) and healthy boys. San Francisco (CA): Society for Pediatric Radiology Meeting; 2012.

32. Fleckenstein JL, Canby RC, Parkey RW, et al. Acute effects of exercise on MR imaging of skeletal muscle in normal volunteers. AJR Am J Roentgenol 1988;151(2):231–7.

33. Barger AV, DeLone DR, Bernstein MA, et al. Fat signal suppression in head and neck imaging using fast spin-echo-IDEAL technique. AJNR Am J Neuroradiol 2006;27(6):1292–4.

34. Mito S, Ishizaka K, Nakanishi M, et al. Comparison of fat suppression techniques of bilateral breast dynamic sequence at 3.0 T: utility of three-point DIXON technique. Nihon Hoshasen Gijutsu Gakkai Zasshi 2011;67(6):654–60 [in Japanese].

35. Sijens PE, Edens MA, Bakker SJ, et al. MRI-determined fat content of human liver, pancreas and kidney. World J Gastroenterol 2010;16(16):1993–8.

36. Pykett IL, Rosen BR. Nuclear magnetic resonance: in vivo proton chemical shift imaging. Work in progress. Radiology 1983;149(1):197–201.

37. Ahmad M, Liu Y, Slavens ZW, et al. A method for automatic identification of water and fat images from a symmetrically sampled dual-echo Dixon technique. Magn Reson Imaging 2010;28(3):427–33.

38. Ma J. Dixon techniques for water and fat imaging. J Magn Reson Imaging 2008;28(3):543–58.

39. Le-Petross H, Kundra V, Szklaruk J, et al. Fast three-dimensional dual echo Dixon technique improves fat suppression in breast MRI. J Magn Reson Imaging 2010;31(4):889–94.

40. Cornfeld DM, Israel G, McCarthy SM, et al. Pelvic imaging using a T1W fat-suppressed 3-dimensional dual echo Dixon technique at 3T. J Magn Reson Imaging 2008;28(1):121–7.

41. Gold GE, Reeder SB, Yu H, et al. Articular cartilage of the knee: rapid three-dimensional MR imaging at 3.0 T with IDEAL balanced steady-state free precession–initial experience. Radiology 2006;240(2):546–51.

42. Wren TA, Bluml S, Tseng-Ong L, et al. Three-point technique of fat quantification of muscle tissue as a marker of disease progression in Duchenne muscular dystrophy: preliminary study. AJR Am J Roentgenol 2008;190(1):W8–12.

43. Kinali M, Arechavala-Gomeza V, Cirak S, et al. Muscle histology vs MRI in Duchenne muscular dystrophy. Neurology 2011;76(4):346–53.

44. Hajnal JV, Doran M, Hall AS, et al. MR imaging of anisotropically restricted diffusion of water in the nervous system: technical, anatomic, and pathologic considerations. J Comput Assist Tomogr 1991;15(1):1–18.

45. Schaefer PW, Grant PE, Gonzalez RG. Diffusion-weighted MR imaging of the brain. Radiology 2000;217(2):331–45.

46. Le Bihan D, Breton E, Lallemand D, et al. MR imaging of intravoxel incoherent motions: application to diffusion and perfusion in neurologic disorders. Radiology 1986;161(2):401–7.

47. Turner R, Le Bihan D, Maier J, et al. Echo-planar imaging of intravoxel incoherent motion. Radiology 1990;177(2):407–14.

48. Buxton RB. The diffusion sensitivity of fast steady-state free precession imaging. Magn Reson Med 1993;29(2):235–43.

49. Cui Y, Zhang XP, Sun YS, et al. Apparent diffusion coefficient: potential imaging biomarker for prediction and early detection of response to chemotherapy in hepatic metastases. Radiology 2008; 248(3):894–900.

50. Humphries PD, Sebire NJ, Siegel MJ, et al. Tumors in pediatric patients at diffusion-weighted MR imaging: apparent diffusion coefficient and tumor cellularity. Radiology 2007;245(3):848–54.

51. Stieltjes B, Kaufmann WE, van Zijl PC, et al. Diffusion tensor imaging and axonal tracking in the human brainstem. Neuroimage 2001;14(3): 723–35.

52. Hoon AH Jr, Lawrie WT Jr, Melhem ER, et al. Diffusion tensor imaging of periventricular leukomalacia shows affected sensory cortex white matter pathways. Neurology 2002;59(5):752–6.

53. Gilbert G, Simard D, Beaudoin G. Impact of an improved combination of signals from array coils in diffusion tensor imaging. IEEE Trans Med Imaging 2007;26(11):1428–36.

54. Le Bihan D, Mangin JF, Poupon C, et al. Diffusion tensor imaging: concepts and applications. J Magn Reson Imaging 2001;13(4):534–46.

55. Le Bihan D, van Zijl P. From the diffusion coefficient to the diffusion tensor. NMR Biomed 2002;15(7–8): 431–4.

56. Clark CA, Le Bihan D. Water diffusion compartmentation and anisotropy at high b values in the human brain. Magn Reson Med 2000;44(6):852–9.

57. Mori S, Crain BJ, Chacko VP, et al. Three-dimensional tracking of axonal projections in the brain by magnetic resonance imaging. Ann Neurol 1999;45(2):265–9.

58. Mori S, van Zijl PC. Fiber tracking: principles and strategies—a technical review. NMR Biomed 2002;15(7–8):468–80.

59. Basser PJ, Pajevic S, Pierpaoli C, et al. In vivo fiber tractography using DT-MRI data. Magn Reson Med 2000;44(4):625–32.

60. Noseworthy MD, Davis AD, Elzibak AH. Advanced MR imaging techniques for skeletal muscle evaluation. Semin Musculoskelet Radiol 2010;14(2): 257–68.

61. Sinha U, Yao L. In vivo diffusion tensor imaging of human calf muscle. J Magn Reson Imaging 2002; 15(1):87–95.

62. Toussaint N, Sermesant M, Stoeck CT, et al. In vivo human 3D cardiac fibre architecture: reconstruction using curvilinear interpolation of diffusion tensor images. Med Image Comput Comput Assist Interv 2010;13(Pt 1):418–25.

63. Gullberg GT, Defrise M, Panin VY, et al. Efficient cardiac diffusion tensor MRI by three-dimensional reconstruction of solenoidal tensor fields. Magn Reson Imaging 2001;19(2):233–56.

64. Zhang J, Zhang G, Morrison B, et al. Magnetic resonance imaging of mouse skeletal muscle to measure denervation atrophy. Exp Neurol 2008; 212(2):448–57.

65. Serai SD, Towbin AJ, Podberesky DJ. Pediatric liver MR elastography. Dig Dis Sci 2012;57(10): 2713–9.

66. Tse ZT, Janssen H, Hamed A, et al. Magnetic resonance elastography hardware design: a survey. Proc Inst Mech Eng H 2009;223(4):497–514.

67. Muthupillai R, Lomas DJ, Rossman PJ, et al. Magnetic resonance elastography by direct visualization of propagating acoustic strain waves. Science 1995;269(5232):1854–7.

68. Manduca A, Oliphant TE, Dresner MA, et al. Magnetic resonance elastography: non-invasive mapping of tissue elasticity. Med Image Anal 2001; 5(4):237–54.

69. Dresner MA, Rose GH, Rossman PJ, et al. Magnetic resonance elastography of skeletal muscle. J Magn Reson Imaging 2001;13(2):269–76.

70. Mason P. Dynamic stiffness and crossbridge action in muscle. Biophys Struct Mech 1977;4(1):15–25.

71. Chen Q, Basford J, An KN. Ability of magnetic resonance elastography to assess taut bands. Clin Biomech 2008;23(5):623–9.

72. Brauck K, Galban CJ, Maderwald S, et al. Changes in calf muscle elasticity in hypogonadal males before and after testosterone substitution as monitored by magnetic resonance elastography. Eur J Endocrinol 2007;156(6):673–8.

73. Debernard L, Robert L, Charleux F, et al. Analysis of thigh muscle stiffness from childhood to adulthood using magnetic resonance elastography (MRE) technique. Clin Biomech 2011;26(8): 836–40.

74. Debernard L, Robert L, Charleux F, et al. Characterization of muscle architecture in children and adults using magnetic resonance elastography and ultrasound techniques. J Biomech 2011; 44(3):397–401.

75. Domire ZJ, McCullough MB, Chen Q, et al. Wave attenuation as a measure of muscle quality as measured by magnetic resonance elastography: initial results. J Biomech 2009;42(4):537–40.

76. Papazoglou S, Hamhaber U, Braun J, et al. Horizontal shear wave scattering from a nonwelded interface observed by magnetic resonance elastography. Phys Med Biol 2007;52(3):675–84.

77. Mariappan YK, Glaser KJ, Manduca A, et al. Cyclic motion encoding for enhanced MR visualization of slip interfaces. J Magn Reson Imaging 2009; 30(4):855–63.

78. Mariappan YK, Glaser KJ, Manduca A, et al. Vibration imaging for functional analysis of flexor muscle

compartments. J Magn Reson Imaging 2009;31: 1395–401.

79. Song J, Kwon OI, Seo JK. Anisotropic elastic moduli reconstruction in transversely isotropic model using MRE. Inverse Probl 2012;28(11):115003.

80. Boesch C. Musculoskeletal spectroscopy. J Magn Reson Imaging 2007;25(2):321–38.

81. Boesch C, Machann J, Vermathen P, et al. Role of proton MR for the study of muscle lipid metabolism. NMR Biomed 2006;19(7):968–88.

82. Keeler J. Understanding NMR spectroscopy. Chichester (West Sussex): John Wiley & Sons; 2005.

83. Provencher SW. Estimation of metabolite concentrations from localized in vivo proton NMR spectra. Magn Reson Med 1993;30(6):672–9.

84. Naressi A, Couturier C, Devos JM, et al. Java-based graphical user interface for the MRUI quantitation package. MAGMA 2001;12(2–3):141–52.

85. Boesch C, Slotboom J, Hoppeler H, et al. In vivo determination of intra-myocellular lipids in human muscle by means of localized ^{1}H-MR-spectroscopy. Magn Reson Med 1997;37(4):484–93.

86. Kreis R, Koster M, Kamber M, et al. Peak assignment in localized ^{1}H MR spectra of human muscle based on oral creatine supplementation. Magn Reson Med 1997;37(2):159–63.

87. Bongers H, Schick F, Skalej M, et al. Localized in vivo ^{1}H spectroscopy of human skeletal muscle: normal and pathologic findings. Magn Reson Imaging 1992;10(6):957–64.

88. de Graaf RA. In vivo NMR spectroscopy: principles and techniques. 2nd edition. Chichester (West Sussex): John Wiley & Sons; 2007.

89. Prompers JJ, Jeneson JA, Drost MR, et al. Dynamic MRS and MRI of skeletal muscle function and biomechanics. NMR Biomed 2006; 19(7):927–53.

90. Lodi R, Muntoni F, Taylor J, et al. Correlative MR imaging and ^{31}P-MR spectroscopy study in sarcoglycan deficient limb girdle muscular dystrophy. Neuromuscul Disord 1997;7(8):505–11.

91. Vorgerd M, Schols L, Hardt C, et al. Mitochondrial impairment of human muscle in Friedreich ataxia in vivo. Neuromuscul Disord 2000;10(6):430–5.

92. Park JH, Niermann KJ, Ryder NM, et al. Muscle abnormalities in juvenile dermatomyositis patients: P-31 magnetic resonance spectroscopy studies. Arthritis Rheum 2000;43(10):2359–67.

93. Newman RJ, Bore PJ, Chan L, et al. Nuclear magnetic resonance studies of forearm muscle in Duchenne dystrophy. Br Med J (Clin Res Ed) 1982;284(6322):1072–4.

94. Younkin DP, Berman P, Sladky J, et al. 31P NMR studies in Duchenne muscular dystrophy: age-related metabolic changes. Neurology 1987; 37(1):165–9.

95. Kemp GJ, Taylor DJ, Dunn JF, et al. Cellular energetics of dystrophic muscle. J Neurol Sci 1993; 116(2):201–6.

96. Barbiroli B, Funicello R, Iotti S, et al. ^{31}P-NMR spectroscopy of skeletal muscle in Becker dystrophy and DMD/BMD carriers. Altered rate of phosphate transport. J Neurol Sci 1992;109(2):188–95.

97. Torriani M, Townsend E, Thomas BJ, et al. Lower leg muscle involvement in Duchenne muscular dystrophy: an MR imaging and spectroscopy study. Skeletal Radiol 2012;41(4):437–45.

Managing Radiation Dose from Thoracic Multidetector Computed Tomography in Pediatric Patients

Background, Current Issues, and Recommendations

Robert D. MacDougall, MSc[a], Keith J. Strauss, MSc[b],
Edward Y. Lee, MD, MPH[c,d],*

KEYWORDS

• MDCT • Pediatric imaging • Radiation dose • Thoracic CT

KEY POINTS

- Risk projections for pediatric CT based on effective dose estimates are not appropriate and should be discouraged.
- Size-specific dose estimate (SSDE) is the most appropriate metric for estimating absorbed patient dose in pediatric CT.
- Diagnostic reference ranges (DRR) that include lower and upper limits for SSDE based on patient size should be established to ensure adequate diagnostic quality at appropriate dose levels.
- DRRs can be established based on typical dose levels for adult thoracic CT.
- For the level of radiation dose delivered in pediatric thoracic CT (less than 50 mSv), the immediate clinical benefit of an appropriately ordered CT examination should outweigh the hypothetical, long-term risks from radiation.

INTRODUCTION

Computed tomography (CT) is an established and highly valuable diagnostic tool for thoracic imaging in modern radiology departments. Since its inception, CT has obviated the need for invasive testing in various thoracic disorders, making it particularly useful in pediatric patients. CT continues to evolve both in terms of technology and novel clinical applications. Major advances over the past 20 years include the introduction of multidetector CT (MDCT) from single slice to 4, 16, 64, and up to 320 slices acquired in a single gantry rotation, helical scanning techniques leading to faster scan times, and iterative reconstruction algorithms resulting in improved image quality at lower patient doses. These technical advances have led to increased speed and expanded applications, such as CT angiography (CTA) and coronary CTA. New applications, together with increased access, have resulted in a rise in the number of

[a] Department of Radiology, Boston Children's Hospital, 300 Longwood Avenue, Boston, MA 02115, USA;
[b] Department of Radiology, Cincinnati Children's Hospital Medical Center, University of Cincinnati School of Medicine, 3333 Burnet Avenue, Cincinnati, OH 45229-3026, USA; [c] Division of Thoracic Imaging, Department of Radiology, Boston Children's Hospital, Harvard Medical School, 300 Longwood Avenue, Boston, MA 02115, USA; [d] Magnetic Resonance Imaging, Boston Children's Hospital, Harvard Medical School, 300 Longwood Avenue, Boston, MA 02115, USA
* Corresponding author. Division of Thoracic Imaging, Department of Radiology, Boston Children's Hospital, Harvard Medical School, 300 Longwood Avenue, Boston, MA 02115.
E-mail address: Edward.Lee@childrens.harvard.edu

Radiol Clin N Am 51 (2013) 743–760
http://dx.doi.org/10.1016/j.rcl.2013.04.007

radiologic.theclinics.com

CT examinations performed annually: from approximately 3 million in 1980 to more than 67 million studies in 2006.[1] In children presenting in the emergency department, the use of CT has followed a similar trend, with chest CT increasing more than 435% from 2000 to 2006 in one study.[2] Given the now undisputed clinical value of CT, the continued utilization should not be surprising and any potential detriment from radiation should be considered with respect to the clinical benefit gained from CT imaging.

Although the diagnostic benefits of CT are well known, the risk versus benefit ratio remains a largely abstract concept in the minds of many practicing radiologists. Potential risks to the patient include adverse reactions to contrast material and effects of sedation and general anesthesia in addition to any risks associated with exposure to ionizing radiation. The potential risks associated with ionizing radiation have received heightened attention, suggesting a need for an up-to-date review on this topic. In this article, the authors review the underlying fundamental physics of CT, radiation dose metrics, the basics of health risks associated with ionizing radiation from CT imaging, currently available strategies for managing radiation dose for thoracic MDCT, and recommendations to optimize the diagnostic image quality and radiation dose in the pediatric population.

REVIEW OF FUNDAMENTAL PHYSICS OF CT

A review of basic scanner hardware and CT dose metrics is available elsewhere[3–5] and Nievelstein and colleagues[6] provides an excellent overview of factors affecting radiation dose and protocol guidelines for pediatric MDCT in particular. The basic choices that the operator must consider to properly acquire the scan data used by the scanner to produce images are revisited briefly in this article for convenience. Equally important is the proper choice of image-processing parameters to be used by the scanner, as these settings affect the image quality in the reconstructed clinical CT images. Because image-processing parameters tend to be proprietary to each manufacturer of CT scanners, a detailed discussion is beyond the scope of a general review article, but a brief refresher is included at the end of this section.

Starting at acquisition, CT scans produce tomographic images of anatomy from three-dimensional data sets. Modern scanners use a geometry in which the x-ray tube and detector rotate around the patient at speeds as fast as 0.28 second per rotation as the patient is moved through the CT gantry (ie, along the z-axis) during image acquisition. The number of detector elements along the z-axis (eg, 4, 16, 64, 320)

has been adopted as a classification scheme (eg, 64-slice CT scanner). The thinnest and maximum number of reconstructed images in the transverse plane per gantry rotation occurs when only one detector element in the z-direction is used to create each transverse image. However, because detector elements along the z-axis can be combined to form a thicker effective detector element, fewer and thicker reconstructed transverse images can be created per rotation. The selected number and width of the detector elements in the z-direction determine the collimated beam width: for example, 32 detector elements with a 0.6-mm width correspond to a 19.2-mm beam width in the z-axis direction, whereas 24 detector elements with a 1.2-mm width (combining two 0.6-mm detector elements) corresponds to a 28.8-mm collimated beam width. It should be noted that although some scanners are classified as 40 or 64, slice scanners, such as some Siemens models (Siemens Medical Solutions, Forchheim, Germany), the physical number of detector elements (and thus the collimated beam width) may be less due to a flying focal spot that samples each detector element twice. As beam width affects overall scan time, it is important to know the physical dimensions of the detector configuration.

Scan time is one of the major factors that affects image quality in the pediatric population. Without sedation, it is often difficult for a child to remain still over the course of the acquisition time. The operator should understand the various factors and trade-offs that affect scan time. The collimated beam width (in the z-axis), rotation time, and pitch determine the scan time of the entire study. A larger collimated beam width encompasses a larger scan length along the z-axis per rotation, resulting in a faster scan time. A faster rotation time results in an overall shorter scan time. The acquisition mode (eg, axial or helical), also affects scan time. Axial scans acquire data during a single rotation with a stationary table after which the table moves a prescribed increment and another axial section is imaged. Imaged sections can either be contiguous or separated by a gap. In helical mode, data are acquired continuously for the duration of the scan while the table is moved through the gantry at a constant speed. The distance of table motion per rotation with respect to collimated beam width is the pitch. Higher-pitch values will result in a faster scan time.

Because of faster scan time, higher-pitch acquisitions are less susceptible to patient motion. However, one argument to avoid high pitch values has been that of overscanning, because a small volume of patient tissue, at the beginning and end of the scan range that does not contribute to image information may be irradiated.[7] For a collimation of 64 × 0.6 mm, the length of overranging is approximately 2 cm at the start and end of the scan length for a pitch of 1; overranging increases with higher pitch values. However, this problem has been minimized by state-of-the-art CT scanners that are equipped with adaptive pre-patient collimators capable of blocking most of the unused radiation at the beginning and end of the scan range.[8,9] In this case, there is very little disadvantage to high-pitch scanning. In scanners without adaptive collimators, the radiologist must decide whether a small increase in patient dose is warranted based on improved image quality and lower repeat rates. In the experiences of the authors, there is often a net benefit to reducing the scan time.

The beam quality (average energy of x-rays in the beam at the CT detector) affects the contrast in the reconstructed image. The quantity (number of x-rays in the beam at the detector) affects the quantum mottle or noise properties in the reconstructed image. The tube voltage in kilovolts (kV) applied to the x-ray tube of the x-ray beam affects both quality and quantity of the x-rays emitted from the tube. Beam quality changes because a change in tube voltage affects the energy levels of the x-rays. Quantity changes because tube voltage affects the efficiency of Bremsstrahlung production of x-rays. The tube current (mA) and rotation time of the gantry (seconds) affect the quantity of x-rays emitted by the tube per rotation because both control the total electron flow in the x-ray tube during one rotation of the gantry. The generation of ionizing radiation within the x-ray tube per rotation of the gantry is determined by the selected tube voltage, tube current, and rotation time of the gantry.

The path length of the x-rays through the patient affects both the quality and quantity of the x-rays reaching the detector. For a uniform density object, larger path lengths significantly reduce the quantity due to increased attenuation while the average beam quality (energy) is slightly increased due to selective attenuation of the lower-energy x-rays by the longer path length.

If tube voltage, tube current, and rotation time remain constant, increased pitch reduces the time interval that any location of the patient's body is irradiated within the gantry, which lowers patient dose. However, increasing pitch is an indirect method of lowering patient dose and it is important to understand and separate these two parameters. As stated previously, increasing pitch decreases dose only if all parameters are left unchanged. However, a reduction in dose could equally and more directly be achieved by simply modifying the mA of the scan and leaving the pitch unchanged. Therefore, mA (or dose modulation settings) should be used to change patient dose and pitch should be used to optimize scan time. It is important to know how a particular scanner reacts to adjusting technical parameters, such as pitch. For example, some scanners automatically increase the tube current when the pitch is increased to maintain constant Effective mAs, image quality, and patient dose (eg, Siemens scanners), where

$$Effective\ mAs\ =\ mAs/pitch \qquad (1)$$

The user should exercise caution and understand whether the scanner is automatically adjusting technique factors to maintain dose or image quality when pitch is changed. In any case, tube voltage, tube current, rotation time, and pitch are independently adjustable (whether automatically by the scanner or manually by the user), and selection of pitch should be selected to control overall scan time within the tube current limits (discussed later). Modern CT scanners with higher tube limits, isotropic resolution, and adaptive collimation are also reasons to consider using high pitch for pediatrics.

Selection of tube voltage typically ranges from 80 to 140 kV, although some modern scanners have a 70-kV[10] selection for neonates and applications such as neck imaging and CTA. The selection of tube voltage affects the contrast and noise properties of the reconstructed image. This is quantified by the contrast-to-noise ratio (CNR) of objects in the image. An 80-kV beam is less penetrating, resulting in more quantum mottle in the image for the same Effective mAs. Because the amount of quantum mottle appears in the denominator of the CNR, increased quantum mottle reduces the CNR. However, x-ray energies contained in an 80-kV beam are closer to the k-edge of contrast material (iodine), resulting in a higher signal contrast. Because the contrast appears in the numerator of the CNR, increased contrast increases the CNR. The reverse relationship is true for higher energies (eg, 120 kV). Scan technique factors should be selected to optimize CNR while reducing the radiation dose and the potential for artifacts.[11] This process is discussed in the "Automatic Dose Modulation" section. While one scanner can currently automatically select tube voltage for a scan based on information derived from the projection scan (Siemens Care kV), typically the operator must select the tube voltage manually.

Additional input from the operator before the scan includes the tube current in the manual mode or an image quality index when dose modulation is enabled. As noted earlier, rotation time and pitch also must be set before the scan. When making these selections, it is important to consider the limitation imposed by scanner hardware that limits choices of tube voltage or tube current on large patients. This so-called "tube-loading limit" determines the maximum tube current, and therefore the maximum Effective mAs for a given pitch and rotation time that can be produced by the x-ray tube. For a given scan range and selected scan parameters, if the x-ray tube cannot generate enough x-rays to reach the desired Effective mAs and dose, a scan parameter must be changed to obtain an acceptable level of noise. For example, assume a patient requires an Effective mAs of 150 through the lungs for adequate image quality. For a maximum mA of 500, a rotation time of 0.33 second, and a pitch of 1.2, using Eq. 1, the maximum Effective mAs that can be generated by the scanner is 137. In this case, pitch must be reduced, rotation time must be increased, or tube voltage must be increased so as to achieve an acceptable noise level.

The bowtie filter selection affects the overall radiation dose rate delivered to the patient. **Fig. 1** illustrates how the bowtie filter received its name from its shape. The shape of this filter increases the filter thickness for the x-rays that will travel through a thinner section of the patient anatomy. The x-rays that travel through the thickest portion of patient anatomy travel through the thinnest portion of the filter. Compensating for changes in patient thickness with a uniquely shaped filter reduces artifacts in the reconstructed image. Most scanners select the

bowtie filter based on the selection of the scan field of view (SFOV) by the operator.

The choice of image-processing parameters is critical to the quality of the image displayed on a radiologist review monitor. In general, smooth reconstruction algorithms for viewing soft tissue offer a lower noise level at the expense of lower spatial resolution and edge definition. Sharp reconstruction algorithms offer enhanced detail at the cost of increased noise in the image. The largest reconstructed image thickness that allows adequate anatomic detail should be used in image reconstruction, as image noise decreases rapidly with increasing image thickness. For multiplanar and 3-dimensional reconstructions, the original "thin" data set should be used for reconstruction to avoid artifacts. Additionally, it is important to ensure appropriate default Window and Level (W/L) settings. The reader is advised to work with the vendor's application specialists of their scanner to optimize the selection of image-processing parameters as a function of the type of examination or body part imaged. Last, when evaluating image quality, it is important to use a high-resolution, calibrated viewing monitor. Often, noise and contrast will be reduced on the scanner control monitor.

UNDERSTANDING RADIATION DOSE METRICS
Radiation Dose Metrics for CT

The term "CT dose" can be split into two broad categories: (1) radiation production of the scanner and (2) radiation dose absorbed by the patient. Scanner radiation production is typically quantified in terms of volume computed tomography dose index ($CTDI_{VOL}$) and dose length product (DLP), both of which represent the dose absorbed by a standard size (16 or 32 cm) $CTDI_{VOL}$ phantom. These radiation production metrics are useful in evaluating the appropriateness of scanning protocols but have limited value in directly estimating dose to a patient. However, $CTDI_{VOL}$ is a metric of scanner output so, for a given patient, absorbed dose will be proportional to $CTDI_{VOL}$. Methods of calculating absorbed dose for various patient sizes are discussed in the "Size-Specific Dose Estimate" section. Radiologists tend to be more familiar with the quantity of effective dose (E Dose). Although E Dose is defined in this section, its important limitations are outlined in the following section concerning risk estimates.

CT Dose Index

It is instructive to review the definition of $CTDI_{VOL}$. Although this metric is routinely measured by a qualified medical physicist, the value displayed and exported from a scanner for an examination

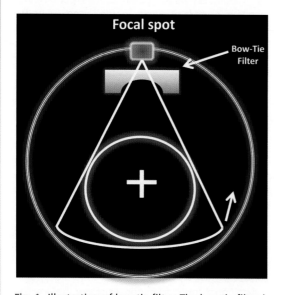

Fig. 1. Illustration of bowtie filter. The bowtie filter is designed to produce a uniform number of photons at the detector by gradually increasing the attenuation of the beam from the center to the periphery as the path length through the patient decreases.

is a calculated value based on the technical factors used during the scan.

$CTDI_{100}$ is the absorbed dose to the CTDI phantom and measured with a 100-mm ionization chamber placed at the peripheral and central holes of a 16-cm or 32-cm CTDI phantom (**Fig. 2**). For the 32-cm phantom, the dose approximately doubles as one moves radially from the center to surface of the phantom due to attenuation by the peripheral layers of the phantom. For the 16-cm diameter phantom, the central and surface doses are approximately equal.

The weighted CTDI ($CTDI_w$) is calculated from measurements of $CTDI_{100}$ at the periphery and center to estimate the single average dose across the radial cross section:

$$CTDI_W = \frac{1}{3} CTDI^{CENTER} + \frac{2}{3} CTDI^{PERIPHERY}$$
(2)

$CTDI_{VOL}$ is the average absorbed dose in the phantom and includes the effect of pitch:

$$CTDI_{VOL} = \frac{CTDI_W}{pitch}$$
(3)

Originally, the 16-cm CTDI phantom was intended to represent the approximate size of an adult head or pediatric abdomen, whereas the 32-cm CTDI phantom was intended for an adult abdomen. However, the application of these phantom sizes to various examinations is not consistent among vendors. As an example, Siemens calculates $CTDI_{vol}$ using the 32-cm phantom for all body protocols and the 16-cm for all head protocols, whereas GE (GE Healthcare Technologies, Waukesha, Wisconsin) uses the 32-cm phantom only for adult body protocols and the 16-cm phantom for pediatric body (based on the SFOV) and all head protocols. The value of $CTDI_{VOL}$ should always be displayed with the size of the CTDI phantom that was used for its calculation and this is widely available on the patient protocol page. Using identical scanning techniques, the $CTDI_{VOL}$ measured with the 16-cm phantom will be approximately twice as high compared with the $CTDI_{VOL}$ measured with the 32-cm phantom.

Dose Length Product

DLP is the product of $CTDI_{VOL}$ and scan length (in units of mGy cm). It describes the CT scanner's radiation output to the CTDI phantom along the entire scan length:

$$DLP = CTDI_{VOL} \times Scan\ Length$$
(4)

Size-Specific Dose Estimate

Both $CTDI_{VOL}$ and DLP are based on the quantity of radiation delivered to a standard cylindrical plastic phantom with a 16-cm or 32-cm diameter. Neither the shape nor density of these phantoms resembles most patients. Because a better estimate of dose delivered to the *patient* was needed, the American Association of Physicist in Medicine's (AAPM) Task Group 204[12] derived a quantity termed the size-specific dose estimate (SSDE) to estimate the average dose delivered to the patient's anatomy within the scan volume of a CT examination. Patient size is calculated in terms of an effective diameter (ie, the diameter of a circle that has the same area as the cross section of a patient). Through the use of conversion factors developed by phantom and Monte Carlo methods, values of $CTDI_{vol}$ can be converted into an SSDE. The SSDE can be calculated *after* the projection scan, but *before* the acquisition of the volume scan. This allows the operator to compare the calculated SSDE of the planned scan to established reference SSDE values within the department and alter the planned scan parameters if necessary to adjust the delivered patient dose (an example of this is discussed later in the Recommendations section).

A couple of current limitations will slow the widespread adoption of SSDE. Until the CT manufacturers calculate and display SSDE on their scanners, each site must develop or purchase a software solution to perform the calculation. TG204 (AAPM, College Park, MD) did not specify the location along the z axis where SSDE should be calculated. Although the umbilicus provides a consistent and easily identifiable landmark to measure, it may not be the optimum location. The average thickness along the z axis may be a reasonable choice for many situations; the calculated SSDE will be highest and lowest at the smallest and largest patient thickness, respectively. This suggests an average

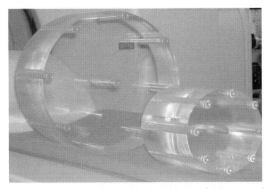

Fig. 2. CTDI phantoms with diameters of 32 cm and 16 cm. Holes at the center and peripheral locations allow insertion of a 100-mm ionization chamber to measure $CTDI_{100}$ and calculation of $CTDI_{VOL}$.

value of the patient's largest and smallest thickness along the scan volume may be appropriate. SSDE calculations contain more error for thoracic as opposed to abdominal CT, as a result of different attenuation properties introduced in the thorax by the presence of air. CT manufacturers will address this limitation; their calculation of SSDE will address both patent size and body part attenuation properties. Until this occurs, defining a "water equivalent" diameter, as opposed to an actual patient thickness, will improve accuracy of patient dose estimates. For the same patient thickness, the chest has a smaller water equivalent diameter than the abdomen.

E Dose

The concept of E Dose states that risk from a radiation dose to particular organs (eg, breast, thyroid) can be expressed in terms of an equivalent whole-body dose. A typical CT scan of the chest/abdomen/pelvis carries more risk of radiation-induced cancer than a typical CT scan of an extremity. By expressing dose as an equivalent whole-body dose that would carry the same risk, one can compare doses to different organs and from different modalities directly as a single value. The calculation of E Dose is simply the sum of absorbed organ doses (H_T) multiplied by a tissue-weighting factor (ω_T):

$$E \text{ Dose} = \sum \omega_T H_T \qquad (5)$$

With ICRP 103[13] weighting factors (eg, $\omega_T = 0.12$ for breasts and 0.01 for skin) as a reference, if the absorbed dose to specific organs is known, a weighted sum results in the E Dose. However, determining specific organs doses from a CT scan is unreasonable for a radiologist or physicist for every examination. DLP to E Dose conversion factors have been estimated to simplify this estimation.[14] If one knows the DLP from the dose protocol page, age of patient, and region of body scanned, the appropriate conversion factor can be applied to get a quick E Dose *estimate*. Considering the multiple sources of error in these estimates (eg, exposed organs, patient size), the E Dose should be expressed to one significant figure. Although the simple method of estimating E dose is enticing, one must not forget that E dose is *not* a patient dose. Rather, it describes the whole body dose to a standard phantom (not resembling a pediatric patient) and with tissue-weighting factors derived from a reference population (not a pediatric population).

BASICS OF HEALTH RISKS ASSOCIATED WITH IONIZING RADIATION FROM CT IMAGING

Over the past decade, information concerning the health effects of ionizing radiation has come largely from two sources: the International Commission on Radiation Protection Report 103 (ICRP 103)[13] and the Biologic Effects of Ionizing Radiation Report on Health Risks from Exposure to Low Levels of Ionizing Radiation (BEIR VII Phase 2).[15]

ICRP 103 delivered guidance for radiation protection based on three fundamental principles: justification, optimization, and the application of dose limits. One objective was the standardization of E Dose calculations and an update to tissue-weighting factors. This objective strives to develop a metric capable of comparing dose from various sources and modalities (eg, radionuclide examinations, projection radiography, and CT). Perhaps as a reaction to the quick adoption and inappropriate use of E Dose from previous reports, the report made great efforts to restrict its use. From Executive summary item (k):

"The collective E Dose quantity is an instrument for optimization, for comparing radiological technologies and protection procedures predominantly in the context of occupational exposure. Collective effective dose is not intended for a tool for epidemiologic risk assessment and it is inappropriate to use it in risk projections. The aggregation of very low individual doses over extended time periods is inappropriate, and in particular the calculation of the number of cancer deaths based on collective E Doses from trivial individual doses should be avoided."[13]

A significant contribution to the understanding of radiation effects on humans has come from the data collected in the Life Span Study (LSS) of atomic bomb survivors on Hiroshima and Nagasaki conducted by the Radiation Effects Research Foundation. A comprehensive analysis of the LSS data over the past decade comes from The National Research Council Committee to Assess Health Risks from Exposure to Low Levels of Ionizing Radiation (BEIR VII Phase 2).[15] The BEIR VII report describes preferred risk models and a methodology for estimating Lifetime Attributable Risk (LAR) for cancer incidence and mortality under various exposure conditions for both leukemia and solid cancers. Several risk models are presented based on LSS data and a linear, no-threshold model.

Tables 12D-1 and 12D-2 in the BEIR VII report are very often misused to create sensational data concerning the future cancer incidence and cancer mortality. Hendee and O'Connor[16] have done an excellent job in this regard of separating fact from fiction. These investigators point out that predicting increases in future cancer induction from a linear no-threshold (LNT) model is hypothetical and speculative, which creates fear and anxiety on behalf of the patient or parents that could lead to a real risk of a deferred examination. Zanzonico and Stabin[17] attempted to quantify, in lives saved, the benefit from medical imaging using ionizing radiation. Although the study did not include pediatric examinations, in every case there was a net benefit of lives saved as a result of medical imaging. These investigators emphasize that the lives saved were real lives, whereas the lives lost that were considered in the net benefit calculation were theoretical lives predicted from the LNT model. However, because children could be at increased risk of developing cancer over a lifetime, it is unclear how these data translate to the pediatric population, although it is not unreasonable to believe that the patient receives a net benefit from an appropriately ordered examination. In any case, adherence to evidence-based appropriateness criteria is a critical component to radiation reduction in the pediatric population.[18]

The most recent update and analysis of LSS data was published by Ozasa and colleagues in 2012.[19] Important findings confirm previous assumptions: a strong dependence of risk on age at exposure and an increased risk of cancer mortality throughout life. **Fig. 3** shows the excess absolute risk versus attained age for an exposure at 10, 20, 30, 40, and 50 years old. Although a linear model provided the best fit to the risk data, values for excess relative or absolute risk in the dose range below 200 mSv remain statistically insignificant, as seen in **Fig. 4**.

When discussing E Dose, one must not abuse the calculated value for the sake of convenience. To summarize, E Dose is a calculated value based on absorbed organ doses to *sex and age averaged phantoms* based on tissue-weighting factors developed from a *reference population*. ICRP 103 states, as previously noted, that it is entirely inappropriate to use these values for individual risk projections or epidemiologic studies. Also worth noting is that even with an accurate method of calculating whole-body equivalent dose to an individual, statistical studies thus far are not powerful enough to detect excess risk in the diagnostic imaging range (below 200 mSv).

A recent article concerning CT scans in *The Lancet*,[20] projecting speculative potential excess cancer risk estimates, created new concerns among patients. In this study, patients first examined with a CT scan between 1985 and 2002 and younger than 22 years of age were studied. Absorbed dose to the brain and red bone marrow were estimated based on UK surveys of common CT technique factors. These estimated doses were used to assess excess risk of radiation-induced brain cancer and leukemia. Estimates for excess absolute risk from one head CT scan include one excess case of leukemia and one excess brain tumor per 10,000 patients. Put into a different context by the investigators, CT scans resulting in a cumulative dose of 50 mGy might triple the risk of leukemia whereas 60 mGy might double the risk of brain cancer.

The AAPM issued a public position statement on radiation risks from medical imaging procedures in response to *The Lancet* article, which states in part[21]:

> *"Risks of medical imaging at effective doses below 50 mSv for single procedures or 100 mSv for multiple procedures over short time periods are too low to be detectable and may be nonexistent. Predictions of hypothetical cancer incidence and deaths in patient populations exposed to such low doses are highly speculative and should be discouraged."*

Second, because the absolute risk for developing these cancers is small to begin with in the absence of radiation, the excess absolute risk is also small. Third, absorbed dose estimates are based on techniques from a UK survey of common CT techniques; individual examination doses were not measured or considered. In addition, it is probably reasonable to assume that today's improved CT techniques have reduced the average absorbed dose to the patient.

A focused discussion of *potential, unproven* risks of ionizing radiation from CT scans creates an additional, real risk to the patient. If the patient refuses a clinically indicated CT examination because of their unwarranted fear of speculative risks of future

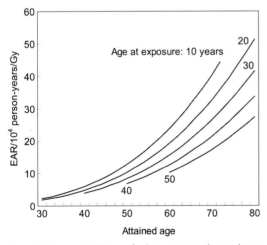

Fig. 3. Demonstration of the strong dependence of excess absolute risk on age at exposure. (*From* Ozasa K, Shimizu Y, Suyama A, et al. Studies of the mortality of atomic bomb survivors, Report 14, 1950-2003: an overview of cancer and noncancer diseases. Radiat Res 2012;177(3):229–43; with permission.)

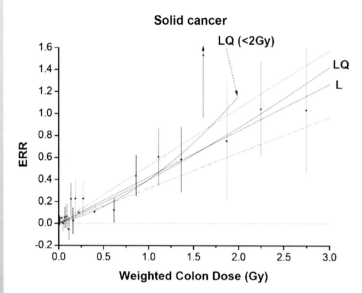

Solid cancer

Fig. 4. Graph showing the uncertainty involved in calculating risk at doses in the dose range of diagnostic CT (<200 mSv). In this figure, as with previous LSS reports, dose to all organs is represented by weight colon dose for analysis of incidence of solid cancer. The term "weighted" indicates a correction for gamma and neutron radiation. For the purpose of providing context for these doses, weighted colon dose (in Gy) can be thought of as effective dose. (*From* Ozasa K, Shimizu Y, Suyama A, et al. Studies of the mortality of atomic bomb survivors, Report 14, 1950-2003: an overview of cancer and noncancer diseases. Radiat Res 2012;177(3):229–43; with permission.)

cancer induction from the radiation dose, the patient may suffer serious harm from the lack of emergent medical treatment. Caregivers must provide the patient with a proper understanding of the potential *large* benefit and *small* risk that results from the medical diagnostic examination.

Despite the current debate and large uncertainties associated with predicting radiation risks from pediatric thoracic CT, it is prudent for all medical professionals to take the necessary steps to ensure that no more radiation dose than that level necessary is used to answer the medical question. This need may be more acute for children because their potential risk is believed to be elevated when exposure occurs at a young age (see **Fig. 3**). The Image Gently Campaign has been successful in raising awareness of the need for special care in pediatric radiology; many useful materials are available for download at their Web site (imagegently.org).

CURRENTLY AVAILABLE STRATEGIES FOR REDUCING RADIATION DOSE FOR THORACIC MDCT

Brenner and Hall[22] in 2001 discussed the relationship between radiation dose from pediatric CT and potential increased cancer risk. The investigators argued that the product of tube current and rotation time, mAs, should be reduced for pediatric CT examinations. Indeed, the mA product must be reduced to 40% (tube voltage unchanged) of its value for an adult patient to deliver a similar radiation dose to an average newborn patient undergoing an abdominal CT scan.[23] Pediatric techniques should be reduced to deliver smaller radiation doses to small children compared with

adult doses. In addition to adjusting the "baseline" dose to pediatrics (discussed in the Recommendations section) the following sections will focus on 4 currently available radiation dose reduction techniques to all patients, including pediatrics: reduced tube potential, automatic dose modulation, organ shields, and iterative reconstruction. Then, the progress made in developing pediatric-specific techniques is outlined.

Lowering Tube Potential

Using a lower tube voltage (eg, 80 kV, 100 kV) enhances the subject contrast of the patient and, if noise is unchanged (increase in mAs), increases the CNR. Yu and colleagues[11] explain the benefits and trade-offs very clearly. A balanced alternative may be the most appropriate. For large structures, such as vessels containing a contrast agent, more noise can be tolerated when it is accompanied by increased contrast. However, for small structures, such as lesions, there reaches a noise level beyond which increased contrast will not enhance conspicuity if the lesion cannot be distinguished from its background due to elevated noise. As tube voltage is decreased, the mAs must be increased to constrain the increase in noise. In practice, the noise level for pediatric examinations should not exceed that of adult examinations, as less noise is required to visualize the small structures and anatomy in pediatric patients.

Automatic Dose Modulation

Strategies for automatically modulating the radiation production of a CT scanner for various patient sizes and attenuation within a given patient are used frequently as a dose reduction tool. The concept based on patient attenuation is referred to as automatic exposure control (AEC), tube current modulation, or dose modulation, along with vendor specific terminology (eg, CareDose 4D, Siemens; Auto/Smart mA, GE; DoseRight, Philips [Philips Medical Systems, Best, The Netherlands]; sureExposure, Toshiba [Toshiba Medical Systems, Tokyo, Japan]). There are three main components; algorithms may use any combination of the three: (1) adaptation to patient size/attenuation, (2) z-axis modulation, and (3) angular modulation. The dose modulation algorithm is managed with a user-defined image quality metric (eg, Quality Reference mAs, Noise Index, Reference Image). Based on the projection scan (eg, Scout, Topogram, Scanogram, or Scanview) the software estimates patient size and attenuation. From this, the algorithm determines the baseline dose level required to meet the desired image quality over the entire scan length. The radiation production required in the lungs comprised mostly of air will be significantly less than that required by the pelvis, with more attenuating bone and soft tissue. The system also typically modulates radiation production over the course of a single rotation, as the x-ray path length through the patient changes with the rotation of the x-ray beam about the patient's elliptical shape. Comparisons of dose modulation algorithms have been discussed in the literature.[24] Tutorials on dose reduction features for different scanner models are available on the Image Gently Web site (www.imagegently.org).

The myriad versions of AEC algorithms across vendors and software platforms make the production of clinical protocols in this article difficult and vulnerable to misuse. A brief and noncomprehensive discussion of the subtleties and variations of these algorithms will illustrate this point. Two vendor algorithms are used in this example.

Siemens CareDose 4D requires input of a Quality Reference mAs from the user. Based on the calculated attenuation of the patient from the localizer, the Siemens algorithm attempts to optimize the tube current from a CareDose "curve" for all other sizes. Older versions of Siemens CareDose 4D used two "reference patients." For child protocols, the input Quality Reference mAs was defined for a 20-kg pediatric reference patient. For adult protocols, the Quality Reference mAs was defined for a 70-kg to 80-kg adult reference patient. Two separate CareDose "curves" exist. The most recent version of CareDose 4D uses a single adult reference patient. Although the shape and position of the CareDose curve can be altered, it may be difficult to optimize image quality and dose for all pediatric patients within a single pediatric protocol. It may be necessary to create subgroups based on weight or size to optimize dose across the range of sizes in the pediatric population. Yu and colleagues[11] published empirically developed pediatric technique charts using the older version of Siemens CareDose 4D on a Siemens Sensation 64 and the table is reproduced in **Table 1**.

The Noise Index (NI) parameter in GE's Smart mA and Auto mA algorithm is fundamentally different from the Siemens approach. NI defines the noise tolerance for a particular examination type. Unfortunately, the appropriate NI is a function of both the examination type and patient size, requiring

Table 1
Empirically developed weight-based technique chart for routine pediatric chest CT examinations on a Siemens sensation 64 (older version of CareDose 4D)

Weight, kg	Tube Potential, kV	QRM[a]	AEC[b]	Pitch	Rotation Time, s	Kernel	Section/ Interval Thickness, mm	Collimation, mm	CTDI$_{vol}$, mGy[c]
<10	80	150	On	1.2	0.33	B40f	3/3	64 × 0.6	2.1 ± 0.2
10–20	100	70	On	1.4	0.33	B40f	3/3	64 × 0.6	3.5 ± 0.3
20–45	120	40	On	1.4	0.33	B40f	3/3	64 × 0.6	5.2 ± 1.2

Abbreviation: AEC, automatic exposure control.
[a] QRM, Quality reference mAs, a name termed on a Siemens scanner.
[b] We used CareDose 4D (Siemens).
[c] CTDI$_{VOL}$ values are based on a 32-cm CTDI phantom and are presented as mean ± SD.
Data from Yu L, Bruesewitz MR, Thomas KB, et al. Optimal tube potential for radiation dose reduction in pediatric CT: principles, clinical implementations, and pitfalls. Radiographics 2011;31(3):835–48; and Articular requirements for the safety of x-ray equipment for computed tomography. Geneva (Switzerland): International Electrotechnical Commission; 2002. Report No.: 60601-2-44 Ed. 2.1.

the operator to select a different NI for each patient size for a given type of examination. Frush[25] presented AEC guidelines for pediatric CT based on a GE MDCT, and this table is reproduced in **Table 2**. Therefore, image noise can be customized for each patient size at the expense of a larger protocol database and with it the potential for operator error in choosing an incorrect protocol.

Organ Shields

Over the past decade, some have advocated[26] breast, thyroid, or gonadal shields, whereas the AAPM[27] recommends a simple reduction of the product of tube current and rotation time, mAs, to reduce dose to surface radiosensitive organs. For all scanners, if used, shields must be placed on the patient only after the projection scan is acquired. Fricke and colleagues[26] reported a 29% reduction in radiation dose to the breast in infants without any perceptible change in image quality after implementation of bismuth breast shields for thoracic scans. Breast shields are easy, relatively inexpensive, and can reduce patient anxiety. It should be noted that it is very difficult to reverse this practice once it is implemented, as repeat patients will expect similar treatment. Although breast dose reduction with shields is acknowledged,[27] others propose[28] a similar dose reduction to the breast without shields by reducing mAs over the entire scan length. First, breast shields waste diagnostic information by blocking radiation that has penetrated the patient in the posteroanterior (PA) dimension from reaching the detector. Second, breast shields cause increased quantum mottle over the entire field of view in phantom studies.[28] Third, the shields may create artifacts and changes to CT numbers.[28] Finally, and most importantly, breast shields may interfere with the proper function of AEC algorithms for certain scanner models even if placed on the patient after the completion of the projection scan. For all these reasons, the AAPM recommends technique reduction as opposed to shields to reduce radiation dose to surface organs.[27]

Some state-of-the-art scanners reduce dose to surface organs (eg, eyes, breast, thyroid, gonads) by reducing the tube current as the tube passes over the surface and increasing it during posterior projections. Unfortunately, the benefits of this organ-based modulation technique are reduced in pediatric patients, as the x-rays in the posterior projections are less attenuated, resulting in smaller reductions in breast dose and possibly higher dose to the lungs, which is equally undesirable.[28]

Iterative Reconstruction

Traditionally, CT images have been reconstructed using a Filtered Back Projection (FBP) algorithm.

Table 2
Automatic exposure control guidelines for pediatric chest and abdomen scans based on a GE multidetector computed tomography scanner

| Zone | Weight, kg | Length, cm | Age | Noise Index | |
				Chest	Abdomen Pelvis
Pink	5.5–7.4	60–67	2.5–5.5 mo	9.5	6.5
Red	7.5–9.4	67–75	5.5–11.5 mo	10.0	7.5
Purple	9.5–11.4	75–85	11.5–22 mo	10.5	8.5
Yellow	11.5–14.4	85–97	22 mo–3 y, 2 mo	11	9.5
White	14.5–18.4	97–109	3 y, 2 mo–5 y, 2 mo	12	10.5
Blue	18.5–23.4	109–121	5 y, 2 mo–7 y, 4 mo	13	11.5
Orange	23.5–29.4	121–133	7 y, 4 mo–9 y, 2 mo	14	12.5
Green	29.5–36.4	133–147	9 y, 2 mo–13 y, 6 mo	15	13.5
Black	36.5–55	>147	>13 y, 6 mo	16	14

Noise index (NI) must be defined for a specific image thickness. A scan performed with an NI for a small image thickness will deliver more dose than the same NI defined for a larger image thickness. Users should use caution when building protocols from published sources to ensure the NI is appropriate for the desired image thickness. On a GE scanner, the simplest way to build a protocol from a published source is to input the NI at the published image thickness and then adjust the image thickness to the desired thickness of the user. In this way, NI will adjust to compensate for the change in image thickness.

   Max (ceiling) should be set to mA in tables depending on region and scanner so that routine mA *is not exceeded*.

   Data from Frush DP. MDCT in children: scan techniques and contrast issues. In: Kalra MK, Saini S, Rubin GD, editors. MDCT [Internet]. Milano (Italy): Springer Milan; 2008. p. 333–54. Available at: http://rd.springer.com/chapter/10.1007/978-88-470-0832-8_26. Accessed January 11, 2013.

The assumptions of the acquisition process inherent in this algorithm produce an imperfect estimation of the scanned volume (ie, CT image) based on the raw acquisition data. Iterative reconstruction algorithms attempt to improve the quality of FBP images through multiple reconstructions aimed at minimizing the error between the forward projection data and a noise model. The first reconstruction is typically based off the FBP image to generate the forward-projection data with subsequent iterations attempting to minimize the error between the forward-projection data and an error matrix. The noise texture in the resulting image can sometimes be adjusted by changing a "strength" parameter that changes the noise model to deliver a more or less "smooth" image based on radiologist preference. **Fig. 5** shows three chest CTs of the same patient with three different radiation doses. Despite the different levels of quantum mottle, diagnostic quality is acceptable in all three images. The example in **Fig. 5** shows the potential reduction of quantum mottle afforded by iterative reconstruction (IR).

Optimization of IR should take place after basic acquisition protocols based on patient size have been established. Doses can be lowered incrementally if the noise content of the IR images is below an acceptable noise "ceiling."

Performance of these iterative algorithms is dependent on the dose level used to form the image and the accuracy of the noise model. Radiologists often notice the different noise texture of IR compared with FBP images, sometimes describing IR images as "plastic" or "foggy" in appearance. Because pediatric dose levels may be lower and the noise model may differ from an adult population, the use of IR algorithms may be more restricted in pediatrics. If used aggressively, they could adversely affect image quality. Careful selection of the reconstruction kernel and iterative reconstruction settings is required. A lower "strength" of IR is not uncommon for children.

Progress Made in Developing Pediatric-Specific Radiation Dose Reduction Techniques

Efforts to manage radiation dose by optimizing acquisition protocols for pediatric patients have been ongoing for quite some time and continue to progress. This section aids to provide a historical context for the recommendations made in the next section. A survey conducted in 2006 showed that technical parameters affecting radiation dose decreased significantly from a previous survey conducted in 2001.[29] During this time, both tube voltage and mAs were effectively reduced to deliver increased image contrast and reduced dose respectively. Weight as opposed to age was adopted to identify pediatric patient size. Developing pediatric techniques has been a slow progression and continues to be an empirically based endeavor. Several notable attempts to develop pediatric CT protocols are listed in the following paragraphs in chronologic order.

Cody and colleagues,[30] in 2003, developed pediatric techniques by selecting protocols that created the same level of quantum mottle in pediatric images as those levels found in adult images. In the same year, Boone and colleagues[31] improved on this approach by matching the CNR in pediatric images to the CNR in acceptable adult images. Although both were novel approaches to quantifying pediatric CT protocols, neither study identified that a greater CNR and lower level of quantum mottle are required in pediatric CT images of the smallest patients in part because of the smaller anatomic structures of the pediatric patients.

Vock and colleagues,[8] in 2007, published a collection of CT protocols taken from various sources reflecting the most current published

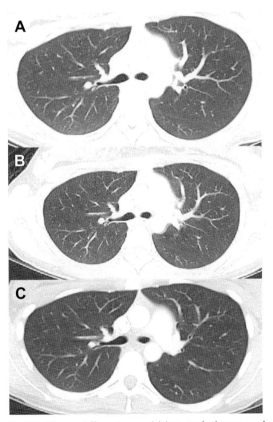

Fig. 5. Three different acquisition techniques and image processing settings for helical routine chest CT. (A) Filtered back projection, kVp = 100, CTDI (32 cm) = 8.16 mGy. (B) Filtered back projection, kVp = 100, CTDI (32 cm) = 4 mGy. (C) Iterative reconstruction (SAFIRE 2), kVp = 100, CTDI (32 cm) = 3.46.

guidelines. Because today's state-of-the-art scanners have more advanced designs than scanners before 2007, these reported techniques would need to be updated to adapt to current technologies but are still a valuable reference of published protocols.

Siegel and Babyn,[32] in 2008, published mA setting for pediatric chest CT based on weight in 5-kg intervals ranging from less than 10 kg to 45 kg. These investigators recommended tube voltage selections of 80 kV for patients weighing less than 45 kg. Although using mass is preferable to using the patient's age, the measured path length through the pediatric patient's imaged anatomy recently was proposed as the most accurate method to characterize patient size.[33]

Frush,[25] in 2008, published scan techniques for pediatric MDCT for three common scanner models that serve as an excellent reference point for sites hoping to develop size-specific protocols. Technical factors are based on color-coded zones corresponding to weight ranges. These factors specify both fixed mA and AEC techniques for GE scanners and fixed techniques for a Siemens scanner. *The reader is cautioned that detailed scan techniques cannot be transferred from one scanner model to another model by the same manufacturer because of the unique design characteristics in each CT scanner.*

Lee and colleagues,[34] in 2010, published a study that evaluated the effects of radiation dose reduction on the assessment of the trachea lumen on expiratory MDCT images of pediatric patients referred for evaluation of tracheomalacia. Their study showed that the radiation dose of paired inspiratory-expiratory MDCT imaging can be reduced by 23% while maintaining similar diagnostic confidence for assessment of the tracheal lumen compared with a standard-dose technique in pediatric patients. Therefore, they recommended a reduced-dose technique for evaluating tracheomalacia in the pediatric population.

Nievelstein and colleagues,[6] in 2010, published guideline pediatric CT protocols for common examinations, including CT of the chest, for scanners from 4 major vendors of both 16-slice and 64-slice capabilities. A notable difference from the protocols published by Frush is a shift to lower tube voltage settings (80–100 kV for patients up to 64 kg as opposed to 120 kV for all patients).

Efforts to establish diagnostic reference level (DRLs) for CT are ongoing. These DRLs are typically based on a percentile (ie, 75%) value of doses from collected survey data, which is affected by various generations of technology and varying national standards of practice. The most notable published data include surveys and DRLs from the United Kingdom, Germany, and Switzerland.[35] The data from all three surveys were summarized in the most recent Swiss survey and are reproduced in **Table 3**. A large range of DRLs exist between countries and most likely between hospitals as well. Because DRLs are based on survey data, they provide a snapshot of "state-of-practice" as opposed to "state-of-art" criteria.

To address the lack of up-to-date pediatric DRLs in the literature, the Quality Improvement Registry for CT Scans in Children (QuIRCC) group was formed in the United States to develop Diagnostic Reference Ranges (DRRs) for pediatric CT scans. The QuIRCC group is a coalition of 6 children's hospitals aimed at developing DRRs based

Table 3
DRLs of three countries: Switzerland (denoted by "this work"), Germany (D), and United Kingdom

Age Group	Quantity	Brain			Chest			Abdomen		
		This Work	D	UK	This Work	D	UK	This Work	D	UK
<1 y	CTDI$_{vol}$	20	33	30	5	3.5	12	7	5	20[a]
	DLP	270	390	270	110	55	200	130	145	170[a]
1–5 y	CTDI$_{vol}$	30	40	45	8	5.5	13	9	8	20[a]
	DLP	420	520	470	200	110	230	300	255	250[a]
5–10 y	CTDI$_{vol}$	40	50	50	10	8.5	20	13	13	30[a]
	DLP	560	710	620	220	210	370	380	475	500[a]
10–15 y	CTDI$_{vol}$	60	60	65	12	6.8	14	16	10	14
	DLP	1000	920	930	460	205	580	500	500	560

Abbreviations: DLP, dose length product; DRL, diagnostic reference level; CTDI$_{vol}$, volume computed tomography dose index.
[a] Values recommended from Reference.[39]
Data from Verdun FR, Gutierrez D, Vader JP, et al. CT radiation dose in children: a survey to establish age-based diagnostic reference levels in Switzerland. Eur Radiol 2008;18(9):1980–6; and Shrimpton PC, Wall BF. Reference doses for pediatric computed tomography. Radiat Prot Dosimetry 2000;90(1–2):249–52.

on SSDE. The DRR is based on a lower limit, below which scans may not be diagnostic, and 75th percentile upper limit, above which dose may be excessive. To date, data for contrast-enhanced abdominal/pelvic scans have been analyzed.[36] The coalition hopes to analyze data for the thorax in the near future.

Many of the recommendations are self-explanatory. A well-trained medical physicist available to help the lead radiologist and technologist communicate with the application specialists and other resource individuals from the vendor is critical to help a department leverage the design capabilities of their scanners to the specific clinical needs of their practice. In step 4, substituting a nonionizing radiation examination (ultrasound or magnetic resonance imaging) for the CT scan is the most effective method of reducing ionizing radiation dose to the patient. When step 5 prevents nonindicated CT scans from being performed, the ionizing radiation dose to the patient is eliminated. Step 9 prevents the patient's radiation dose from needlessly being doubled and limits the patient's tissues that are directly irradiated. Step 10 provides a better experience for the pediatric patient and has the potential for reducing patient dose during some examinations. The discussion that follows amplifies the information in steps 6 to 8 and includes information not addressed in the previous publication (eg, iterative reconstruction).

The appropriate use of AEC ensures that radiation dose is adapted to patient size and is delivered based on the attenuation properties of each region of the patient (ie, more radiation in areas of high attenuation and less radiation in areas of low attenuation). AEC control of radiation production provides significant dose savings. For example, the superior regions of the lung can extend to the highly attenuating shoulder. Distal soft tissue tends to be greater beneath the shoulders and tapering off at the inferior edge of the lung. Attenuation at the lung apices is increased due to soft tissue structures at the same axial position (eg, liver). An example of a routine chest scanned in AEC mode (Siemens CareDose 4D) is shown in **Fig. 6**. A fixed technique would have resulted in one of two outcomes: compromised image quality at the level of the shoulders or unnecessary dose throughout the lung region.

Regardless whether AEC is turned on, the goal of the imaging team should be to produce consistent, diagnostic image quality at a reasonable dose to

Recommendations

In 2010, the Image Gently Steering Committee published "Ten Steps You Can Take to Optimize Image Quality and Lower CT Dose for Pediatric Patients."[37] These steps are outlined here.

1. Increase awareness and understanding of CT radiation dose issues among radiologic technologists.
2. Enlist the services of a qualified medical physicist.
3. Obtain accreditation from the American College of Radiology (ACR) for your CT program.
4. When appropriate, use alternative imaging modalities that do not use ionizing radiation.
5. Determine if ordered CT is justified by the clinical indication.
6. Establish baseline radiation dose for adult-sized patients.
7. Establish radiation doses for pediatric patients by "child-sizing" CT scanning parameters.
8. Optimize pediatric examination parameters
   a. Center patient in the gantry
   b. Reduce dose during projection scans
   c. Advantages of axial versus helical modes
   d. Reduce detector size in z direction during acquisition
   e. Adjust product of tube current and exposure time
   f. When to adjust tube voltage
   g. Increase pitch
   h. Manual versus automatic exposure control
9. Scan only the indicated area: scan once
10. Prepare a child-friendly and expeditious CT environment

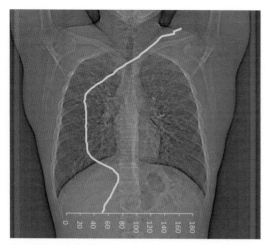

Fig. 6. Dose modulation for pediatric chest CT. The tube current is highest at the shoulder and lung apices and decreases throughout the lungs, composed mainly of air.

the patient (steps 6–7 of the previous publication). To this end, DRRs should be established based on the image quality expectations of the radiologist(s). It may be simpler to work with an experienced radiologist "champion" dedicated to managing patient dose rather than building a consensus among a large group. DRRs can be used to prospectively modify scanning parameters before a patient is scanned and/or retrospectively when performing audits to ensure compliance with dose levels and to investigate outliers. **Fig. 7**

shows data from routine chest CTs performed at a large pediatric hospital. Generating reports such as the table shown in **Fig. 7** allows examinations falling outside established DRRs to be visually identified. These examinations should be investigated.

The following optimization process is recommended. It consists of some steps that should be completed before, during, and after patient scanning has been completed.

Steps Before Scanning:

1. Create a development team consisting of a technologist, radiologist, and medical physicist to direct the quality management aspects of patient care with respect to CT scanning. If the department does not have a working relationship with an experienced, qualified medical physicist, this deficiency should be corrected.

2. The development team should create a working relationship with the application specialists of the scanner(s) within the department. The design capabilities of the department's scanners must be understood. As one practical example, create an understanding of the x-ray tube-loading limits. Calculate the maximum Effective mAs that can be achieved with current settings: for a tube limit of 500 mA and pitch of 1.5, rotation time of 0.5 second, the maximum Effective mAs is 167. Is this sufficient for the prescribed tube voltages that will be used clinically? As a second practical example, "At what point will increased pitch have an effect on

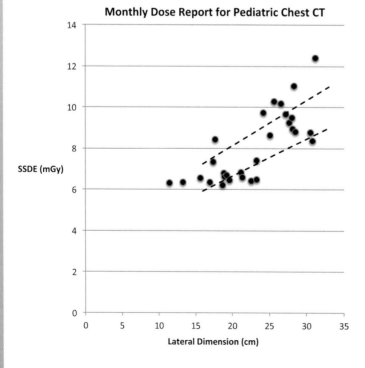

Fig. 7. Example of a dose report based on SSDE and patient diameter. The desired SSDE range generated using **Table 4** is marked by the dashed lines. Such a report should be generated on a routine basis (eg, monthly) to monitor appropriateness of techniques and investigate studies that fall outside the desired dose range.

z-axis resolution?" "When will shorter rotation times result in fewer projections and decreased image quality?" "Are there adaptive shields for helical over-scanning?"

3. Establish baseline estimates of the patient's radiation dose for commonly performed clinical scans for *adult-sized* patients. This is completed by the calculation of SSDE by that Qualified Medical Physicist (QMP) from the annual dosimetry results performed by the QMP on the department's scanner(s). These calculations provide the adult SSDE found in the eighth row of data of **Table 4** sixth column.

4. Establish patient radiation dose estimates, SSDE, guidelines within the department for pediatric patients of various sizes. The data in **Table 4** recommend 7 pediatric SSDE values (guidelines) for patients (sixth column) that range from newborns to adults. In each row of the table, a range of PA and Lateral thicknesses, of weight, and of age are provided. **Table 4** recommends that the estimated patient dose for the newborn is 65% of the estimated patient dose of the adult patient. These recommended patient doses will result in increased CNR as the patients diminish in size. Experienced pediatric radiologists may be comfortable with smaller pediatric patient dose estimates relative to the adult-sized patient than those recommended in the table. Radiologists with less experience interpreting pediatric images may require higher estimated pediatric patient doses (eg, SSDE values for the smallest patients that are equal to the SSDE for adult patients). The development team in consultation with the department's radiologists should select appropriate ratios of pediatric to adult patient doses. To aid in implementation and consistency of scanning within a DRR, it is possible to construct a "technique chart" with acceptable values of $CTDI_{VOL}$ for a range of patient sizes. Because SSDE and $CTDI_{VOL}$ can be calculated from each other if the patient size is known, it is possible to develop a technique chart, developed from SSDE DRRs, but based on $CTDI_{VOL}$. The technologists is able to view the prescribed $CTDI_{VOL}$ after the localizer image and can correct the technique (for example, changing the Quality Reference mAs or NI) if the prescribed $CTDI_{VOL}$ falls outside the acceptable range. An example of such a technique chart is shown in **Table 5**. This method of modifying protocols "on the fly" to ensure appropriate patient doses is useful once a new piece of equipment is installed and the AEC settings have not been optimized. Once the protocols are optimized, it may be possible to discontinue use of the technique chart.

Steps During Each Scan:

5. Use 80 kV for the smallest patients and 100 kV for medium-size patients. Use **Table 4** as a guideline.

6. Select pitch and rotation time with respect to the trade-off between scan time and potential detriment to image quality and radiation dose. Typically, the reduction in repeat rate from faster scanning outweighs any benefits achieved by slower scans and hence a higher pitch, short rotation time may be preferred.

7. Choose a reconstructed slice thickness that balances an acceptable level of axial resolution, (eg, thinner thickness), with reasonable level of quantum mottle (eg, larger image thickness) to minimize image noise at an acceptable radiation dose. Ensure the acquisition collimation will provide adequate thickness of reconstructed images. On modern scanners, the "scan thin, view thick" approach is the preferred method.

Table 4
Recommended reference patient doses

LAT Dim, cm	AP Dim, cm	Weight, kg	Age, y	kV	SSDE
15–17	10–12	3.5–10	NB–1	80	0.65 × Adult
17–19	12–14	10–14	1–3	80	0.70 × Adult
19–22	14–15	14–20	3–6	80	0.75 × Adult
22–25	15–17	20–30	6–9	100	0.8 × Adult
25–27	17–19	30–40	9–12	100	0.85 × Adult
27–29	19–20	40–50	12–14	100	0.9 × Adult
29–32	20–22	50–60	14–17	100	0.95 × Adult
32–35	22–24	60–70	17–20	120	Adult

Correlation of age to AP and LAT dimensions and weight can be found in References.[33,40]
Abbreviations: AP, anteroposterior; Dim, dimension; LAT, lateral; SSDE, size-specific dose estimate.

Table 5
Example of technologist technique chart based on SSDE diagnostic reference ranges developed within a hospital

LAT Dim, cm	SSDE Range	CTDI, 32 cm	CTDI, 16 cm
15–17	3.9–5.2	1.7–2.3	3.5–4.6
17–19	4.2–5.6	1.9–2.6	3.9–5.2
19–22	4.5–6.0	2.2–2.9	4.4–5.9
22–25	4.8–6.4	2.5–3.3	5.1–6.8
25–27	5.1–6.8	2.9–3.9	6.0–8.0
27–29	5.4–7.2	3.3–4.4	6.8–9.0
29–32	5.7–7.6	3.7–4.9	7.6–10.1
32–35	6.0–8.0	4.3–5.7	9.0–11.9

By prospectively changing scan parameters after the localizer image, patients can be scanned consistently at appropriate dose levels.

Abbreviations: CTDI, Computed Tomography Dose Index; Dim, Dimension; LAT, Lateral; SSDE, Size Specific Dose Estimate.

8. Set AEC parameters required to achieve scans with an acceptable level of image noise and at an acceptable patient radiation dose, using the reference SSDE values in **Table 5**. Using data provided in TG204, the selected tube voltage in step 5, selected pitch and rotation time of step 6, the QMP in consultation with the application specialists and design engineers from the CT scanner manufacturer should be able to configure the AEC settings to "child-size" the tube current to deliver the estimated patient dose recommended in **Table 4**.

9. Consider a "fixed" manual technique for the smallest patients if the AEC cannot be configured to provide the recommended SSDE in **Table 4**.

10. After the establishment of basic protocols, apply iterative reconstruction algorithms if available following the guidelines of the manufacturer's application specialists. Start at a lower "strength" and experiment with varying levels. The effectiveness of some iterative reconstruction algorithms is intimately tied to radiation dose. Too aggressive application of iterative techniques can result in "plastic" or "waxlike" appearance in reconstructed images.

Steps Post Scanning:

11. The QMP should periodically read the dose reports created and sent to PACS with all modern CT scanners. Note the CTDI phantom used along with kV and effective mAs to compare against other examinations and DRLs. The QMP should report any unusual results to the development team to allow any required corrective action. An audit process to detect and investigate examinations that fall outside the established reference SSDEs should be established. This could consist of technologists retrospectively reviewing dose reports if dose-tracking software is not available in the department.

12. The development team should adopt, implement, and maintain a comprehensive quality control program to monitor and manage the ongoing quality of the CT program. The American College of Radiology has published[38] a reasonable program that must be adopted to maintain the ACR's accreditation. This program contains daily, weekly, and monthly quality control tests to be performed by technologists. Annual quality control tests must be performed by the QMP. The development team must annually audit the department's protocols for appropriateness.

SUMMARY

Four sections in this review article provide an overview of the basic technical understanding of CT imaging that a practicing radiologist should understand to optimize pediatric thoracic CT with respect to radiation dose. Fundamental physics and dose metrics associated with MDCT are reviewed. By no means comprehensive, an understanding of the concepts outlined in the sections "Review of Fundamental Physics of CT" and "Understanding Radiation Dose Metrics" will provide the knowledge required to understand and interpret radiation dose in the literature and dose reports, as well as dose delivered to the patient as a result of changing technique parameters on the scanner. The section "Basics of Health Risks Associated with Ionizing Radiation" discusses the small potential, projected risks of CT scans, which are typically outweighed by the large benefit of receiving a timely diagnosis and delivery of needed treatment. The section "Currently Available Strategies for Reducing Radiation Dose for Thoracic MDCT" summarizes recent research in technique optimization for pediatric thoracic CT. Building on these results, section 5 presents practical recommendations to optimize technique factors and establish reasonable dose levels for common thoracic examinations.

REFERENCES

1. National Council on Radiation Protection and Measurements. Ionizing radiation exposure of the

population of the United States. Bethesda (MD): National Council on Radiation Protection; 2009. Report No.: NCRP report no. 160.

2. Broder J, Fordham LA, Warshauer DM. Increasing utilization of computed tomography in the pediatric emergency department, 2000–2006. Emerg Radiol 2007;14(4):227–32.

3. The Measurement, Reporting, and Management of Radiation Dose in CT [Internet]. College Park (MD): American Association of Physicists in Medicine; 2008. Report No.: 96. Available at: http://www.aapm.org/pubs/reports/RPT_96.pdf. Accessed January 11, 2013.

4. McNitt-Gray MF. AAPM/RSNA physics tutorial for residents: topics in CT radiation dose in CT. Radiographics 2002;22(6):1541–53.

5. Cody DD, Mahesh M. Technologic advances in multidetector CT with a focus on cardiac imaging. Radiographics 2007;27(6):1829–37.

6. Nievelstein RA, Van Dam IM, Van der Molen AJ. Multidetector CT in children: current concepts and dose reduction strategies. Pediatr Radiol 2010;40(8):1324–44.

7. van der Molen AJ, Geleijns J. Overranging in multisection CT: quantification and relative contribution to dose—comparison of four 16-section CT scanners. Radiology 2007;242(1):208–16.

8. Vock P, Stranzinger E, Wolf R. Dose optimization and reduction in CT of children. In: Tack D, Kalra MK, Gevenois PA, editors. Medical Radiology. Heidelberg: Springer; 2012. p. 419–36.

9. Christner JA, Zavaletta VA, Eusemann CD, et al. Dose reduction in helical CT: dynamically adjustable z-axis x-ray beam collimation. AJR Am J Roentgenol 2010;194(1):W49–55.

10. Gnannt R, Winklehner A, Goetti R, et al. Low kilovoltage CT of the neck with 70 kVp: comparison with a standard protocol. AJNR Am J Neuroradiol 2012; 33(6):1014–9.

11. Yu L, Bruesewitz MR, Thomas KB, et al. Optimal tube potential for radiation dose reduction in pediatric CT: principles, clinical implementations, and pitfalls. Radiographics 2011;31(3):835–48.

12. Size-specific dose estimates (SSDE) in pediatric and adult body CT examinations [Internet]. College Park (MD): American Association of Physicists in Medicine; 2011. Report No.: 204. Available at: http://www.aapm.org/pubs/reports/RPT_204.pdf. Accessed January 11, 2013.

13. The 2007 recommendations of the International Commission on Radiological Protection. ICRP publication 103. Ann ICRP 2007;37(2–4):1–332.

14. Deak PD, Smal Y, Kalender WA. Multisection CT protocols: sex- and age-specific conversion factors used to determine effective dose from dose-length product. Radiology 2010;257(1):158–66.

15. Committee to Assess Health Risks from Exposure to Low Levels of Ionizing Radiation, National Research Council. Health risks from exposure to low levels of ionizing radiation: BEIR VII Phase 2. Washington, DC: The National Academies Press; 2006.

16. Hendee WR, O'Connor MK. Radiation risks of medical imaging: separating fact from fantasy. Radiology 2012;264(2):312–21.

17. Zanzonico P, Stabin MG. Benefits of medical radiation exposures. Health Physics Society Web [Internet]. 2009 [cited 2013 Mar 28]. Available at: http://www.ehs.utoronto.ca/Assets/ehs+Digital+Assets/ehs3/rad/Benefits+of+Medical+Radiation+Exposures.pdf. Accessed January 11, 2013.

18. Linet MS, Slovis TL, Miller DL, et al. Cancer risks associated with external radiation from diagnostic imaging procedures. CA Cancer J Clin 2012;62(2): 75–100.

19. Ozasa K, Shimizu Y, Suyama A, et al. Studies of the mortality of atomic bomb survivors, Report 14, 1950-2003: an overview of cancer and noncancer diseases. Radiat Res 2012;177(3):229–43.

20. Pearce MS, Salotti JA, Little MP, et al. Radiation exposure from CT scans in childhood and subsequent risk of leukaemia and brain tumours: a retrospective cohort study. Lancet 2012;380(9840):499–505.

21. AAPM Public & Media. CT scans are an important diagnostic tool when used appropriately [Internet]. [cited 2013 Jan 11]. Available at: http://www.aapm.org/publicgeneral/CTScansImportantDiagnosticTool.asp. Accessed January 11, 2013.

22. Brenner DJ, Hall EJ. Computed tomography—an increasing source of radiation exposure. N Engl J Med 2007;357(22):2277–84.

23. Strauss KJ, Goske MJ, Frush DP, et al. Image gently vendor summit: working together for better estimates of pediatric radiation dose from CT. AJR Am J Roentgenol 2009;192(5):1169–75.

24. McCollough CH, Bruesewitz MR, Kofler JM. CT dose reduction and dose management tools: overview of available options. Radiographics 2006; 26(2):503–12.

25. Frush DP. MDCT in children: scan techniques and contrast issues. In: Kalra MK, Saini S, Rubin GD, editors. MDCT [Internet]. Milano (Italy): Springer Milan; 2008. p. 333–54 [cited 2013 Jan 11]. Available at: http://rd.springer.com/chapter/10.1007/978-88-470-0832-8_26; 2008. Accessed January 11, 2013.

26. Fricke BL, Donnelly LF, Frush DP, et al. In-plane bismuth breast shields for pediatric CT: effects on radiation dose and image quality using experimental and clinical data. AJR Am J Roentgenol 2003; 180(2):407–11.

27. AAPM Position Statements, Policies and Procedures. Details [Internet]. [cited 2012 Dec 29]. Available at: http://aapm.org/org/policies/details.asp?id=319&type=PP&current=true. Accessed January 11, 2013.

28. Duan X, Wang J, Christner JA, et al. Dose reduction to anterior surfaces with organ-based

tube-current modulation: evaluation of Performance in a Phantom Study. AJR Am J Roentgenol 2011; 197(3):689–95.

29. Arch ME, Frush DP. Pediatric body MDCT: a 5-year follow-up survey of scanning parameters used by pediatric radiologists. AJR Am J Roentgenol 2008; 191(2):611–7.

30. Cody DD, Moxley DM, Krugh KT, et al. Strategies for formulating appropriate MDCT techniques when imaging the chest, abdomen, and pelvis in pediatric patients. AJR Am J Roentgenol 2004; 182(4):849–59.

31. Boone JM, Geraghty EM, Seibert JA, et al. Dose reduction in pediatric CT: a rational approach. Radiology 2003;228(2):352–60.

32. Siegel MJ, Babyn PS. Pediatric body CT. Philadelphia: Lippincott Williams & Wilkins; 2008.

33. Kleinman PL, Strauss KJ, Zurakowski D, et al. Patient size measured on CT images as a function of age at a tertiary care children's hospital. AJR Am J Roentgenol 2010;194(6):1611–9.

34. Lee EY, Strauss KJ, Tracy DA, et al. Comparison of standard-dose and reduced-dose expiratory MDCT techniques for assessment of tracheomalacia in children. Acad Radiol 2010;17(4):504–10.

35. Verdun FR, Gutierrez D, Vader JP, et al. CT radiation dose in children: a survey to establish age-based diagnostic reference levels in Switzerland. Eur Radiol 2008;18(9):1980–6.

36. Goske M, Strauss K, Coombs L, et al. Diagnostic reference ranges for pediatric abdominal CT. Radiology 2013. [Epub ahead of print].

37. Strauss KJ, Goske MJ, Kaste SC, et al. Image gently: ten steps you can take to optimize image quality and lower CT dose for pediatric patients. AJR Am J Roentgenol 2010;194(4):868–73.

38. Requirements.pdf [Internet]. [cited 2013 Jan 14]. Available at: http://www.acr.org/Quality-Safety/Accreditation/~/media/ACR/Documents/Accreditation/CT/Requirements.pdf. Accessed January 11, 2013.

39. Shrimpton PC, Wall BF. Reference doses for paediatric computed tomography. Radiat Prot Dosimetry 2000;90(1–2):249–52.

40. Growth Charts. Homepage [Internet]. [cited 2013 Jan 14]. Available at: http://www.cdc.gov/growthcharts/. Accessed January 11, 2013.

Index

Note: Page numbers of article titles are in **boldface** type.

Radiol Clin N Am 51 (2013) 761–766
http://dx.doi.org/10.1016/S0033-8389(13)00086-9
0033-8389/13/$ – see front matter © 2013 Elsevier Inc. All rights reserved.

Moving?

Make sure your subscription moves with you!

To notify us of your new address, find your **Clinics Account Number** (located on your mailing label above your name), and contact customer service at:

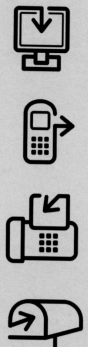

Email: journalscustomerservice-usa@elsevier.com

800-654-2452 (subscribers in the U.S. & Canada)
314-447-8871 (subscribers outside of the U.S. & Canada)

Fax number: 314-447-8029

Elsevier Health Sciences Division
Subscription Customer Service
3251 Riverport Lane
Maryland Heights, MO 63043

*To ensure uninterrupted delivery of your subscription, please notify us at least 4 weeks in advance of move.

ELSEVIER